NEGOTIATING RISK

NEGOTIATING RISK

BRITISH PAKISTANI EXPERIENCES OF GENETICS

Alison Shaw

Berghahn Books
New York • Oxford

First published in 2009 by
Berghahn Books
www.berghahnbooks.com

Library of Congress Cataloging-in-Publication Data

Shaw, Alison, 1957-
Negotiating risk : British Pakistani experiences of genetics / Alison Shaw.
p. ; cm.
Includes bibliographical references and index.
ISBN 978-1-84545-548-4 (alk. paper)
1. Medical genetics--Great Britain. 2. Consanguinity--Great Britain. 3. Pakistanis--Great Britain. I. Title.
[DNLM: 1. Consanguinity--Great Britain. 2. Consanguinity--Pakistan. 3. Genetic Screening--psychology--Great Britain. 4. Genetic Screening--psychology--Pakistan. 5. Culture--Great Britain. 6. Culture--Pakistan. 7. Genetic Diseases, Inborn--ethnology--Great Britain. 8. Genetic Diseases, Inborn--ethnology--Pakistan. 9. Risk Assessment--Great Britain. 10. Risk Assessment--Pakistan. QZ 50 S534n 2009]

RB155.S435 2009
616'.042--dc22

2008051053

British Library Cataloguing in Publication Data

A catalogue record for this book is available from the British Library
Printed in the United States on acid-free paper

ISBN 978-1-84545-548-4 hardback

This book is dedicated to the memory of Husnain, Fatima and Mariam.

CONTENTS

LIST OF FIGURES

ACKNOWLEDGEMENTS

This book is based on research initially supported by Brunel University and subsequently funded by a grant from the Wellcome Trust, U.K. I am grateful to my colleagues at Brunel for their interest and encouragement in the early stages of this project. This research would not have been possible without the cooperation of the Department of Clinical Genetics in Oxford, most especially Dr Jane Hurst, with whom it has been a privilege to work, and Dr Susan Huson, now at the Department of Clinical Genetics in Manchester, who initially invited me, as an anthropologist, to observe the work of clinical geneticists: it was this that eventually led to the ideas for this project being formulated. I am deeply grateful to the families who agreed to be part of this study for sharing their experiences of genetics referrals with me. I have incurred academic debts to the colleagues who have read sections of this book or discussed with me aspects of chapters presented at academic seminars. Martin Richards of the Centre for Family Research at the University of Cambridge took an interest in this project from the outset and read and commented on each chapter as I wrote it. I am grateful also to the geneticists who checked some of the technical sections. I alone am responsible for any errors that may remain.

Some passages in this book have been published in journal articles not listed in the bibliography. In particular, portions of Chapter 7 appear in A. Shaw and J.A. Hurst. 2008. 'What is this genetics, anyway': Understandings of Genetics, Illness Causality and Inheritance Among British Pakistani Users of Genetic Service. *Journal of Genetic Counseling,* 17(4): 373–83, and in A. Shaw and J.A. Hurst. 2009. 'I don't see any point in telling them': attitudes to sharing genetic information in the family and carrier testing of relatives among British Pakistani adults referred to a genetics clinic. *Ethnicity and Health,* 14(2). Parts of Chapters 1 and 3 have also appeared in A. Shaw. 2006. British Pakistani arranged transnational cousin marriages: critique, dissent and cultural continuity. *Contemporary South Asia,* 15: 209–20.

INTRODUCTION
EXPLORING GENETIC RISK

In 2003, I received an enquiry from a British Muslim woman, Khadija, living in the north of England, whose daughter had fallen in love with a first cousin while on holiday in India visiting her mother's sister's family. The daughter now wanted to marry this cousin, but her father, Khadija's husband, objected strongly because of the genetic risks; as a professional in education, he was aware that rates of learning disability are higher among British Pakistanis than other ethnic groups and that research suggests 'consanguineous' marriage or marriage between people 'of the same blood', usually second or first cousins, explains this observation. He had therefore resolved that his own children would not be married within the family. That his daughter now wanted to marry a first cousin seemed too much to bear: he did not want her to 'ruin her life' by caring for a child or children with mental or physical handicaps. He also feared his daughter would be increasing the risk of depressive illness in her children by marrying her mother's sister's son, because Khadija's mother had suffered an episode of depression and this cousin would be carrying some identical genetic characteristics. Khadija, however, was sceptical that consanguineous marriage would increase the risk of depression; as a professional in the mental health services, she is aware that depression is common in all populations regardless of parental consanguinity. She felt inclined to support the match because of her daughter's love for her cousin, but was unsure how significant the genetic risks are. She had seen my report on the Wellcome Trust website (Shaw 2003a) and wanted further information to help the family resolve a dispute that was threatening to divide father, mother and daughter.

I told Khadija that research from Birmingham, England, in the 1990s showed that deaths and serious illnesses occurred more frequently among the children of consanguineously married Pakistani couples than among the children of non-consanguineous couples, and up to three times more often in families with a history of consanguineous marriage, but whether you consider this a low or high risk depends (among other things) on how you look at the research figures. A doubled or tripled risk sounds high, but in absolute terms the figures are comparatively small. Any couple has a risk of somewhere between 2 and 3 per cent of having a child with a serious congenital or genetic condition. This assessment combines many smaller risks, including risks for the more common recessively inherited disorders (those caused by inheriting a mutation in the same gene from each parent) such as thalassaemia or cystic fibrosis, which vary slightly with family or ethnic origin. If the couple are first cousins, they have, in addition, a risk of having a child with a recessive disorder, deriving from the probability that they will share a mutation inherited from a common grandparent. This gives them, overall, a 4–6 per cent risk of having a child with a congenital or genetic problem, or a 94–96 per cent chance of having an unaffected child. With complex consanguinity in the family, such as where parents and grandparents are also first cousins, the risk increases again, to around three times the background risk (to 6–9 per cent) but this can also be expressed as an over 90 per cent (or 91–94 per cent) chance of having an unaffected child. Whether this is a risk worth taking is a personal decision, a balance of many different factors, of which genetic risk is only one.

Khadija's daughter, I suggested, could ask her family doctor for a referral to a genetics clinic. To establish whether or not there is a risk for any specific genetic condition, a trained genetic counsellor would draw up a family tree, ask for details of any illnesses in the family and detail any history of consanguineous marriage. They would probably also recommend a blood test to check if the daughter is a carrier of thalassaemia, a serious haemoglobin condition that requires regular life long blood transfusions and other medical treatments, as risk for thalassaemia is part of the background risks indicated by this family's origin in India. Carriers of thalassaemia have a mutation in a gene linked with the condition but which does not cause them to be ill; in fact, being a carrier of thalassaemia confers resistance to malaria. It is only by inheriting two copies of the gene, one from each parent, that a child can be affected with the condition, so, if the daughter is not a carrier, the couple need worry no more; if she is, then they could check her cousin's carrier status too. If both of them prove to be carriers, they would have a one in four chance of having an affected child and in this case could consider the options of prenatal genetic diagnosis or termination of an affected pregnancy – but the first step would be a carrier test. With a more accurate assessment of genetic risk in this situation, those involved would be in a better position to consider its significance in the context of the proposed marriage. Khadija later told me that their clinical genetics appointment had been reassuring: the family history revealed no known genetic condition in the family, her daughter's blood test for thalassaemia had shown she was not a carrier and the marriage was going ahead.

Putting consanguinity and genetic risk in social and cultural context

Khadija's story illustrates some of the direct personal and emotional implications of the contemporary discourse of genetic risk associated with cousin marriages, which, in the popular imagination at least, can also link such marriages with risk not just for recessive conditions but for complex phenomena such as depression. The elevated genetic risk with consanguineous marriages constituted the 'foreshadowed problem' (Malinowski 1922: 9) that the research this book draws from was designed to address. I was introduced to this issue while observing the work of clinical geneticists, who, at their regular meetings, discuss cases of children and adults referred for a genetic diagnosis or genetic risk assessment (Shaw 2000b; Shaw et al. 2003). Sometimes these cases concerned children of Pakistani backgrounds. Clinicians would note whether or not the parents were related because, although parental consanguinity does not rule out other genetic or non-genetic causes of birth abnormality, it makes a recessive genetic diagnosis more likely.

For me, this focus on parental consanguinity was striking, because the genetic risk of cousin marriages had not been a dominant concern for the British Pakistanis among whom I had done fieldwork in the 1980s and again in the 1990s, although consanguineous and particularly first cousin marriage was common (Shaw 2000a, 2001). In fact, my impression was that for those I knew – unlike for Khadija and her husband – genetic risk was a minor if not irrelevant concern among the factors involved in the arrangement of marriage, suggesting a differently constituted perception of risk (Shaw 2000b). Yet, for many of those involved in public health and health service provision in the U.K., the conclusions of the Birmingham study about the contribution of 'inbreeding' (consanguineous marriage) to infant mortality and morbidity present an unambiguous message. Reporting on the health of nearly 5,000 Birmingham babies, from all ethnic groups, over a period of five years, the study showed that although Pakistanis comprised only 20 per cent of the study population they contributed to 40 per cent of the serious illnesses observed, including intellectual and physical disabilities. More specifically, consanguineously married Pakistani couples were three times more likely to have children with serious problems than those not married in the family. The study suggested that if people stopped marrying cousins, infant mortality and severe morbidity would be reduced by half (Bundey and Alam 1993).

The public health implications of Pakistani consanguineous marriages have been debated at intervals in the U.K. since the 1990s, in public meetings and in the national media. In a recent British Broadcasting Corporation television 'Newsnight' report (November 2005), for example, a Member of Parliament described cousin marriages as a public health issue and argued that prevention by discouraging such marriages is preferable to using state resources to support affected people and their carers. The discourse of genetic risk in consanguineous marriage has also featured in recent public and professional debate elsewhere in Europe, in Norway and Denmark for instance, in relation to Pakistani Muslim and other minorities. By and large, the views and experiences of British Pakistanis affected by genetic conditions are missing in these debates. This book aims to fill this gap. How do British Pakistanis themselves perceive the epidemiological discourse of genetic risk in consanguineous marriage? For those with a family experience of a particular condition, what does a genetic diagnosis mean and what does the identification of genetic risk imply for risk communication within the family, particularly where marriages with close kin, such as first cousins, continue to be practised? Such questions have more than a local, national or European significance. Consanguineous marriage is favoured in parts of North Africa, the Middle East, and South Asia; currently about one-third of all births occur within populations in which consanguineous marriage is common and the epidemiological discourse of genetic risk has global dimensions (see, for example, http://www.consang.net).

This book draws on fieldwork with people from over sixty families of Pakistani origin in the U.K. who were referred to a genetics clinic for or following the diagnosis of a genetic condition or because of concerns about genetic risk. It also incorporates the views and experiences of families with older children with disabilities not currently attending genetics clinics, to whom I was introduced during the fieldwork. As I argue in this book, a central problem with the discourse of genetic risk in consanguineous marriage is that it focuses attention on the marriage pattern as if it were inherently problematic, in so doing obscuring the fact that risk is always perceived and experienced in a social and cultural context and diverting attention from the social and ethical issues associated with genetic risk generally and with any specific genetic diagnosis.

My starting point is Mary Douglas's insight that risk perception is socially and culturally shaped. Douglas observes that modern risk assessment differs from other ways of ascertaining danger because it is rooted in the mathematical study of probabilities and is thus akin to gambling (1992: 14). Nonetheless, she continues, risk identification can be studied for what it reveals of a society's social and political structure and its values, using approaches similar to those with which anthropologists have analysed beliefs about purity and pollution (Douglas 1966, 1985, 1992; Douglas and Wildavsky 1982). Modern forms of risk assessment are, she argues, related to the emergence of modern industrial society, in which risk discourse serves to build a moral community. 'The neutral vocabulary of risk', Douglas writes, 'is all we have for making a bridge between the known facts of existence and the construction of a moral community' (1992: 26). In fact, in a modern complex society, the language of risk becomes the perfect political tool with which to construct a shared culture or a moral community. As Douglas puts it, 'The idea of risk could have been custom-made. Its universalizing terminology, its abstractness, its power of condensation, its scientificity, its connection with objective analysis, make it perfect' (ibid.: 15). Risk identification has this role because, despite its apparent neutrality, it implies a moral judgement on the perpetrators of 'risky behaviour' and so is always moral and political. Thus, a risk concerning the behaviour of those at society's 'margins' is often perceived and managed differently from risks that apply to those at the 'centre' (Douglas 1992). In other words, rather than accepting expert assessments of genetic risk uncritically, Douglas would invite us to consider why it is that modern society singles out some risks for attention rather than others. From this perspective it is clear that the particular salience of current U.K. and European debates over managing genetic risk in consanguineous marriages, for example, is inextricably linked to the status of the minorities there that practise such marriage; such debates are likely to take a different form in Pakistan or the Middle East, where cousin marriage is common. In a modern complex society, the language of risk is 'custom-made' for perpetuating ideas that differentiate one social group from another. In the culture of a 'risk society' (Beck 1992), to ignore expert assessments of health risks, such as by smoking or having unprotected sex, is to be ignorant, deluded or irresponsible; indeed, the very fact of being 'at risk' stigmatises people by placing them in the margin between health and illness.

Drawing on these insights, this book seeks to provide a socially, historically and culturally grounded analysis of the professional and public discourse of consanguinity and genetic risk and its impact on how British Pakistani users of genetic services respond to and negotiate the implications of specific risks associated with particular clinically identified genetic conditions. I delineate different contexts of risk perception, in epidemiology, in the media, in the genetics clinic and in local British Pakistani understandings, and argue that, across these different contexts, responses to an identified genetic risk are less a matter of weighing probabilities than of evaluating different kinds of socially situated and culturally mediated knowledge. I do not deny the reality of genetic risk, but seek to show how social and cultural processes determine why some genetic risks are highlighted for attention rather than others and why people may nonetheless continue with activities that are deemed to be risky within official epidemiological or public health discourse.

In making this argument, this book contributes to social science research concerned with exploring the differential social impacts of the so-called 'new' genetics and of how people in receipt of genetic risk information negotiate the implications of this knowledge (Richards 1993; Conrad and Gabe 1999). It also seeks to contextualise concerns with genetic risk in general and associated with consanguineous marriage in particular. In so doing, it also contributes to a growing body of anthropological literature concerned with producing culturally and sociologically grounded analyses of contemporary situations involving risks of very different kinds (Douglas and Wildavsky 1982; Douglas 1992; Caplan 2000). The first three chapters explore the more public aspects of the discourse of consanguinity and genetic risk: the role of ideas about genetic risk in relation to epidemiological and lay understandings of ethnic differences in health outcomes (Chapter 1); the historical origins of the current discourse of consanguineous marriage as genetically risky (Chapter 2) and the role that ideas about potential biological harm play in relation to the other considerations involved in a British Pakistani marriage proposal (Chapter 3). The next four chapters draw from my clinical ethnography to explore the more private or personal dimensions of the experience of genetic risk: the meanings that a genetic diagnosis has for doctors and for their patients (Chapter 4); how adults attending a genetics clinic negotiate the implications of an identified risk for a subsequent pregnancy (Chapter 5); the issues raised for parents by the diagnosis of a fatal condition (Chapter 6) and the implications of a genetic diagnosis for communication about genetic risk with other members of the family (Chapter 7). The final chapter (Chapter 8) summarises the main findings concerning British Pakistani families' experiences of genetics, particularly regarding marriage, reproduction and healthcare, and draws out some of implications of these findings for the delivery of genetic services to a culturally diverse population.

Genetics as a modern discourse of risk

Talk about risk of all sorts, not just about the specific genetic risks of consanguineous marriage, is a feature of contemporary life, as regular television, radio and newspaper reports of accidents, environmental disasters, acts of terrorism and outbreaks of illness testify. We could say that exposure to risk discourse is itself a hazard of modern living. Sociologists such as Anthony Giddens (1991) and Ulrich Beck (1992) have theorised that the current preoccupation with identifying and managing risk is a distinctive feature of modern society. The anthropologist Mary Douglas argues that the modern preoccupation with risk is a contemporary means of dealing with danger, which is a perennial feature of human society (Douglas 1985, 1992; Douglas and Wildavsky 1982).

Risk talk is not, of course, merely a matter of discourse, but reflects real dangers to human health and safety. Such hazards have been present throughout human history, but, as Ulrich Beck argues in his book *Risk Society*, contemporary risk is different in being by and large the product of modern lifestyles. We should not assume that 'pre-modern' hazards such as plagues or famine were never caused by human activity, or that environmental toxins or carcinogens are always the products of human rather than natural environmental hazards, but many contemporary risks are indeed the consequences of human technological development or have increased over earlier levels as a consequence of environmental changes caused by technological advance (Beck 1992: 19, 21). Much sociological writing about risk deals with the dangers presented to human health and the environment by new technology, such as the nuclear industry (Krimsley and Golding 1992; Sagan 1993).

A further element of contemporary risk discourse is that risk identification demands a particular kind of risk management, one that is often informed by economic and psychological assessments of alternative management strategies (Douglas 1985; Giddens 1991; Beck 1992). Statistical assessments of risk, as calculations of possible happenings, are used to inform future behaviour and shape public policies in such areas as health and insurance, constituting, for Ulrich Beck, a distinctively modern 'colonisation of the future' (1992: 109–12). Such risk assessment is increasingly a matter of institutional responsibility, through explicit policies of management or containment. The U.K. public health programmes – initially aimed at eliminating disease through sanitation – now largely represent preventive medicine informed by scientific assessments of health risks and concerned with the efficient management of public resources (Busfield 2000).

The identification of genetic risk shares some of these features of the modern preoccupation with risk, for it too demands the management of real possibilities for harm to health. According to modern genomic science, we all are, and always have been, at risk of unknowingly inheriting or acquiring *de novo* (anew, or by chance) changes called mutations in the sequence of information carried in the deoxyribonucleic acid (DNA) that is contained in every cell of our bodies. Changes in DNA sequence are now understood to constitute a central mechanism of evolution, generating the variation on which natural selection operates – an understanding only made possible by the rediscovery in the early twentieth century of Gregor Mendel's work on the inheritance of characteristics such as tallness and shortness in pea plants.

Contemporary genetic theory proposes that each one of us is at risk of mutations or changes in the DNA in our approximately 30,000 genes. Mutations occur unevenly within and between populations as a result of both genetic and environmental factors, and do not necessarily cause illness; some turn out to be linked with disease while some may prove advantageous in evolutionary terms. Thalassaemia and sickle-cell anaemia, for instance, are more prevalent among people with ancestral origins in the malarial areas of the world – which explains why there are more thalassaemia carriers among people of South Asian, Afro-Caribbean and Mediterranean origins – while a Northern European ancestry indicates risk for cystic fibrosis, a serious respiratory disorder, because being a carrier of this recessive mutation is thought to confer resistance to tuberculosis. We cannot know for sure whether or not mutation rates in the human genome have increased over time as a result of environmental and technological changes, but we do know that the influence of genetic inheritance on human health and mortality was previously disguised by high rates of illness and death from other causes, as it still is in many parts of the world. In this sense, the identification of genetic risk and the 'problem' of managing it are the creation of modern knowledge.

Since the development in the 1970s of what were then new techniques for submicroscopic DNA analysis, many individual genes or changes in DNA sequence have now been identified, dramatically increasing our knowledge of how genetics affects human health. This so-called 'new' genetics, which enabled the sequencing of the entire human genome by 2003, has been described as heralding major advances in preventive medicine and, eventually, in the scope for therapeutic treatments. Despite some significant expansions in clinical provision, the promised medical advances have, to date, been more modest than the media and scientific hype would have us believe. Nonetheless, the advances in scientific and clinical genetic knowledge that have occurred raise questions about managing genetic risk that are inevitably shaped by political, socio-economic, cultural and moral concerns. In the developed world and, increasingly, in parts of the developing world, genetic risk management is being incorporated into public health policies as preventive medicine, but how this is occurring is a matter of local, national and international politics and resources.

Genetic risk and ethnicity

Within multi-ethnic Britain, the uneven distribution of genetic variants raises difficult questions for policymakers about where most effectively to deploy resources. For example, about one person in twenty-five of Northern European ancestry is a carrier of cystic fibrosis, compared with approximately one in fifty Pakistanis (although the risk of affected children may be roughly equal, because of the effect of parental consanguinity), while estimates for beta thalassaemia indicate that up to one in ten people of 'Asian' ancestry (more precisely, South Asian, mostly Indian and Pakistani) may be a carrier, compared with one in 1,000 'White British' or people of Northern European ancestry (Marteau and Anionwu 1996: 124). Should routine carrier screening for common genetic conditions be offered to everyone in a population, or should it be offered selectively, only to people from ethnic groups with higher estimated carrier frequencies for particular recessive condition, as calculated from ethnic differences in the incidence of affected births?

One problem with targeted screening concerns the assumption that ethnicity indicates particular genetic risks, since people's biological heritage is usually complex and marriages often occur across so-called ethnic boundaries. Some programmes targeting specific ethnic groups for specific conditions have been very successful, if success is measured by uptake of screening and a reduction in the number of births of affected children (rather than by the exercise of informed choice over whether or not to be screened, to proceed with prenatal diagnosis and proceed to end an affected pregnancy; see Bradby 1996: 304–5; Marteau and Anionwu 1996: 123–35). Screening for Tay–Sachs disease, a fatal and currently untreatable recessive neurological condition involving mental and physical disabilities, was initiated in the 1970s among sections of the Ashkenazi Jewish population in the United States and is now performed in many parts of the world and has virtually eliminated the condition. In fact, Tay–Sachs disease now affects more non-Jewish than Jewish infants, so ethnicity is now a poor indication of risk for this condition (Marteau and Anionwu 1996: 131).

However, very specific circumstances seem to have contributed to the success of these programmes. The first community-based Tay–Sachs carrier screening programme, an early example of 'co-operative consenting eugenics' (Duster 2003: ix), involved anonymous premarital carrier testing in a Jewish community in the Washington DC/Baltimore area (ibid.: 46–47). A similar programme began in

1984 among New York's Hasidic Jewish community, in which marriages were routinely arranged through brokers. To avoid any negative effects on their self-image, test results would not be given to the tested individuals, but would be made available to the marriage brokers, who would then avoid a match between carriers (Richards 1996b: 263). The result was a dramatic reduction in Tay–Sachs births 'without recourse to abortion' (Wilkie 1994: 114). Religious orthodoxy, the fact that these programmes were voluntary and community-led and the structurally privileged position of American Jews may also have contributed to the success of the Tay–Sachs carrier screening (Bradby 1996: 307; Duster 2003: 50).

In contrast, other targeted screening programmes are now recognised as having been unqualified disasters, notably the screening in the United States of Afro-Americans for sickle-cell trait, to identify carriers of sickle-cell disease, a blood condition. This story illustrates a major theme in policy debates on risk management: the potential for risk identification to strengthen prior social distinctions, with the result that those who are already disadvantaged suffer more (Douglas 1992: 34). In some states, people of African descent were refused marriage licences if they had not taken sickle-cell carrier tests, and untested children were refused school entry (Kevles 1985; Duster 2003). The very idea that people of African descent might 'carry' a genetic condition served to perpetuate a racialised perception of them as intellectually and physically inferior to whites (Rose et al. 1984; Jones 1994; Bradby 1996: 303–6). It remains a matter of debate whether the stigma of a 'spoiled self-identity', if not overt discrimination, can be avoided when healthy carriers of recessive conditions are identified (Goffman 1990; Bradby 1996: 304–6).

Universal rather than targeted screening might seem to offer a solution to the problem of stigmatisation. In Cyprus, mandatory carrier testing since 1984, combined with facilities for terminating affected pregnancies, has almost eliminated thalassaemia (Modell and Petrou 1994). One again, this programme emerged under quite specific social conditions, including the proliferation of both U.S.- and U.K.-aided facilities (both Greek and Turkish) on the island, local awareness of the disorder and a powerful social consensus supporting carrier screening. Apparently the Greek Orthodox Church will not marry those whose carrier status is unknown, and carrier couples will use prenatal diagnosis and abortion to avoid the births of affected children (Richards 1996b: 262–63). In more heterogeneous populations, the uptake of voluntary screening for conditions such as thalassaemia and cystic fibrosis in routine prenatal care is often uneven, reflecting considerable divergence in risk awareness (Richards and Green 1993; Marteau and Anionwu 1996). For example, more Cypriots than Indians and Pakistanis chose to participate in a thalassaemia screening programme in London, probably because of their greater prior awareness of the condition (Weatherall 1985; Petrou et al. 1990). Since then a nationwide campaign has raised awareness of thalassaemia, screening for which is offered universally in parts of the U.K.

Risks for thalassaemia, Tay–Sachs disease, sickle-cell disease and cystic fibrosis have thus been associated with particular 'ethnicities' and with some targeted screening programmes; indeed, ethnic identity is generally (and sometimes misleadingly) thought to evoke a particular biological heritage and thus a particular risk for a specific genetic condition. With targeted screening programmes in mind, doctors in genetics and other medical professionals have sometimes asked me why British Pakistanis do not use carrier matching schemes to prevent the births of children with recessive conditions, or why they do not systematically use premarital or pre-conception screening for recessive conditions, similar to anonymous premarital carrier testing for Tay–Sachs among orthodox Ashkenazi Jews, for instance. The problem with this question is that the elevated risk for recessive disorders associated with consanguineous marriage is not a risk for any specific condition. Consanguineous marriage redistributes recessive mutations in a population, slightly increasing the prevalence of many, mostly extremely rare, conditions and concentrating commoner conditions such as thalassaemia or cystic fibrosis within certain families. This means that the added risk of recessive disorders within a consanguineous population does not necessarily indicate risk for any particular condition, except where there is already a general population risk (as for thalassaemia for South Asians), unless there is a family history of a particular condition (Bennett et al. 2002; Shaw and Ahmed 2004). Instead, as in the U.K. the elevated recessive risk can be 'managed' through routine surveillance of pregnancy and birth.

Managing reproductive risk

The people recruited to this study were mostly young married adults referred to a genetics clinic for problems with childbearing or infant health: after prenatal detection of a foetal abnormality, recurrent miscarriage, or an unexpected infant death, or after a health professional or relative had observed a medical problem or unusual physical features, often combined with learning difficulties, in a baby or older child. Some genetic problems can be detected prenatally, especially if there is a known family history, for this will alert prenatal or paediatric staff to check for signs of the condition or offer a particular genetic test. Others only become evident if a child fails to reach a developmental milestone or loses a particular ability. In such cases, the genetics referral often occurs in tandem with other routine and specialist referrals to the National Health Service (NHS) for therapeutic or surgical corrections for the child's problems. In the hospital region of this study, the medical disciplines were well integrated and it seemed that relatively few potential 'genetic' cases slipped through the net of referral by a general practitioner, health visitor, paediatrician or obstetrician.

For my study participants, the NHS provisions for pregnancy, childbirth and infant health represented a significant improvement over the facilities available in rural Pakistan and Azad Kashmir. Nonetheless, some babies of all ethnic backgrounds are born with serious problems. Approximately 2 per cent of babies born each year have a congenital abnormality at birth (Office for National Statistics). In the U.K. today, the generally low rates of fertility and perinatal and infant mortality, combined with now routine investigations of the causes of infant death or infant health problems detected through regular infant health surveillance, have made the added risks of infant mortality and morbidity due to recessive conditions, as a consequence of the elevated risk of recessive conditions associated with consanguineous marriage, particularly apparent. The fertility rate of British Pakistanis (4.0) is also high in comparison with the U.K. average (1.7) (Berthoud 2001). It is therefore not surprising that some of the people in my study considered genetic conditions were present only in Britain and absent in Pakistan. As one father of boys with a muscular problem put it, 'What I don't understand is why we don't have these disorders [i.e. genetic disorders] over there [in Pakistan].'

The dominant recent Western biomedical view of birth and developmental problems is that they represent 'errors of nature', requiring surveillance and intervention (Geertz 1983). In the U.K., this combines the use of prenatal technology (particularly since the Second World War, alongside liberalised abortion laws) with routine paediatric assessments, child development reviews and appropriate specialists referrals, including to genetics clinics. Such provisions are, in turn, linked with structural demands to monitor trends in and causes of birth anomaly. Since 1964, after the thalidomide disaster, the Office for National Statistics has operated a register (the National Congenital Anomaly System) for birth anomalies in England and Wales. Some regions operate local registers, such as the Congenital Anomaly Register for Oxfordshire, Berkshire and Buckinghamshire (CAROBB), established in 1991, which relies on prenatal departments, obstetricians, paediatricians, geneticists and other key specialists to register anomalous births, for the analysis of local trends and for monitoring the efficacy of prenatal screening.

Reproductive surveillance and management since the 1960s uses the key technologies of amniocentesis and ultrasound scanning in the clinic, and, more recently, chromosome and molecular genetic tests in the laboratory (Richards 1975, Chard and Richards 1977, 1990). Amniocentesis, first used in the U.K. and the U.S.A. in the 1950s to test for rhesus incompatibility (maternal–foetal blood group incompatibility), has been used in the U.K. since 1967, mainly to enable prenatal diagnosis of chromosomal conditions, about half of which are Down syndrome. It was used from 1973 to sample alphafetoprotein levels (in amniotic fluid) for the prenatal diagnosis of neural tube defects such as spina bifida (which leads to stillbirth or neonatal death) and is now sometimes used for molecular genetic tests (Farrant 1985; Davis 1993; Rapp 2000: 27–28). Carried out after fifteen weeks of pregnancy, amniocentesis involves inserting a fine catheter through the abdomen in order to extract a sample of the amniotic fluid surrounding a baby in the womb. Since some of the baby's cells are present in amniotic fluid, they can then be examined in the genetics laboratory. Amniocentesis carries a 1 per cent risk of spontaneous abortion, but is usually justified with reference to the roughly equivalent risk of Down syndrome in a baby born to a woman aged forty.

Ultrasound scanning has made amniocentesis and other invasive procedures safer, by guiding the insertion of needles, for instance. It works by using sound waves generated by a transducer placed against a pregnant woman's skin to create an image of the foetus. Originally developed to detect enemy submarines during the First World War, 'the implications for foetuses as pseudo-submarines were not immediately picked up' (Oakley 1984: 156). After the war, ultrasound was used in shipping and in the metallurgical industry, and only by chance was turned to obstetric use, as Ann Oakley describes in her history of the medical care of pregnant women. In 1955, Ian Donald, Regius Professor of Midwifery at the University of Glasgow, had read about ultrasound in the Glasgow metalworking industry and arranged to borrow metal flaw-detecting equipment to help him diagnose abdominal tumours in women; sometimes these tumours turned out to be pregnancies. Later, in the early 1960s, the technique was applied to obstetrics and used for early prenatal diagnosis (Oakley 1984: 156) It is now routinely used for the prenatal diagnosis of gross abnormalities, such as anencephaly (undeveloped skull and brain) and diaphragmatic hernia (a breach in the diaphragm that means the stomach is displaced up into the chest), and as an aid in managing pregnancy and childbirth by allowing medical staff to check how many foetuses are present and to assess foetal position, size, heartbeat and so on (Taylor 1998: 17–19). In particular, the 'dating scan' is now a routine part of prenatal care (Press and Browner 1997). Although it is generally considered safe, there are some continuing uncertainties, the main risk being that of a false positive diagnosis ('positive' being a clinical misnomer that refers to an affected pregnancy or child), which might result in the termination of an unaffected pregnancy (see also Price 1996; Rapp 2000: 28–29).

In the 1980s, chorionic villus sampling (CVS) was added to the prenatal repertoire. Also performed under ultrasound, it involves extracting from the chorion (the structure from which the placenta develops) a sample of foetal cells, which can then be examined for chromosomal or submicroscopic genetic abnormalities. CVS can be carried out earlier than amniocentesis, enabling an earlier termination of an affected pregnancy (a later termination, such as following amniocentesis, is done rarely: it requires feticide, an induced labour and birth by vaginal delivery), but, following the observation made by the Oxford Congenital Abnormality Register that some babies born following early CVS had malformed fingers and toes, the technique is not now used before eleven weeks (Firth 1991). Since the 1980s and 1990s, maternal serum screening has been used to estimate risks of having a child with neural tube defects or Down syndrome; women may then be offered tests such as amniocentesis and ultrasound (Rapp 2000: 30–31).

Genetic testing and the expansion of clinical genetics

The genetic aspects of reproductive surveillance and management rely, in part, on prenatal diagnostic techniques, but genetic tests are just one component of prenatal surveillance and have many other uses besides prenatal diagnosis. Since DNA is contained in every cell of the body, genetic tests can be performed on cell samples obtained from unborn and newborn infants, children or adults by techniques that include amniocentesis, CVS, needle and syringe or biopsy from a newborn's umbilical cord or from other tissue, or buccal swab (taking a sample of cells from the mouth). Thus procured, cells may be sent for analysis to the local genetics laboratory – known by the clinical geneticists in my study as 'cyto' (literally, 'cell'), in an abbreviation of cytology (the study of cells) or cytogenetics (the study of a cell's genetic structure) – or sent to another U.K. hospital laboratory or to a research laboratory elsewhere in the U.K. or the world.

Genetic tests are essentially of two sorts: chromosomal or submicroscopic. Chromosome analysis, or karyotyping, a technique attributed to French geneticist Jerome Lejeune in 1959 (Kevles 1985), is now routine in the local genetics laboratory. It involves preparing cells to make the thread-like structures that are chromosomes visible through a microscope. Laboratory scientists 'grow' more cells by creating the conditions for cells to replicate by chromosome doubling (mitosis), and then 'arrest' cell growth at a point when the chromosomes can be seen down a microscope. They then photograph the chromosomes and construct a 'map' by arranging the chromosome pairs in size order. The resulting karyotype is a laboratory-produced and in this sense artificial image of chromosomal structure.

Following laboratory protocols, these images are examined to see if all twenty-three pairs of chromosomes (twenty-two pairs plus the sex chromosomes, either as an X and a Y or as two X chromosomes) are present and in the correct arrangement. In the 1960s, chromosome karyotypying was the main technology supporting the work of obstetricians and paediatricians investigating causes of birth anomaly and miscarriage. Today, it remains the standard first-line genetic investigation to check for deletions, additions or rearrangements to chromosome structure that might explain birth anomalies or recurrent miscarriages.

Submicroscopic investigations of the finer genetic structure of a cell, which is invisible through a microscope, may be performed if a chromosome test result is negative. These tests use molecular analysis to observe small alterations in DNA sequence undetectable by chromosome karyotyping. Molecular techniques include the polymerase chain reaction (PCR), for making multiple copies of sections of DNA, and fluorescent *in situ* hybridisation (FISH), which is a molecular probe for detecting submicroscopic alterations in DNA sequence. The use of molecular technology has dramatically expanded the scope for genetic counselling and carrier testing, and has sometimes indicated routes to possible treatments. As one senior clinical geneticist told me: 'It used to be that all we could say to people was "we think this is an inherited condition, so it might be best if you don't have another child", but now it's much more complicated, since for many conditions we can offer tests to establish risks in another pregnancy and even in the wider family.'

Clinical genetics is now a complex medical speciality, nationally and internationally, with twenty-seven regional U.K. genetics centres, each with a professional structure of clinicians (consultants and registrars) who are physicians with specialist training in clinical genetics; laboratory scientists who carry out chromosome and mutation analysis; and counsellors (clinical nurse specialists or genetic associates) who have specialist training and expertise in the social and psychological aspects of living with genetic conditions. News of the discovery of particular genes associated with rare disorders is a regular feature of work within this discipline: during my fieldwork, genes for four rare disorders were discovered by molecular techniques for conditions diagnosed within my study sample, making genetic prenatal and carrier tests available to the families concerned. When it first became an established medical sub-speciality in Europe and America after the Second World War, clinical genetics was mainly concerned with managing 'anomalous' births (Shaw et al. 2003). Today, clinical geneticists also see clients for diagnosis and risk assessments for single-gene adult disorders such as breast cancer (BRCA1 and BRCA2) and Huntington's disease. Nevertheless, I would contest the view that genetic counselling 'has moved out of the reproductive arena' (Resnick 2003: 246), because much of the work in this speciality still concerns reproduction and is located within structures for the surveillance and management of pregnancy and infant health.

Genetics in society and geneticisation

Much has been written by social scientists and philosophers about the potential impacts of the use of 'new' genetic techniques on clinical and wider social processes. The sociologist Abby Lippman (1992), for instance, describes as geneticisation the process of assigning an underlying genetic cause to problems with reproduction and health and, she argues, thus prioritising genetic explanations over other understandings of health and illness. For Lippman, geneticisation gives a new twist to the medicalisation of life to which Ivan Illich refers in his discussion of the rise, since the nineteenth century, of Western biomedical knowledge, practice and control (1992: 230). Dorothy Nelkin and M. Susan Lindee (1995), in a rather similar way, describe the increasing use of genetic technology as entailing genetic essentialism, by which they mean reductive or determinist explanations of human behaviour that overlook the importance of environmental factors or gene–environment interactions.

Informed by the history of the eugenics movements, many commentators have noted the potential for genetics to be put to harmful rather than beneficial uses, in perpetuating the idea that human difference is rooted in DNA and for discrimination on grounds of essentialist or determinist assumptions about race, ethnicity or social class (Kevles 1985; Lippman 1992; Duster 2003). There is, however, a problem with arguments about geneticisation that seem to equate the increasing use of genetic technology with an increasing acceptance of determinist or essentialist genetics. Molecular genetic technologies are increasingly used in clinical medical genetics and in other professional domains, such as in forensic use, across the globe, but it does not necessarily follow that widespread use entails a widespread acceptance of genetic essentialism or determinism by those who work or engage with these technologies. Thus, while the weaker form of the geneticisation thesis quite accurately reflects technological change, the stronger form remains open to empirical exploration. We need to examine the meanings that are in practice attached to the use of genetic technologies in the contexts in which they are employed (see also Hedgecoe 1998). From the use of molecular techniques in clinical genetics, for instance, does it really follow that medical and behavioural problems are necessarily being 'reduced' to underlying sequences of DNA and prioritised over other understanding of illness?

An emerging body of work is offering more nuanced accounts of what a genetic diagnosis is and how genetic knowledge is constituted in clinical practice (Latimer 2006; Shaw 2003b; Shaw et al. 2003). Clinical geneticists are professionally committed to identifying an underlying change in chromosomal structure or DNA sequence (genotype) related to a particular set of presenting features (phenotype), such as medical symptoms, ultrasound scan or biochemical test results, and clinical observations of physical features. However, a genetic diagnosis does not rest on the use of genetic test results alone but requires clinical skill and considerable specialist knowledge and expertise (Shaw 2003b). Likewise, recent studies show that the patients who attend genetics clinics do not necessarily interpret genetic risk information in deterministic ways (Featherstone et al. 2006; Svendsen 2006; Rozario and Gilliat-Ray 2007). Such studies point to the culturally mediated agency of individuals in negotiating the implications of genetic information, indicating that genetic knowledge is not everywhere accorded the same meaning. People's prior ideas about kinship, inheritance and the causes of illness are likely to shape their responses to genetic information in important ways (Featherstone et al. 2006). This theme recurs throughout this book in my discussion of the meanings of genetic diagnosis among both genetics clinic doctors and their British Pakistani patients, challenging the assumption that geneticisation in its stronger form is inevitable.

What is a genetic diagnosis?

Research participants sometimes asked me to explain what genetics is. Individuals in the general population are often unsure of the meanings of terms such as genetics and genes, or have misconceptions about them that can have serious clinical implications (Lanie et al. 2004). This section offers an introduction to these concepts as they are used in clinical genetics. Doctors in this speciality sometimes describe genetic material or DNA as being like a building manual for the body, or a set of instructions for the body's structure and functions. Chromosomes may be likened to pages or chapters of a book and genes (as smaller units of DNA contained along the chromosomes) are likened to the words on a page, although Lily Kay (2000) considers that this literary image needlessly elevates the status of DNA over that of other living processes and elements. Alternatively, chromosomes may be described as thread-like structures or strings containing genetic material, and genes as being like beads on a string of DNA, although recent research is challenging the idea of the gene as a discrete entity (Pearson 2006).

In clinical genetics, diagnosis is about defining problems such as infertility, infant death or long-term difficulties with physical or mental health as arising from alterations in DNA sequence (like spelling errors in words) or from larger chromosomal rearrangements (like missing, repeated or switched pages). A genetic diagnosis can thus explain a problem and may indicate a line of treatment, but the prospects for changing the DNA (via gene therapy) remain generally remote because the DNA structure of all bodily cells is laid out at conception. According to genetic theory, DNA is present in two copies, one inherited from the mother, one inherited from the father, in every cell of the body except the gametes (the eggs and sperm), which contain a single set of DNA. At conception, the maternal and paternal DNA from the gametes combines to make a new foetal cell, which then divides countless times in the formation of a baby. The idea of an equal genetic contribution from the parents at conception, via the male and female gametes, is crucial to genetic theory although it can be at odds with people's everyday understandings of biological inheritance. The idea that genetic material is contained in every cell of the body is also unfamiliar to many people, even those educated to graduate level (Lanie et al. 2004). Among my research participants, my accounts of genetics sometimes produced amusement and even outright and slightly embarrassed laughter. As one Pakistani Muslim husband commented, 'In our culture, in our religion, it's not like this.' Since genetic theory also concerns human reproduction, it can at times be hard to discuss openly between unrelated men and women, even in the more neutral clinical setting of a medical consultation.

Mendelian genetics

The models of inheritance used in clinical genetics draw upon Gregor Mendel's hypothesis of two 'elements', which, as he observed in 1866, governed each particular visible characteristic (which we would now call the phenotype), such as height in pea plants. These elements, which we would now call genes, become separated from each other in the formation of gametes (sperm and eggs). Following the laws of probability (or chance), these elements recombine when an egg and sperm unite in sexual reproduction, yielding four possible combinations of elements.

> For example, if two cross-fertilizing plants each contained one element for tallness and another for shortness, the frequency of possible combinations among their offspring would be: a tall element with a tall; a short element with a short; and two tall-with-shorts. The tall–tall combination would yield a tall plant; the short–short a short one. But though a tall–short union might have been expected to produce a plant of intermediate height, Mendel observed that it regularly yielded a tall plant. To account for this phenomenon, Mendel theorized that the element for tallness must always overwhelm that for shortness. He called such elements 'dominants' and gave the name 'recessives' to elements that did not express themselves except when combined with each other. (Kevles 1985: 42)

This model provides the basis for contemporary understandings of the inheritance of single-gene conditions as either 'dominant' or 'recessive' (recessive conditions are more common). Currently around 4,000 conditions are known to be inherited according to Mendelian principles (Online Mendelian Inheritance in Man (OMIM) http://www.ncbi.nlm.nih.gov/omim/). The distinction between dominant and recessive inheritance is important because it has different implications for the assessment of genetic risk. Doctors in genetics also distinguish X-linked and chromosomal conditions, with particular implications for risk assessment.

Recessive conditions arise when a child inherits two copies, one from each parent, of a mutation that in a single copy would have no significant health risk. A family history of a recessive condition is not necessary for there to be a risk of recessive disease. We all carry single copies of a few potentially harmful recessive mutations and, as 'carriers', we may pass them on through the generations without an affected child being born. It is only by inheriting a mutation in the same gene from each parent that a child is affected. Thus, a recessive diagnosis means the person's parents are unaffected carriers of a single copy of the mutation, a fact they may be unaware of until after the condition is diagnosed in their child. The diagnosis implies a reproductive risk for the parents of one in four, or a 25 per cent chance, of having an affected child each time they conceive. This is because only one of each parent's two copies of all their genetic material goes to form each gamete (egg or sperm), in a process determined by chance, which gives a probability of fifty per cent that any particular gamete contains the mutation. There are four resulting possible combinations when the egg and sperm combine, as shown in Figure I.1: a child receives a gene with the mutation from each parent, a child receives the mutation from the mother and the unchanged copy from the father, or vice versa, or the child receives a gene without the mutation from each parent. This yields a one in four chance of having an affected child, a two in four chance of a child being an unaffected carrier, like the parents, and a two in four chance of a child being neither a carrier nor affected. Recessive inheritance can explain how a particular condition can affect a child without being apparent in

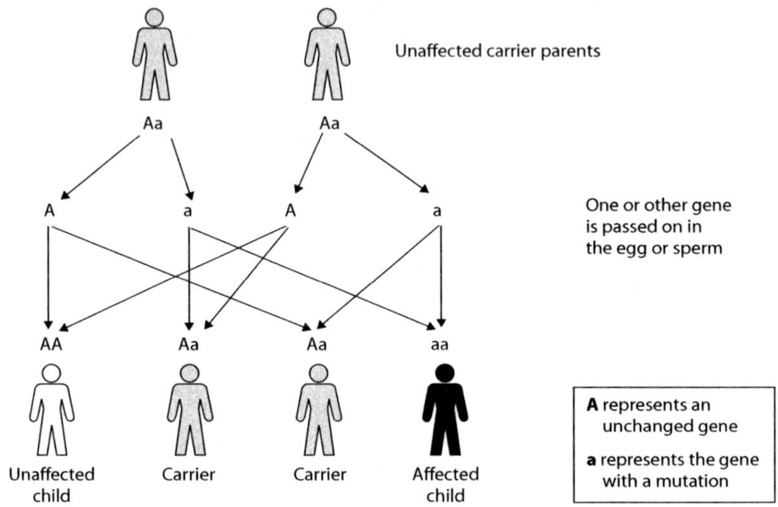

Figure I.1 Autosomal recessive inheritance

either parent. Unaffected siblings and children of carrier parents may also be carriers. A recessive diagnosis has particular implications for the wider family where consanguineous marriage is practised because marriages between people who are unaffected carriers are more likely.

Dominant conditions are caused by a mutation in a single gene that has a 'dominant' effect, overriding any compensatory effects of the presence of the unchanged copy. The effects of some dominant conditions can range from mild to severe, even within one family (clinicians talk of a condition 'not running true' across the generations), or else may only become apparent in early or late adulthood. Dominant conditions may 'run in families' but may also arise *de novo,* that is, as new mutations. A diagnosis implies that one or other parent might also carry the mutation and have the condition. Reproductive risk assessments following a diagnosis in a child usually therefore include clinical examination of the parents and other children. If a parent has the condition, the chance of their having another affected child is fifty per cent (see Figure I.2). (This diagnosis raises the possibility that a parent or sibling of the affected parent also has the disorder.) If a clinical examination demonstrates that neither parent has the condition, the mutation will be presumed to have arisen *de novo* and the couple will be told they are unlikely to have another affected child. There is a small additional risk implication with consanguineous marriage, in that two dominant mutations could be fatal to a foetus.

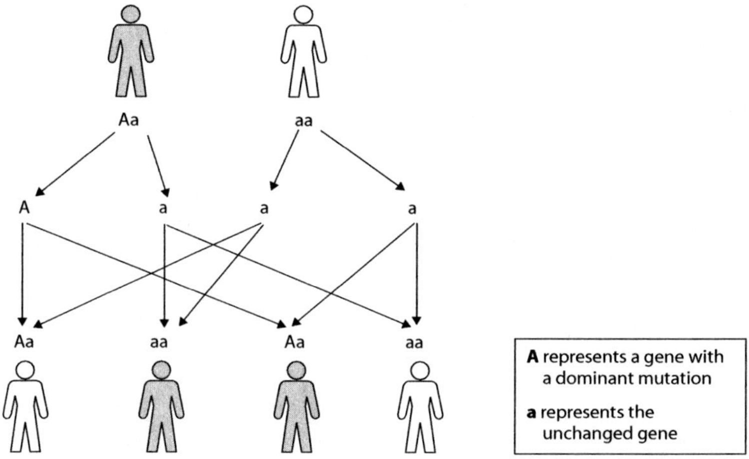

Figure I.2 Autosomal dominant inheritance

Chromosomal conditions involve not changes in single genes but rearrangements of chromosome structure, usually as deletions or additions of chromosome sections or alterations from the normal chromosome number. Down syndrome, for instance, involves having three copies of chromosome 21; sex chromosome conditions involve having a missing or extra X or Y chromosome. These rearrangements can occur for the first time (*de novo*) during the production of the maternal and paternal gametes. A *balanced translocation* is a chromosome rearrangement that involves part of one chromosome breaking off and exchanging places with a section of another chromosome. Generally, it does not cause health problems for the person carrying it, because all their genetic material is present, only rearranged (approximately one in 500 people carries a balanced translocation), but it implies a reproductive risk because the child of a person with a balanced translocation can inherit an *unbalanced translocation,* with serious health consequences. When the chromosome pairs in a balanced translocation separate to form gametes, some of the resulting gametes will contain an excess of material associated with one chromosome and a deficiency in material associated with another. A child of a person with a balanced translocation can thus inherit either an unbalanced translocation, a balanced translocation like the parent's or the usual chromosome complement.

X-linked conditions comprise a third category of single-gene conditions, which are caused by mutations in a gene on the X chromosome and may be recessively or dominantly inherited. We all have twenty-three pairs of chromosomes, of which twenty-two pairs are called the autosomes (many recessive and dominant conditions are also sometimes described as autosomal) and one is called the sex chromosomes. Females have two X chromosomes and males have one X and one Y chromosome.

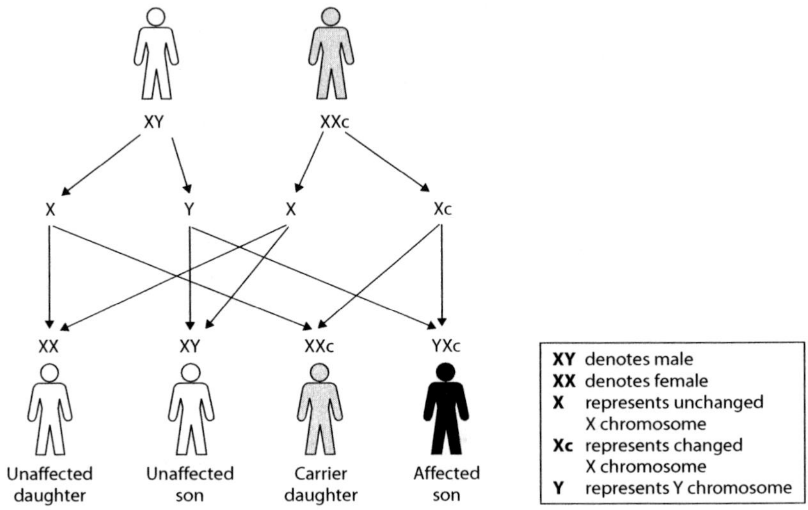

Figure I.3 X-linked recessive inheritance

Recessive X-linked conditions usually only affect boys, because boys do not have a second X chromosome to compensate, but can be passed on by females, who are usually unaffected because their second X chromosome compensates for the effect of the mutation (see Figure I.3) (Pembrey 1996: 65–67).

Limitations of Mendelian genetics

While most of the diagnostic work performed in clinical genetics concerns single-gene or chromosomal conditions, an important proviso is necessary because Mendelian genetics in fact accounts for a very small proportion of the total genetic contribution to human behaviour. Most human traits, including common medical conditions such as diabetes, asthma, eczema, heart disease, many cancers, anxiety and depression, are complex, which means that they have a genetic component likely to shape susceptibility through the interaction with environmental factors of many genes, each having a small effect. Mendelian models are of little use in understanding these processes: complex trait genetics relies on measuring the amount of observed variation in a trait attributable to genetic as opposed to environmental effects, usually from very large population samples. In fact, to explain the inheritance of complex traits, Mendelian models will probably have to be replaced by models that recognise the importance of both heredity and environment. Such models may be more easily accommodated within people's everyday or intuitive understandings of inheritance, in different cultural contexts, than the somewhat counter-intuitive theory of Mendelian inheritance (see, for example, Edwards 2000; Lock 2005).

It is therefore important to underline the specificity and limitations of Mendelian genetics. Although Mendelian models dominate in the teaching of genetics in schools and to the public, 'post-genomic' genetic research (in the era following the sequencing of the human genome) increasingly concerns complex conditions, with media hype and government initiatives focusing on expectations for genetic testing for common complex conditions and for extending genetic services for such conditions into primary care. The reality is that most genetic testing still concerns Mendelian conditions, but it would be very misleading to suggest that Mendelian principles and models of risk be extended to the understanding of the inheritance of complex conditions because the precise contribution of genetic effects to complex traits is currently poorly understood and likely to be very small. Evidence suggests that consanguineous marriage elevates the risk for common complex conditions through the additive effects of recessive alleles, but this must be considered together with what is known of the interaction of genetic with environmental effects (see, for example, Rudan et al. 2003).

Diagnostic uncertainty

Much contemporary discussion of genetic risk is based on the assumption that risk assessment is grounded in stable diagnostic categories. Social constructivist approaches to the assumptions and investigative protocols of science, such as Bruno Latour and Steve Woolgar's (1979) analysis of laboratory life, have detailed the ways in which scientific facts are constituted. As a form of knowledge, scientific facts gain legitimacy by means of protocols and practice performed within hierarchies of power (see also Pickering 1992; Knorr-Cetina 1999). Similarly, a genetic diagnosis can be viewed as a socially constructed product, the result of the clinical and scientific work of identifying an underlying change in DNA sequence or chromosome structure (a genotype) that relates to a particular constellation of signs and symptoms (phenotype).

In clinical genetics, sometimes a particular diagnosis is easily made, with clinical observations and genetic tests yielding relatively unambiguous results. Often, though, as I demonstrate in this book, the process of attributing a particular genotype to observed features is slow, uncertain and incomplete, particularly with respect to the rare recessives that comprised the majority of conditions observed in this study. Genetics clinic doctors cannot always easily rule out non-genetic causes such as infection or birth trauma in the process of differential diagnosis; they must then establish the inheritance pattern, considering, if relevant, the possible significance of a family history of consanguinity.

In a review of the sixty-six Pakistani families seen during the study period for which full medical details were available (Hurst 2005), clinicians observed sixty-nine different conditions (three families were affected by two different conditions), and of these fifty-seven were considered genetic. Of the genetic conditions, most

(44/57, or about 77 per cent) were considered recessive, each one classifiable according to the bodily system it mainly affects (metabolic, neurological, renal, skeletal, etc.) and each typically very rare. There were also some (9/57, or about 16 per cent) autosomal dominant conditions and a few (4/57, or about 7 per cent) chromosomal conditions. This confirms the observation that genetic conditions of all types occur among British Pakistanis (as among other groups) alongside the elevated risk for recessive disorders associated with consanguineous marriage. Yet a quarter of the recessive diagnoses were classified as probable or possible rather than certain; this reflects the fact that, despite recent expansions in the clinical diagnostic repertoire, a genetic diagnosis cannot always be established with certainty but may be provisional, subject to revision in the light of future research and new clinical knowledge, a fact that has important implications both for clinical risk assessment and for affected families.

Genetics, kinship and inheritance

According to genetic theory, blood relatives share some of their DNA – in fact, the extent of shared DNA can be precisely calculated: parents each contribute half their nuclear DNA (contained in the nucleus of every cell) to a child, so an individual shares fifty per cent of their nuclear DNA with each parent and sibling, 25 per cent with their grandparents, their parents' siblings and their siblings' children and 12.5 per cent (or 1/8) with their first cousins, and so on. The diagnosis of a genetic condition therefore implies not just a model of illness causality as rooted in the structure of every cell of the body (and thus at odds with models that imply external agents, such as infections, accidents or spiritual causes) and future reproductive risks for the individual or couple but also quite particular risks for kin, risks that are dependent on the amount of shared DNA and the particular inheritance pattern of the condition (as recessive, dominant, etc.). Thus, a key theme in recent commentary on the new genetics concerns its implications for kinship through its potential to transform the ways in which we think about our connections to others.

On the basis of work with American adoptees and people with breast cancer, Kaja Finkler (2000, 2001) argues that kinship is being medicalised by means of genetics. While Ivan Illich uses 'medicalization' to describe the rise of modern biomedicine by means of its various investigative techniques, such as the 'techniques of the survey' (epidemiology) and clinical scrutiny of the physical body (1992: 230; see also Foucault 1973, 1979), Kaja Finkler implies something different: that kinship itself is becoming pathological by means of genetics. The fact of their shared DNA, she writes, makes blood relatives of breast cancer sufferers into potential patients, and in so doing makes kinship itself pathological. In this, she follows Davis-Floyd's use of medicalisation to describe the transformation of a normal process such as childbirth into one that must be managed by doctors (Davis-

Floyd 1992; see also Oakley 1984). However, she also regards kinship as becoming 'reduced' to genetics and uses the term medicalisation in much the same way as Dorothy Nelkin and Susan Lindeee use the term geneticisation.

A key problem with arguments of this type is that they seem to be driven more by critical polemic than by empirical observation (Hedgecoe 1998). They also contain a fundamental flaw by assuming that people are blank slates on which a genetic theory of risk will be rigidly inscribed. As anthropologists have observed in relation to sociological theories of risk in contemporary societies, there exist a wide range and variety of alternative forms of knowledge outside the domains of experts or scientists (Caplan 2000). While a concern with risk management offers citizens new opportunities for engaging with expert knowledge, the specialised nature of much contemporary science is also exclusive. Scientists and their publics can inhabit very different social and cultural worlds and may have different material and ideological interests in any given scientific project (Irwin and Wynne 1996). The same observation may also be made of clinicians and patients in genetics clinics genetic processes, in that, as I show in this book, patients' prior understandings of kinship and inheritance may differ from those of the clinicians they consult, and these models can influence their negotiation of genetic diagnostic and risk information in important ways.

Alternative models of inheritance

From a cross-cultural perspective, ideas about inheritance vary and may reflect differing constructions of social kinship and understandings of the 'natural' facts of procreation. In some matrilineal Melanesian societies, descent and lineage identity are constructed through females. A person's closest male relative is thus considered to be their mother's brother rather than their mother's husband, who is a relation by marriage, rather than by descent. Correspondingly, ideas about biological reproduction emphasise the mother's rather than the father's role in procreation. In the famous so-called 'virgin birth' debate over whether fathers in the Trobriand Islands have any physiological connection with their children, Bronislaw Malinowski claimed that among the Trobriand islanders biology was not thought to underpin social paternity. He wrote that, according to Trobriand procreation ideas, 'The mother makes the child out of her blood' and 'without doubt or reserve ... the child is of the same substance as its mother' (Malinowski 1929: 3), but critics objected that Trobriand fathers could not really be ignorant of physical paternity (Leach 1967; Spiro 1968; see also Franklin 1997). Subsequent scholarship suggests that we view Trobriand reproduction as a cultural process to ensure the reproduction of the line of descent through women. Sexual intercourse between a husband and wife facilitates the entry of the ancestral spirit, *baloma,* into a woman's body and a foetus forms from ancestral spirit combined with maternal blood (Weiner 1976: 31). Such ideas do not imply that the father is a genitor or the mother a genitrix; both mother and father contribute, in different ways, to the nurturing of a child, but neither can be thought of as making a generative contribution to the child equivalent to the modern medical idea of genetic substance.

Elsewhere, in North Africa and the Middle East, around the Mediterranean's eastern and southern shores, as well as in parts of South and East Asia, a system of patrilineal descent constructs ancestry and social identity through men and the decisive generative contribution to a child may be viewed as male rather than female. In Pakistan and among British Pakistanis, identity as a member of a *birādarī* or kinship group is generally considered to be transmitted through men, by means of blood (*khūn*) (Jeffery 1979; Donnan 1988; Shaw 2000a). In addition to social identity, a child's physical and intellectual qualities may also be regarded as transmitted across the generations from father to child, as Monika Böck and Aparna Rao report for many parts of South Asia (Böck and Rao 2000). According to John Baily, Gujarati musicians in the UK believe their musicality is passed down over the generations through the blood of their male ancestors (Baily 1993.4, quoted in Böck and Rao 2000: 6). A belief that ancestors are reborn in the form of children is common in many parts of India (Bharadwaj 2003).

The idea of the father's generative agency is often linked to the idea of semen as concentrated blood (Shaw 2000a: 218). Moroccan and Egyptian procreation theories include the idea that a man's ejaculate contains preformed foetuses, which then grow in a woman's womb, a notion that has origins in debates within early European medicine (Inhorn 1994, 2003). The potency of the male contribution to the formation of a child is often expressed through the analogy of seed and soil, with the metaphor of the male seed (*bīj*) and the female earth (*zamīn*) recurring across 'almost all of northern and central India, and in some parts of eastern India' (Dube 1986; Böck and Rao 2000). Adoption and third-party gamete donation may therefore be disapproved of unless they occur among close kin, for otherwise the child 'would not be of the same blood' (Fischer and Lyon 2000: 316–19; Shaw 2000a: 217; but see also Shaw 2006). In Egypt, third-party gamete donation is unacceptable because it is *harām* (forbidden) in Islam, and because it interferes with patrilineality (Inhorn 2003: 105–11).

In other words, the type of kinship system in which people live has potentially far-reaching implications for their understanding of genetic theories of inheritance and thus risks for particular genetic conditions (Richards and Ponder 1996; Modell 1997; Meiser et al. 2001). It has been suggested, for instance, that the assimilation of genetic knowledge is 'relatively effortless' for patients from Western European backgrounds, because Western Europe and American kinship is bilateral and descent is understood to occur from both the mother's and the father's side, thus largely corresponding to the descent models used in clinical genetics, whereas it will be more difficult for people with non-Western origins, whose kinship structures and models of inheritance are at odds with genetic theory (Meiser et al. 2001).

One problem with this hypothesis is the assumption that Euro-American social knowledge of inheritance broadly conforms to genetic theory. It is recognised that the concept of social kinship being mapped upon 'natural' genetic facts underpins Euro-American ideas about kinship (Schneider 1968), but in practice people's everyday models of kinship and inheritance often diverge. For instance, Euro-American kinship often tends towards patrilineality, in surname conventions (in which a child's second name is that of the father and a married woman's that of her husband) and in ancestry claims (such as to a Scottish clan identity). These conventions tend to obscure lines of descent through females, despite a tradition of documenting family history via the family tree (Bouquet 1996). A belief in the primacy of male ancestry also runs strongly through the breeding of animals such as racehorses: a racehorse's speed and ability are believed to be inherited from the male (the stallion), while the female (the mare) is accorded a more passive role (Cassidy 2002). Moreover, recent research on Anglo- or White British people's everyday understandings of inheritance reveals that they draw from a range of models, and these may be sharply at odds with bilateral kinship or genetic theory, instead reflecting family observations of patterns in the transmission of inherited characteristics. These include the idea of same-sex resemblances, whereby daughters resemble their mothers and sons resemble their fathers, and the idea of characteristics that skip generations, showing up not in children but in grandchildren (Richards 1996b; Richards and Ponder 1996). An important question for this study therefore concerns the ideas about inheritance, illness causality and risk that British Pakistanis bring to their genetics consultations and the extent to which these might diverge from genetic theory.

Kinship, religion and cultural difference

The fact that genetics clinic patients may have understandings of kinship and inheritance that diverge from genetic models and may influence their perception of genetic risk in clinically significant ways can also be viewed as a matter of culture, in which cultural variation or difference either facilitates or presents particular challenges for genetic counselling. In this context, culture refers to sets of ideas that tend to be shared by members of a particular social or ethnic group, concerning, for instance, kinship and the mechanisms, social importance and control of reproduction (Clarke and Parsons 1997; Meiser et al. 2001). This definition of culture and cultural difference, however, should be treated with caution to avoid stereotyping people of a particular social or ethnic group on the basis of the ideas or traits associated with it (Strathern 1997). Yet knowledge of cultural difference is sometimes used to prejudge individual beliefs, rather than to provide a possible working hypothesis among others, to be discarded if necessary. For example, in relation to religious beliefs about the permissibility of prenatal diagnosis or termination of pregnancy among Muslims, a recent national confidential inquiry into thalassaemia screening showed that health professionals tend to assume that there is no point offering Muslim women prenatal diagnosis because Islam forbids termination of pregnancy (Modell et al. 2000). This assumption negates the principle of informed choice that underpins genetic counselling provision and also, as I show in Chapter 6, represents a crude caricature of Islamic teachings.

Another 'cultural issue' concerns the particular ways in which the dynamics of South Asian kinship may be perceived as potential constraints on individual negotiations of genetic risk. Academic and popular accounts tend to define South Asian families in somewhat stereotypical ways, for instance, as ones in which marriages are strategically arranged, with the interests of senior family members overriding those of young adults, and in which patterns of authority and decision-making reflect clear-cut hierarchies of age and gender, with the result that the interests of senior kin or the wider may significantly constrain individuals' or couples' access to genetic information and the decisions they make in the light of an identified genetic risk. On the other hand, the close-knit structure and communication patterns of the extended family, even when it is geographically dispersed, might in principle facilitate cascade screening (identifying 'at-risk' kin and offering them carrier testing). My exploration of the complexities of these aspects of risk communication within the wider family, in Chapters 6 and 7 in particular, questions the assumption that risk communication within the so-called extended South Asian family is necessarily easier than within other British families.

Questioning the Western philosophical assumption that autonomy represents the individualistic exercise of rights and choice, feminist theorists have proposed that autonomy be understood as relational, because it is exercised in a social and moral context, and represents the outcome of interactions with others with whom ongoing relationships must be sustained (Mackenzie and Stoljar 2000). To offer an American example, parents' decisions about whether or not to end a pregnancy following the diagnosis of foetal abnormality can be significantly influenced by siblings' attitudes to abortion (Wertz et al. 1992). On the other hand, social anthropologists have argued that relationality (the fact that individual persons exist within social and moral collectivities) takes fundamentally different forms in different cultural contexts, with important implications for how new reproductive and genetic technologies are being deployed in non-Western settings and for attempts to indigenise bioethics – that is, to introduce medical ethics within local contexts (Simpson 2004).

In this book, I discuss some of the challenges presented, in multi-ethnic Britain, by people's varying responses to genetic risk information and negotiations of the practical ethical issues associated with it. In particular, I argue for a nuanced, contextualised approach to understanding how British Pakistani adults negotiate the implications of genetic risk or of a positive diagnosis in pregnancy (showing an affected pregnancy or child). Ethnographic research in other contexts of identified risk has detailed how reproductive decisions are made in a social and moral context

(Sobo 1995; Bujra 2000). In this book, I document the varying influences on reproductive decision-making, where there is an identified genetic risk, of such factors as a couple's marital and reproductive history, the information given by medical doctors and the authoritative knowledge of senior kin, other close relatives, religious leaders such as *imāms* (Muslim priests) and *pīrs* (saints) and other religious sources, as well as the influence of the wider medical and popular discourse of genetic risk in consanguineous marriage.

In relation to the use of amniocentesis in America, Rayna Rapp (2000) argues that pregnant women and their partners faced with a 'positive' diagnosis become 'moral pioneers', navigating the relatively uncharted territory into which a positive diagnosis leads. For almost all of my informants, their religion constituted a complete guide to how they should conduct their lives, and their religious faith was rooted in the Qur'an (considered the Word of God delivered to the Prophet Mohammad) and the Sunna and Hadith (the sayings of the Prophet authenticated by Islamic scholars); these are the sources that underpin the Shariah (Islamic law), which regulates the daily life of a practising Muslim. However, my observations also suggest that, even where religious belief derives from these textual sources, opinions differ over their interpretation, and what determines an acceptable or unacceptable action is rarely fixed, but is subject to reinterpretation in the light of experience. In other words, assumed cultural or religious differences constitute an unreliable guide to how delicate practical ethical issues such as in relation to genetic risk in pregnancy are or should be handled, an issue to which I shall return in the concluding chapter.

The fieldwork: locations, people and participant observation

This book draws on fieldwork with families referred to the genetics clinic held in the antenatal department of the general hospital in High Wycombe, a town in the south of England that is known locally to be a centre of furniture-making and textiles, although these businesses are less prominent today. The town is situated in a district of the same name with a population of 162,105 (Census 2001), of whom 10,527 (6.5 per cent) are Muslim and 9,727 (6 per cent) are Pakistani. The Muslim population of the High Wycombe district, located mostly in the town, is the second largest in the 'South-East' outside London (as defined in the Office for National Statistics regional categories), after Slough, also in Buckinghamshire, in comparison with census districts across the U.K. About one Pakistani family per month was referred to the genetics clinic, and over five years I recruited over fifty families to my project.

One clinical concern that emerged when designing this study was that there might be Pakistani families with diagnosable genetic conditions in High Wycombe who have not been referred to the relevant services, reflecting an underuse of genetic services, as reported from elsewhere in the U.K. (Roberts et al. 1996).

During the fieldwork, some of my research participants introduced me to other local Pakistani families with older children with disabilities who were not currently attending the genetics clinic. As I learnt, these families had all had some previous contact with the genetic services, as a result of routine referrals following clinical observation of a neonatal or developmental abnormality, suggesting that local services were not significantly underused.

The High Wycombe district includes some very affluent areas of upper- and middle-class residence, with some of the postcode areas of the district ranking among the 'top ten' for the U.K. The Pakistanis in my study did not live in these postcode areas but were mostly concentrated within certain residential districts of the town, mainly Cressex and Castlefield, but also in Downley to the north and Totteridge and Micklefield to the east. Pakistanis first came to the town in the 1950s and 1960s, in response to local labour shortages, as is true of other areas of Pakistani settlement in the U.K. The pioneer settlers were mostly unmarried men or men with wives and children who remained, at that time, in Pakistan. Family reunion occurred later, in the 1970s and 1980s, and as a result the Pakistani population locally and nationally is young and growing, with a high fertility rate in comparison with the national average. The Castlefield area, particularly around Green Street, is where the first Pakistanis settled and is still considered the heart of the Pakistani settlement, the local view being that most of its Pakistani residents are from Mirpur district of Azad Kashmir. Yusuf Ali, an elderly Mirpuri-origin grandfather who came to Britain in 1958, recalled that, 'In 1963, there were less than a thousand Pakistanis in the High Wycombe.' 'Castlefield and Cressex – that's where it started,' Mohammad Ibrahim, a twenty-eight-year-old British-born store-worker told me:

> My father, he is retired now – he came here when he was eighteen years old [i.e. in 1952]. He went to Birmingham first, but he knew someone [here]. You know how it was, it was getting industrialised. That's why Pakistanis came to Wycombe. And because it is near to Heathrow airport. Most people here are from Kashmir, from Azad Kashmir, from Mirpur.
>
> Q: But you, your family, you're not from Mirpur?
>
> No. I am from Sargodha, and I am from the city. I have had a lot of problems understanding the Mirpuris. Their language is very different, even from the Panjabi I speak.

Ibrahim's comment, 'I am from Sargodha', indicates the importance of origins in Pakistan to the identity of even British-born Pakistanis, and Ibrahim's observation that the majority of the town's Pakistanis have family origins in Azad Kashmir was borne out in my fieldwork. Farook Anwar's family, for instance, is 'typical' in this respect. Farook is a twenty-seven-year-old, British-born, college-educated computer programmer. His father, an ex-factory worker who has recently undergone major heart surgery, came to Britain in 1973, and went first to Rotherham in Yorkshire before moving south to High Wycombe. He is from Azad Kashmir (the 'free' or Pakistan-held territory of Kashmir) and, more specifically, from Thara, after which a grocery store in Castlefield is named. Thara is a large village in the sub-district of Dadial in Mirpur district. Other Azad Kashmiri families in High Wycombe are from such places as Dadial, Chakswari and Lahri ('Mangla colony'). In Mirpur, the new towns of Dadial, Chakswari and New Mirpur were build in the 1960s with the intention of rehousing the 100,000 or so people whose homes (and the old town of Dadial) were submerged by the construction of Mangla dam (Imran and Smith 1997). These parts of Kashmir were just out of the areas directly affected by the devastating earthquake of October 2005, which killed more than 87,000 people in Muzaffarabad and Balakot in Pakistan-controlled Kashmir, although some High Wycombe families lost close relatives in this disaster.

The large proportion of people from Azad Kashmir within my research sample reflects their majority among the town's Pakistani population, and, although reliable national data on regional origins are hard to come by, may also make them 'typical' of the majority of British Pakistani families in the U.K., or at least in such places as Leeds and Bradford, which have large Pakistani populations. However, my study sample also included families from villages around the small town of Dina in Jhelum district in northern Punjab, just south of the border with Mirpur; from Gujar Khan in northern Punjab; from other parts of the Punjab such as Faisalabad and Sargodha, and, in one case, with origins in the North-West Frontier. Such regional diversity is also represented within the Pakistani populations of other British towns and cities (see, for example, Dahya 1972–73; Werbner 1990; Shaw 2000a). Pakistani migration to Britain has always included people from the urban and educated middle classes, and this was also true of my research sample. Some families had close kin based in the cities in Pakistan, as well as in the United States, elsewhere in Europe and in the Middle East (see also Jeffery 1976; Charsley 2003). Ibrahim, introduced above, has relatives in Sargodha, Karachi and Canada. Nighat Sadiq, a graduate from a college in the United States where her parents live, who is married to a British-raised cousin whose father was one of the pioneer Pakistani settlers in High Wycombe, describes herself as from Faisalabad, a centre of textile manufacturing in the Punjab known there as the 'Manchester of Pakistan'. I also met representatives of Pakistan's political elite currently living in High Wycombe. All but one of the families in this study were Sunni Muslims, including one household belonging to the Ahmadiyya sect, while just one family followed Shi'a Islam.

Despite being located within an affluent part of southern England, the town's Pakistani population shares many of the socio-economic characteristics of Pakistani settlements elsewhere in the U.K. National labour force surveys and 2001 Census data show the Pakistanis to be worse off, comparatively, than other ethnic minority groups. Far fewer (by almost fifty per cent) Pakistanis and Bangladeshis are in the U.K. labour force than Indians (Hindus and Sikhs), despite their comparable numbers: there are approximately one million Indians in Britain and approximately one million Pakistanis and Bangladeshis (respectively 750,000 and 250,000). This is partly explained by the youth of Britain's South Asian Muslim population (mainly Pakistanis and Bangladeshis) in comparison with Indians: because family reunification occurred later, there are fewer adults in the labour force. The interaction of gender norms with socio-economic circumstances has also had an effect, for fewer Muslim women work for a regular wage outside the home, although the number of young employed Muslim women is increasing (Ballard 1990, Dale et al. 2002; Peach 2005). The proportion of Pakistani high-ranking professionals is also low in comparison with other groups.

Such broad comparisons disguise important socio-economic differences within the Pakistani population, which are linked to social class and family background as well as to the vagaries of local economies in Britain. My study population included families who would number among the most economically disadvantaged of all British Pakistanis: these tend to be of rural, uneducated and mostly Kashmiri origins, who, in the first generation, had poor social class resources in U.K. terms. In some parts of High Wycombe, Pakistani male unemployment is high and there is local concern about young men's involvement in crime and drug dealing, all of which concerns are documented for the north of England, particularly following the riots in Oldham in May 2001, which spread to Burnley, Leeds and Bradford. On the other hand, other families run local businesses, in the *halāl* meat and grocery trades, clothing wholesaling, rental property and taxi services, in some cases initially facilitated by redundancy pay from factory closures (see also Werbner 1990, Kalra 2000; Shaw 2000a). Among the now adult sons and daughters of pioneer-generation factory workers, there are those in professional occupations, such as lawyers, doctors, nurses and teachers, and those who work in local stores and businesses and for the local authority across such departments as housing and social services.

A majority of my study participants were relatively young married couples living with parents, in-laws and unmarried siblings in houses that they or their families owned. Some couples lived in nuclear family units, in houses or flats they owned or were renting from the local authority, but they usually had extended family in the same or a nearby street and often spent time and shared meals with them. During the fieldwork, two couples moved out of the parental home to council flats, but a third couple turned down a flat they considered too far away from the parental household. These residential patterns reflect a preference for living near kin reported for other areas of Pakistani settlement (e.g. Shaw 2000a).

Most families in this study, like other British Pakistanis, have strong kinship connections elsewhere in the U.K., chiefly in the Midlands and the north: in Birmingham, Bradford, Leeds, Huddersfield, Rotherham and Middlesbrough, for instance. Like Pakistanis elsewhere in the U.K., they can also be understood not as 'immigrants' but as 'transmigrants' – people connected to two or more societies simultaneously (Glick Schiller et al. 1995). They belong to two- or three-generational transcontinental families (Kelly 1990) and typically maintain active links with kin in Pakistan as well as in such places as the U.S.A., Canada, the Middle East and other parts of Western Europe. Many families have some ongoing financial commitments in Pakistan, which, while varying in intensity from family to family and across the generations, are also important in understanding the socio-economic position of Britain's Pakistani population. Typically, the older generation feels more strongly the obligation to support kin such as elderly parents or widowed sisters in Pakistan, but some young Pakistan-raised men married to British-raised women regularly remit part of their earnings to parents or other kin. During my fieldwork, one British-raised woman and her Pakistan-raised husband, a first cousin, returned to the city in Pakistan, so that the husband could join his brother and father in a business there.

Transnational kinship is sustained across the generations with varying intensity in various forms: through the use of telephone and Internet; by means of visiting kin in Pakistan (see also Cressey 2006) to ensure children 'do not forget their language and culture', as one mother put it; visits to sick or dying relatives; and the continuing, though sometimes disputed, practice of returning the bodies of the deceased for burial in Pakistan (the deceased may alternatively be buried in the Muslim sections of local cemeteries; see Chapter 6). These kin connections are perhaps most centrally reinforced by and themselves underpin the practice of transnational marriages, mostly involving first cousins, among the second and third generations. Most study participants were relatively young couples in which one partner was a British-raised son or daughter of pioneer-generation migrants, while their spouse was raised and educated in Pakistan. While most immigrant spouses to the U.K. are South Asian, Pakistan sends more marriage migrants – men and women, in roughly equal numbers – than India and Bangladesh combined (Home Office 2001). The result is a greater diversity of Pakistani-origin users of the U.K. health (and other) services than in earlier phases of settlement; as one senior clinical geneticist remarked, 'The tables have turned: in the 1970s and 1980s, it was common that wives didn't speak much English, compared with husbands, but now it is sometimes the other way round.'

Doctors unfamiliar with this diversity among Pakistani Muslim patients might assume that their attitudes to such issues as genetic testing or termination of pregnancy can be deduced from their age, generation, use of the English language or style of dress – whether a woman is wearing the *hijāb*, a *burqā* or more Western-style clothing, for example. Yet these characteristics rarely map in any simple way on to attitudes to genetic risk. Many of the people I met during the fieldwork defied any easy categorisation, such as the father from a landowning family in rural Faisalabad who quoted Shakespeare during his consultation with the clinical geneticist, called his wife 'the boss', lent and gave me books of Urdu poetry and was equally skilled at mimicking Pakistanis speaking English badly and imitating the English upper classes.

Research with people identified through the NHS, even where it does not involve clinical procedures, requires the formal ethical approval of an NHS research ethics committee and this project required potential participants to be given written information about the project, detailing their involvement and reassuring them of confidentiality. The subject of genetic risk, especially in its association with consanguineous marriage, pregnancy loss or abnormal births, is a delicate issue that raises difficult social and emotional issues for parents, and fear of gossip and its consequences in a relatively close-knit community can inhibit discussion of these issues with anyone other than close and trusted kin and friends. However, very few of the men and women invited to participate in this project declined the invitation. This may have been in part because of my association with the medical profession, since I was introduced to most potential participants by the consultant responsible for the clinic. It probably also helped that I asked all research participants (including those not recruited through the clinic) to sign a consent form and assured them that their real names would not be used any forthcoming publications. In her work with infertile couples attending an IVF clinic in Egypt, Marcia Inhorn notes that, rather than inhibiting rapport between researcher and informant, the process of seeking informed consent was useful in putting people at ease: 'once they realised that the interviews were private, confidential, and ultimately anonymous', many informants were grateful to the opportunity to talk, in confidence, about this painful and private subject (2003: 6, 2004). While I took care not to share people's personal details with other research participants, I was often asked how other families managed living with a child with a particular genetic condition or negotiated the implications of a diagnosis of a problem in pregnancy, and I hope that this book goes some way to filling an information gap and facilitating communication about Pakistani Muslim experiences of these issues. The process of seeking informed consent also served to reinforce my role as researcher, even where my use of participant observation included activities that would otherwise be difficult to distinguish from counsellor, advocate or translator.

Nevertheless, my fieldwork did involve elements of counselling, advocacy and interpreting. As Patricia Jeffery and Roger Jeffery note of their fieldwork in Uttar Pradesh, North India, there are some correspondences between therapy and social research: 'The therapist's facilitating agency is akin to that of the researcher who asks people to talk about their lives, listens intently, and (generally) refrains from making overt judgments, and who takes the whole exercise seriously and carefully registers what people say' (1996a: 22). My listening to women and men's accounts of their experiences, especially in the interviews I conducted in participants' own homes or in some place other than the clinic, clearly had a therapeutic function for at least some participants, particularly those who spoke of the hidden pain and anguish of pregnancy loss. After I had listened, at length, to his wife's account of a stillbirth, one father told me he had encouraged her participation in the research in the hope that this might help her, because she had not wanted to talk to the hospital's bereavement counsellor. Two other women were also seeing a local South Asian counsellor in connection with pregnancy loss. Some interviews proved to be very harrowing, as women broke down in tears recalling the births of infants with fatal disabilities.

In my observations of clinical consultations, I was mainly an observer, listening or taking notes on the conversation, but I have learnt to speak Urdu and because of this also sometimes acted as an interpreter in the genetics clinic and as an advocate for men or women who asked me to raise or remind them of something they wanted to discuss in the clinic. My involvement undoubtedly influenced clinical proceedings, altering the power dynamics of clinician–consultant interaction. For example, during one consultation, a husband who had initially said he did not need an interpreter turned to me for an explanation, in Urdu, of how recessive inheritance works; after I had offered one, his wife, who had until then remained silent, felt empowered to interject, in Urdu, with a question of her own, which I then put to the consultant.

Usually, husbands and wives together consented to their involvement in the project and attended their clinical appointments together. On other occasions, a child or children would be brought to the clinic by one parent or by a grandparent, or else an aunt, aunt and uncle or sister rather than a husband might accompany a woman to a clinical appointment. The home visits gave me opportunities to talk to both parents and often to other relatives. I also supplemented clinic observation and interviews with more informal regular contact with a subset of families; this part of the fieldwork sometimes included accompanying women alone, with their husbands or with other relatives to appointments in the paediatric and antenatal departments of the local general hospital or in specialist departments of the Oxford hospitals. These different research settings offered insights into the wider context in which genetic risk is experienced and the influence of context on patients' access to information.

I interviewed men and women, sometimes together and sometimes separately, but overall I conducted more one-to-one interviews and had more informal contact with women than with men. This is partly a reflection of gendered propriety for in a Muslim society such as Pakistan contact between unrelated men and women is regulated by the ideals of *parda* (segregation by sex) and to an extent these considerations extended to me, as a woman, although I am not a Muslim and not of Pakistani origin. Moreover, pregnancy and childbirth are usually considered 'female' topics, shameful and embarrassing for a man to discuss, even with his wife, and especially with another woman. During one interview, a husband excused himself from the room, leaving me to discuss the details of her pregnancy loss with his wife. During the clinical process of constructing a genetic family history, men would sometimes defer to their wives when asked for information about illness, pregnancy loss or causes of death in the family. Men also tended to defer to their wives when I requested a home-based interview, since women were more usually at home; it took more persistence to fix suitable times in an evening or at a weekend to talk with husbands, particularly if they worked long hours away from home.

Yet husbands' voices and views, as well as the views of other family members, are not absent from this book. In the prenatal or genetics clinic, couples would sometimes discuss subjects such as termination of pregnancy with a consultant or counsellor that they had not broached at home. Some of my interviews in people's homes were primarily conversations with the husbands because I had already spoken with their wives on earlier occasions. Several fathers narrated experiences of abnormal births or infant deaths just as harrowing as those given by women. Other men focused rather more on 'public' issues, such as the discourse of genetic risk and consanguineous marriage or educational and social provisions for children and young adults with disabilities; many fathers of older children with disabilities had direct experience through their day-to-day involvement with medical, educational and social service providers, even though the burden of day-to-day care generally falls on women.

People who had attended clinic appointments sometimes treated the home visits as opportunities for themselves and other family members to ask questions about the clinic consultation and clinical processes: 'The doctor said the chromosomes test was normal, so why did the consultant want to do another blood test? When would the laboratory have the results? Is there a cure for the disorder?' I answered these questions if I could, rather as if I were a genetic nurse or counsellor on a home visit, and sometimes arranged to return with a genetic nurse or counsellor if this seemed more appropriate. One couple asked me to translate into Urdu the clinic letter that confirmed their child's diagnosis, and, when I did so, told me that this was the first time they had heard the syndrome name. Such specific details often do not 'sink in' after a first clinical appointment or even for a long time afterwards, as Katy Featherstone and colleagues note for the white Anglo-British families in their recent South Wales research (Featherstone et al. 2006). In this case, though, the parents' assimilation of the diagnosis was undoubtedly complicated by language and the lack of interpreting provision. Thus, my research involved me in clinical processes in ways I had not anticipated at the start of the fieldwork. I was subsequently issued with honorary clinical contracts from two hospitals acknowledging the roles I had in clinical processes.

Undoubtedly my presence influenced clinical processes in some way, and in ways that I hope improved some patients' access to genetic services and ability to make informed decisions about genetic risk and other medical matters. Sometimes I telephoned a hospital department on behalf of and at the request of study participants who were not confident English speakers, helped arrange hospital appointments and accompanied people – both those fluent in English and those less so – to their appointments. Sometimes, genetics clinic doctors asked me to be present and interpret, if necessary, in consultations involving people who had not been recruited into my fieldwork study. I consider that it would have been unethical not to interpret when translation was needed, or not to take a mother's clinical question back to the consultant if I could not answer it myself. Working in this way also gave me insights into the difficulties of accessing medical information and translating genetic information into Urdu or Panjabi (Shaw and Ahmed 2004) and into how service users' understandings of inheritance and illness potentially conflict with genetic and medical models. Such insights might have been closed to me had I not taken on these roles. Indeed, with some families, I would have been unable to discuss the implications of diagnostic and risk information if I had not had a part in facilitating their access to this information in the first place.

My roles in the fieldwork were also related to my own position as a white, middle-class, middle-aged female and a 'doctor' (though not medical) linked with the clinical genetics service. Several informants said they thought an enquiry or request to a medical or other statutory department made by me would be more likely to have a successful outcome than if they made it. Yet my identity as a *gori* (white woman) did not exclude an additional identification with Pakistanis, through my ability to speak Urdu, familiarity with Pakistani ways of life and previous fieldwork that had taken me to some of the areas in Pakistan that High Wycombe Pakistanis are from. On meeting people for the first time, I would usually be asked either 'How did you learn Urdu?' or 'Have you been to Pakistan?' One potential research participant asked me, over the telephone, 'Are you Pakistani?' and, to my response that I was not, asked, 'Is your husband Pakistani?' Not believing my answers, she said she would meet me at her clinical appointment in order to check this out! On another occasion, at a wedding I attended, a group of girls aged about ten years old asked me if I was Pakistani, and were quite puzzled when I said I was English: 'But you speak Pakistani,' they retorted, thus illustrating the constructed and situational rather than inherent nature of ethnic identities. Some of my friends have introduced me to others as '*ādhi* (half) Pakistani'. Through these different components of belonging and not belonging, within both the clinicians' professional world and the worlds of their patients, I negotiated my role as a participant observer of clinical processes.

Once, during a couple's prenatal appointment following an earlier birth of a child with a confirmed recessive genetic condition involving major limb abnormalities, the husband asked me for my advice: given their recessive recurrence risk, should he and his wife proceed with amniocentesis in this pregnancy, risking a spontaneous abortion? In keeping with the clinical ethic of non-directive counselling, I replied that this was their decision. As the consultation proceeded, it became clear that the next ultrasound scan would be more informative about the pregnancy, and that the couple could postpone a decision about amniocentesis until after the next scan. As we were walking to the car park afterwards, I said it seemed to me right to wait until they had more information, and our conversation ended with phrases that Pakistani Muslims often use in these situations and in which there is some comfort: that in the end, whatever one decides, not everything is under human control, that such matters are ultimately in the hands of God.

CHAPTER I
MEDICAL AND PUBLIC PERCEPTIONS OF CONSANGUINEOUS MARRIAGE AND GENETIC RISK

'Is marrying your first cousin just too dangerous?' a prime-time BBC television 'Newsnight' report asked viewers on 16 November 2005. The report then stated that, while 'most people would find the idea of marrying a first cousin shocking', 'at least 55 per cent of British Pakistanis are married to first cousins' and these marriages carry a risk of 'some rare but very serious illnesses'. It went on to produce some striking figures: British Pakistanis are thirteen times more likely to have children with genetic problems than the general population and, according to one Bradford paediatrician, 140 different recessive conditions have been observed among Bradford Pakistanis, compared with perhaps twenty or thirty among whites. The programme provided a vehicle for the view of a Member of Parliament that cousin marriage is a public health issue that raises questions about the use of the resources of the NHS. Considering marrying a cousin to be a 'risky lifestyle', akin to having unprotected sex, drinking alcohol excessively or smoking cigarettes, and claiming that 'much of the Pakistani community is in denial about the problem', Ann Cryer called for public debate and for the government to consider making cousin marriages illegal: 'Anyone who seeks to excuse the passing on of terrible illness due to cultural traditions needs to know that that sort of culture is unacceptable in the twenty-first century' (Cryer 2005).

The programme's presentation of British Pakistani views included remarks from Neila Butt, a television presenter married to a first cousin from Pakistan, who spoke about the social and emotional advantages of cousin marriages, Myra Ali, a young woman who has a fragile skin condition caused by a mutation inherited from both of her parents, who advised, 'Don't marry cousins,' and a father who had called off his daughter's marriage to a first cousin as a result of a public awareness campaign on this issue. Neila Butt and Myra Ali had already featured in an earlier BBC television documentary, 'Marrying My Cousin', broadcast late at night in March 2005, which had offered a more rounded view of cousin marriages and did not constitute a main news feature.

Those of my Pakistani friends who watched the 'Newsnight' programme included several British-born adults and youngsters who were very alarmed by the figures. Other young people married to cousins took a more critical view, wondering if the figures could be true since, they pointed out, a great many first cousin marriages do not result in children with disabilities. On hearing about the programme, a pioneer-generation grandfather, Arshad Ali, was indignant: 'We have heard it before, but I don't believe this thing.' And others regarded this report as yet another of the politically motivated attacks on British Muslims that have occurred in the tense political climate since 11 September 2001 and following the London bombings of 7 July 2005.

Arshad Ali's remark, 'We have heard it before', reflects the fact that the genetic risk of Pakistani consanguineous marriage has been a topic of medical professional concern in Britain for some decades. Medical and health policy debate and media discussion have returned to this issue at intervals since the 1970s and 1980s, when the pioneer-generation men were joined by their wives and dependent children and new children were born once families were settled. Concern about the possible adverse biological consequences of consanguineous marriage has arisen from epidemiological research detailing 'ethnic' differences in health, specifically in rates of infant death and serious illness. The research shows that higher rates of infant mortality and childhood morbidity among British Pakistanis can be attributed in large part to recessive conditions associated with parental consanguinity. Yet, as I argue in this book, the focus on consanguineous marriage as a public health issue raises some difficult issues. One is that it potentially stigmatises all those already married within the family. 'What's the point of saying it's because you are cousins?' asked Khalida, who is related to her husband in two ways – their fathers are brothers and their mothers are sisters – when we were discussing the recessive diagnosis she had been given following an infant death, 'You can't un-marry the person you are married to.' Another is that it can cause considerable but sometimes unwarranted anxiety among couples who are married or are considering marriage, to the extent that some couples consider separating or not having children on grounds of perceived risk.

A policy to ban or at least discourage any future cousin marriages on grounds of genetic risk would surely be regarded as a breach of human rights. It is difficult to imagine that U.K. politicians would propose banning or discouraging childbearing by women over forty years old on the grounds that risk for Down syndrome increases from about one in a hundred births at age forty to one in fifty births (a 2 per cent risk) at age forty three, and insist instead on childbirth at the biologically optimum age of the early twenties. In this case, the socio-economic and emotional advantages of having children later in life would most probably be seen as outweighing the biological risks, while to legislate on age of childbearing would surely be regarded as breaching a woman's right, explicitly recognised in the British NHS policy on maternity services, to make an informed reproductive choice, drawing on appropriate screening and prenatal service provisions.

This chapter presents some of the evidence for the contribution of parental consanguinity to adverse birth outcome among British Pakistanis and also explores the debate over the adverse biological consequences of cousin marriage as a risk discourse in order to situate the 'problem' of cousin marriages in contemporary British social and political context. The first part details how the public discourse of cousin marriages as genetically risky marks out a minority population by means of 'the neutral vocabulary of risk' (Douglas 1992), even while it represents an epidemiological concern to explain the higher rates of illness, death and disability among British Pakistani children than among the majority white population and to manage the problem in the most appropriate ways. The second part of this chapter considers the stigmatising effect of this discourse in popular images of cousin marriage, noting some parallels with similar discourses elsewhere in Europe, before beginning to explore how adults of Pakistani origin referred to the genetics clinic in High Wycombe understand genetics and genetic risk.

Ethnicity and health differentials

The major causes of death (heart disease, cerebrovascular disease, respiratory disease and cancers) and serious illness (heart disease, hypertension and stroke) are broadly the same across the U.K., but 'ethnic' differences in death rates and the prevalence of particular diseases show that 'ethnic minorities' tend to have higher rates of death and chronic illness than the majority white population (Marmot et al. 1984; Nazroo 1998). Defining ethnicity, however, has been and continues to be quite problematic. In some studies, ethnicity is defined by birthplace in such countries 'outside the U.K.' as the Caribbean, West and South Africa, East Africa and the Indian subcontinent (India, Pakistan, Bangladesh and Sri Lanka), but this excludes as ethnic minorities people born elsewhere in Europe or in Australia, New Zealand or the U.S.A. and also excludes British-born people with 'ethnic minority' parents.

The Fourth National Survey of Ethnic Minorities assigned ethnicity according to a person's 'country of family origin' and included measures of self-assessed health by ethnicity (Nazroo 1997). Its results show that among all ethnic groups, British South Asians have the highest rates of ischaemic heart disease and diabetes, and that among the South Asians, Pakistanis and Bangladeshis experience greater overall disease and disability. They are over 40 per cent more likely to suffer long-term chronic illnesses, such as heart disease, diabetes, high blood pressure and rheumatic disorders, which limit their daily activities and the work they can do (ibid.). Their age pattern of illness is also different, with early-onset heart disease and type 2 diabetes affecting South Asian adults at a younger age than white adults (Simmons and Powell 1993).

Socio-economic status and, more specifically, the interaction of material deprivation with ethnicity are key factors in understanding these differences

(Nazroo 1997). Patterns of material disadvantage associated with ethnicity show that Afro-Caribbeans, Pakistanis and Bangladeshis are, to varying extents, worse off than white and Indian groups (Modood et al. 1997) and these patterns broadly mirror patterns of ethnic differences in health outcomes (Nazroo 1997, 1998: 717–19). This picture is not a straightforward reflection of social class but is complicated by ethnicity in that, even within the same occupational category, people from ethnic minorities are more likely to have lower incomes and more stressful working conditions, such as poorer job security, more unsocial hours and lower-grade jobs than whites, and these factors may affect health in important ways (Nazroo 1997; Bhopal et al. 1999; Davey-Smith et al. 2000a). Thus, 'differences in self-rated health between ethnic groups reduce to non-significance after adjusting for social class, local area deprivation and standard of living' (Chandola 2001).

There are also the effects, positive in some circumstances, of areas of ethnic minority residence on adult health (Smaje 1996; Halpern and Nazroo 2000). Adult health is also influenced by the effects of socio-economic circumstances in early life, a well as by mothers' health, which can have an impact on foetal development and birthweight (Barker 1998; Davey-Smith et al. 1998). As George Davey-Smith notes, 'In many cases, members of minority ethnic groups will, independent of their social circumstances in adulthood, be more likely to bear the long-term effects of their mothers' having been deprived during pregnancy and also to have themselves been deprived in childhood' (2000: 1696). Racism, too, affects the health of ethnic minority groups through its socio-economic and psychological effects as well as through its impacts on access to health services. The health of people from ethnic minority groups also relates more broadly to their particular migration histories or that of their parents. Long-term illness or disability, for example, is often a reflection of the conditions and type of work done by migrants and can in turn influence a person's or a household's socio-economic status and material well-being (see, for example, Kleinman 1995), as well as their psychological and self-assessed health, besides often taking a significant toll on women as carers (Harriss 2004). These complex interactions between social and biological processes are not amenable to sweeping generalisations about the role of, for instance, culture or genetics in influencing differential health outcomes but require careful examination of social and biological data (Davey-Smith 2000). This point also applies to attempts to disentangle the effects of parental consanguinity, socio-economic factors, inter-generational and other genetic factors on ethnic differences in rates of infant mortality and morbidity.

Infant mortality and morbidity

In much of the existing ethnicity data on infant mortality, ethnicity is recorded as the mother's country of birth, yet infants born to British-born Pakistani mothers probably account for at least half of the babies born to women with family origins in Pakistan. Bearing this in mind, research since the 1980s has shown significantly higher death rates in babies between twenty-eight weeks of pregnancy and the first week of birth (perinatal mortality) and in the first four weeks of birth (neonatal mortality) among Pakistanis compared with other ethnic groups (for example, Balarajan et al. 1989; Chitty and Winter 1989; Bundey et al. 1991). Between 1982 and 1985, perinatal mortality in England and Wales was recorded as 18.8 per thousand for the babies of Pakistan-born women, compared with 12.0–13.4 per thousand for other ethnic groups. For the same period, the death rate of infants after four weeks of birth (postneonatal mortality) in England and Wales was also highest among the infants of Pakistan-born mothers. Among Pakistani infants, mortality from congenital malformation was 2.5 times higher than the national rate but the incidence of sudden infant death syndrome was lower (Balarajan et al. 1989; Balarajan and Soni Raleigh 1992). In 1990, the rate of stillbirth in England and Wales was approximately double for Pakistan-born mothers, at 9.1 per thousand, compared with U.K.-born mothers, at 4.4 per thousand (Parsons et al. 1993). For 1996, infant deaths and stillbirths from congenital abnormalities were markedly higher among babies of Pakistan-born mothers (Davey-Smith et al. 2000b).

As noted above for ethnic differentials in health more generally, there is compelling evidence that these differences can be explained with reference to effects of social class and material deprivation, compounded by effects relating to ethnic background (Nazroo 1997). Pakistan-born mothers may, in general, experience more difficulties in making early and effective use of maternity services than British-born Pakistani mothers. Some medical professionals view British Pakistani patients, particularly those who do not speak much English, as needlessly 'demanding' service users and may sometimes withhold services or information on these grounds; in one reported example this resulted in infant death (Ahmad 1996: 78). During my fieldwork, I telephoned a hospital paediatric surgical ward on behalf of the non-English-speaking mother of an infant due to undergo a second major surgery, to check when the family was expected at the hospital. On the previous occasion, the anaesthetist conducting a pre-operation check of the little girl had advised the parents to take her home overnight, to ensure she had a good night's sleep before the operation, telling them to return early the next morning. The family reasoned that if the same arrangements were likely this time, the infant's father might not need to take an extra day off work. The response I received was totally unexpected: 'That's a bit demanding.' In fact – as I told the person at the end of the phone – the family were not being demanding but were simply seeking information; in fact, they could have requested that the operation date be changed, as it actually coincided with Eid (a major Islamic festival), but they considered their daughter's operation was more important (and, in view of the uncertainty of the hospital schedule, the baby's father did take an extra day off work). In my experience, Pakistani families are very grateful for the services offered, appreciative of the constraints on doctors' time and don't like to make a fuss. The origins of the idea that Pakistani patients are demanding users of hospital services seem to reflect a form of racist stereotyping (see also Bowler 1993; Gunaratnam 2001); it may also reflect sometimes serious difficulties in communication and the fact that extra time is needed for achieving good communication where patients have poor English or interpreters are used.

British Pakistani women's use of prenatal services may also be restricted by exclusion from routine or specific testing programmes. There is evidence of medical staff not offering Muslim women the option of terminating a pregnancy, on the assumption that termination is unacceptable on religious grounds (Modell et al. 2000). Such assumptions might also explain the observation that Pakistani women's first antenatal appointments tend to be booked (by GPs) later than those of pregnant women of other ethnicities; as a result, fewer abnormalities will be detected early, when termination is generally more acceptable (Ahmad 1996: 79). Yet, as I discuss in Chapter 6, opinion on the acceptability of termination within Islam varies, with some Muslim scholars arguing that termination is acceptable before the 'animation' of the foetus. Moreover, some British Muslim couples take the view that termination for severe foetal abnormality is primarily a medical or personal matter rather than a religious issue (see also Ahmed et al. 2006a, b). Open and clear communication about what prenatal services can offer – about, for instance, what an amniocentesis or other prenatal test is for – is crucial if Pakistani Muslim women (and women generally) are to make informed decisions about and effective use of prenatal care. However, my fieldwork indicates that communication remains an ongoing problem, despite initiatives designed to address it: doctors may be unable easily to access bilingual professionals or unwilling to use interpreters for reasons of cost or practicability or because they think 'Asian' women should be speaking English (Ahmad 1996; Ahmed et al. 2005; Hundt et al. 2006).

The consanguinity thesis

What, then, are the particular effects of parental consanguinity in explaining the elevated mortality and morbidity among infants and children of Pakistan-born mothers, and can they be disentangled from the broad backdrop of socio-economic and other effects on ethnic minority health? From a population genetics perspective, consanguineous marriage redistributes recessive mutations in a population, concentrating them in particular consanguineous families, and in so doing increasing the risk of recessive conditions – those caused by inheriting two copies of an identical mutation – within these families (Modell and Kuliev 1991; Bittles 2001). As evidence from consanguineous populations worldwide indicates, some of these conditions will be lethal (Bittles et al. 1991); thus, among British Pakistanis, infant mortality is higher than within the general population and includes some lethal congenital malformations known to be autosomal recessive conditions, indicating an effect of parental consanguinity (Young and Clarke 1987; Chitty and Winter 1989; Bundey and Alam 1993). Other recessive conditions associated with parental consanguinity cause not infant death but long-term physical or intellectual problems, or both. These visible long-term conditions are of particular concern to health-service providers in the U.K.; facilities exist to support children with long-term problems, many of whom might not otherwise have survived, but such provisions place a financial burden on the NHS. Over a lifetime, the costs of supporting one person with thalassaemia will amount to hundreds of thousands of pounds. Among Pakistanis, these conditions include not just thalassaemia but a great many other conditions that are rare in the general population, including forms of deafness, blindness, cerebral palsy and moderate to severe learning difficulties.

How big is the added risk associated with parental consanguinity? Empirical studies indicate that parental consanguinity approximately doubles the background risk, to unrelated couples, of having a child with a lethal or long-term congenital or genetic abnormality (Teebi and El-Shanti 2006). A recent handbook on clinical genetics states that the empirical risk of lethal or long-term congenital and genetic disorders diagnosed by one year for children of unrelated parents is 2.0–2.5 percent, increasing by 1 per cent to give a total risk of about 3.0–3.5 per cent for children of first cousins once removed or second cousins, and doubling to give a total risk of between 4.0 and 4.5 per cent for children of first cousin couples (Firth and Hurst 2005). This means that most (about 94.5 per cent) of the children born to first cousins and most (97 per cent) of the children born to first cousins once removed and second cousins will be healthy, providing there is no history of recessive conditions in the family and no history of previous consanguineous marriages among the parents and grandparents. If, however, a couple related as first cousins also have additional consanguineous links in their parents' and grandparents' generations, and perhaps in previous generations too, then the risk of a lethal or serious long-term problem in a child will be higher, sometimes much higher. This fact offers the mostly likely explanation for the strikingly higher rates of serious illness or death reported for sections of the British Pakistani population and publicised in the 'Newsnight' report.

The Birmingham birth study

A study conducted in Birmingham, in the Midlands of England, from the late 1980s sought to assess the risk of adverse birth outcome associated with consanguineous marriage by observing whether consanguineously married couples have more babies with autosomal recessive diseases or polygenic malformations (caused by more than one gene) than non-consanguineously married couples. Sarah Bundey and Hasina Alam traced over five years the health of 4,934 babies from all ethnic groups (Bundey and Alam 1993). Their initial results on perinatal and neonatal mortality showed that recessive disorders accounted for about half of the lethal malformations observed, indicating that both parents in these cases must carry identical recessive mutations. The other lethal malformations observed included heart malformations unrelated to parental consanguinity (Bundey et al. 1991; Bundey 1992). Their later report on postneonatal deaths and long-term ill-health showed that Pakistani children had significantly greater post-neonatal mortality than children of Northern European parentage, largely due to recessive disorders. Overall, although Pakistanis comprised only 20 per cent of the study population, they contributed to 40 per cent of the observed morbidity, this 'excess' mostly due to rare recessive conditions. The birth prevalence of recessive conditions was 0.28 per cent among children of Northern European parents compared with 3.00–3.33 per cent among the British Pakistani children (Bundey and Alam 1993: 209).

The researchers noted that 69 per cent of the couples in the Pakistani sample were consanguineously married and, moreover, that 68 per cent of the consanguineously married Pakistani mothers knew of other consanguineous marriages in their families (ibid.: 210). In contrast, only 0.4 per cent of the parents of Northern European origin were related. In surviving children, the numbers of chronic illness and disabilities needing constant care, mostly consisting of 'unexplained neurological problems with mental retardation', were far higher among the children of consanguineously married Pakistanis than among the other ethnic groups, and three times higher for the consanguineously married compared with the non-consanguineous Pakistani couples (ibid.: 209). The authors suggested that '48% of serious problems in Pakistani children were due to certain, probable or possible recessive diseases,' most of them very rare, 'whereas the percentage for the other ethnic groups was only 3.6' (ibid.: 215). They concluded:

> It is useful, although depressing, to learn that the empirical risk of death or serious diseases in the offspring of consanguineous UK-born Pakistanis is about 1 in 10. Nearly half of these are mentally retarded but one third either had a treatable condition or one that could be recognized prenatally. It is interesting that the offspring of non-consanguineous Pakistanis are at low risk for serious disease ...
>
> As we found no evidence that socio-economic factors distinguish the Pakistanis who practise consanguinity from those who do not, we considered that the excess of ill health amongst Pakistani children with consanguineous parents could be entirely explained by the practice of inbreeding. If we compare their rates to those of the offspring of non-consanguineous Pakistanis and all Bangladeshis and Indians we find that the relative increased risk for mortality and morbidity for inbred Pakistanis is 3.2 [i.e. approximately threefold] and that the risk attributable to inbreeding is 0.6. Thus, if the Pakistanis ceased to marry relations, their childhood mortality and morbidity would decrease by 60% (ibid.: 215–6).

The conclusions and implications of the Birmingham birth study have generated some heated debate among health professionals, particularly the conclusion that infant deaths and serious childhood illness could be more than halved if cousin marriages were to stop. Marrying within the family has been crucial to the establishment of the Pakistani Muslim presence in Britain, and (as I show in Chapter 3) it continues to be important for many younger British-raised Pakistanis. Yet few medical professionals would deny any additional genetic risk in marrying cousins, even if the precise empirical contribution of consanguinity to adverse birth outcome can be debated.

The Birmingham study might have inflated slightly the number of Pakistani children born with fatal or long-term congenital and genetic problems by attributing to parental consanguinity conditions actually caused by the non-genetic factors known to affect birth outcome, such as inequalities in accessing medical, prenatal and genetic services and poverty. As noted above, there are some inequalities in access to and use of services (see also Ahmad 1996, Roberts et al. 1996). On the other hand, a recent study of families affected by deafness shows no significant differences between white parents and children and Pakistanis in their uptake of hospital services, despite their different risk profiles, and also indicates that genetics clinics in Bradford are well attended by Pakistanis (Yoong et al. 2005).

The diagnosis of a condition as genetic is, as I show in Chapter 4, usually the result of a careful examination and consideration of clinical features plus any relevant family history, with or without the use of a genetic test. Rare recessive disorders are particularly difficult to diagnose with certainty. By including probable and possible recessive conditions, the Birmingham birth study might have slightly inflated the mortality and morbidity attributable to recessive disease, but this is unlikely unless the parental consanguinity was used as a proxy for an autosomal recessive diagnosis. Poverty, however, can be ruled out as a cause of an autosomal recessive condition because such conditions (if accurately diagnosed) are genetic. And, while marriage patterns affect the distribution of recessive mutations, such mutations generally occur independently of the health effects of poverty and social class. In fact, the Birmingham study did, in effect, control for occupational class by noting that, while Pakistanis (and Bangladeshis) were concentrated in 'lower' occupational categories, Pakistanis in all the occupational classes practised consanguineous marriage. Thus, although the non-genetic factors affecting adverse birth outcome are likely to correlate with the lower social class (particularly with occupation), they are unlikely to account for the higher mortality and morbidity of children born to consanguineously married parents within the Pakistani sample overall. In other words, the Birmingham study currently offers clinical geneticists the most accurate estimates of the empirical risks of consanguineous marriage within a British Pakistani population

It might be objected that the Birmingham study's findings are specific to Birmingham Pakistanis in the late 1980s and early 1990s and therefore inapplicable elsewhere. To an extent this is true. It is generally accepted that first cousin marriage without any prior consanguinity in the parents or grandparents approximately doubles the risk of serious illness and death (i.e. gives a total risk of about 4–4.5 per cent). Similar risks are reported for Pakistanis in Norway, where they comprise the largest non-European minority population, at about 19,000 people (Stoltenberg et al. 1997; Stoltenberg 1998). The distribution of recessive mutations (and thus the profile of genetic disease) varies in different populations (regardless of ethnicity), while the precise contribution of parental consanguinity to adverse birth outcome in different populations worldwide can be hard to disentangle from population-specific genetic and non-genetic effects (Bittles 2001). What is particularly important is the extent or degree of consanguinity that is brought to a marriage. As we have seen, the Birmingham birth study indicates a risk of just under 10 per cent. Most of this elevated risk can be attributed to additional consanguinity noted for the majority of the consanguineously married couples in that study. Many of these families are from northern Punjab and Azad Kashmir, where cousin marriage has been practised for generations (see, for example, Ballard 1990). A higher risk may therefore be relevant for couples not simply related as first cousins but where there is additional consanguinity traceable back to a relatively recent common ancestor, but less relevant for cousin couples from families where there is little or no previous consanguinity.

Evidence from several social studies suggests that consanguineous marriage remains popular within many British Pakistani families (Chapter 3). Research from a range of clinical specialities points to some of the medical correlates. For example, a recent nationwide study of children with conditions involving progressive intellectual and neurological deterioration found unexpectedly high numbers of cases in districts such as Bradford, where there is substantial Pakistani settlement. Of the 736 cases analysed, 66 per cent were children born to white parents and 19 per cent born to Pakistani parents, yet the U.K. census shows that Pakistanis under the age of sixteen years comprise only 1.8 per cent of the U.K. population; thus, the incidence of these problems among Pakistani children is thus disproportionately high – by about 10 per cent (Devereux et al 2004). The same study indicates that in the three districts with the largest number of reported cases and where consanguinity was known, almost a third of the children were born to consanguineous parents and the majority of these were Pakistani.

Health policy and genetic research on rare recessive conditions

In principle, much of the elevated risk of consanguinity-related deaths and illness can be managed through appropriate health provisions reflecting the contemporary public health imperative to do something about reducing a risk once it has been identified. The Birmingham study's authors themselves recommended better provisions for the early pre- and post-natal detection of health problems in Pakistani children, wider genetic counselling services, including offering pre-conception and prenatal counselling to other relatives within the extended family, and education about the risks of consanguinity, in which: 'Advice could be given that consanguineous marriage should only be planned for individuals no closer related than second cousins and also that both prospective partners should be tested for the carrier state of thalassaemia' (Bundey and Alam 1993: 216).

In the debates that ensued, two related positions can be identified. The dominant one, discussed at public meetings about the genetic aspects of consanguinity – for example, in London in 1991 (15 January), Leeds in 2000 (14 and 15 December) and London in 2002 (4 February) – as well as in international contexts, is that the problem in the UK should be managed primarily through the clinical genetics services (http://www.consang.net; Modell and Darr 2002a). A recent elaboration of this view suggested a multidisciplinary strategy for consanguineous marriages in the U.K.: that existing genetic, obstetric, paediatric and primary care should be tailored to deliver culturally-sensitive genetic services, within which primary care provision could include a form of surveillance to identify families at risk (Modell and Darr 2002b). On the other side, there is a public health view that the risks of consanguineous marriages should become the focus of a much wider media and public health campaign to educate young people, discourage such marriages and encourage premarital carrier testing (*Asian Eye*, March 2005). This view is taken by some medical staff, including paediatricians and GPs who see children affected with recessive conditions whose parents were unaware of the increased risks, and is usually backed up by arguments about the costs to the state of supporting children with long- term medical and intellectual problems.

In 2000, the Birmingham Health Authority launched a public health campaign, justified by Bundey and Alam's research findings, to raise awareness of the genetic consequences of consanguineous marriage. The project was reported in the media, including in the BBC television news and a national paper (Haslam 2001), and targeted community groups and religious leaders. Subsequently, a heated exchange occurred between key representatives of the family-based service provision approach and advocates of the public health campaign, at a meeting held at the Royal Society of Medicine in 2002. Advocates of the Birmingham campaign argued that to avoid addressing the matter as a public health issue for fear of stigmatising a minority on the basis of its culture is itself discriminatory, while representatives of the service provision approach retorted that a more narrowly targeted focus on those already affected by recessive conditions would avoid generating unnecessary anxiety among those who only have theoretical risks.

In recent genetic research, parental consanguinity has become a tool for discovering the genes involved in rare recessive conditions and, potentially, illuminating our understanding of the metabolic pathways of normal and abnormal cell function, and perhaps, ultimately, providing useful therapies.

Mainstream research usually supports research on common complex disorders or single-gene disorders affecting the majority population. Research on rare recessive disorders is patchier and clinicians are often dependent on the goodwill of particular research groups to provide mutation analysis for affected families (Richards 1996a: 52; Parker et al. 2004). But researchers have realised that consanguineous families affected by particular recessive conditions can be a valuable research resource, because in large consanguineous families it may be possible to identify genes by a technique called autozygosity mapping; sometimes using just one consanguineous family is sufficient, providing there is more than one affected member (Lander and Botstein 1987; Mueller and Bishop 1993; Jackson et al. 1998).

In recognition of this, the National Autozygosity Mapping Resource (NAMR) collaboration has collected and stored (by freezing) blood samples from consanguineous families affected with recessive or probably recessive genetic disorders, in the expectation of making relevant samples available to researchers investigating particular recessive conditions. This recruitment of consanguineous families into scientific projects of gene discovery suggests a qualification to Waqar Ahmed's statement that the clinical 'fascination with consanguinity within the NHS owes more to racism that to science' (1996: 68). Consanguinity here is serving genetic science in ways that may inform clinical service provision with particular benefits for consanguineous families.

This point is also relevant beyond the U.K., for instance in the Middle East, where it has been suggested that funds should be increased for medical genetic research into consanguinity-related disorders (Teebi and El-Shanti 2006). One of the first successful linkage studies concerned a consanguineous Pakistani family from High Wycombe. Blood samples from affected and unaffected family members eventually enabled British scientists to identify the leptin gene, involved in obesity, and to develop effective therapeutic treatment (O'Rahilly et al. 2003). Since then, consanguineous families from the Mirpur region of Pakistan living in Bradford, Leeds and Manchester have enabled researchers to identify genes involved in a number of medical conditions, some of which are of wide scientific interest (Brown et al. 1996; Bond et al. 2002, 2003; Cox et al. 2006; Woods et al. 2006). The expectation is that molecular analysis will thus expand diagnostic and therapeutic possibilities for specific rare recessive disorders, particularly those affecting consanguineous families worldwide.

From a clinical genetics perspective, there is now a degree of consensus in North America and Europe that a specific policy regarding consanguineous marriage is unnecessary, even though awareness of the elevated risks is growing and consanguineous couples may, increasingly, request or be given a genetics referral simply on the basis of their consanguinity. In America, cousin marriage remains illegal in thirty-one out of fifty states for reasons dating from the nineteenth and early twentieth century and reflecting concerns about the integration of religious minorities (Ottenheimer 1996). Some contemporary cousin couples have been too frightened to marry or have children because of the misleading but dominant popular belief, also promulgated by some clinicians, that the children of cousins will inevitably be mentally or physically handicapped (see also http://www.cousincouples.com). In order to correct such misconceptions, the National Society of Genetic Counsellors' guidelines state that no additional pre-conception screening or counselling is necessary for consanguineously married couples beyond that already indicated by their ethnicity and 'beyond a thorough family medical history with follow-up of significant findings' (Bennett et al. 2002). These guidelines do not note the added concerns for first cousins where there is additional consanguinity, but the general counselling guidelines are valid: that such couples should be offered screening 'as indicated by their ethnicity' and family history, and increasingly, too, tests are available for some of the rare recessive conditions that a family history might indicate.

Health campaigns and media highlights

Against a background of discussion of the implications for the NHS and for genetic research of the recessive genetic risks associated with consanguineous marriage, it is difficult in the U.K. today to describe the risks of consanguineous marriage without implying a criticism of cousin couples. Public perceptions of risk are not neutral: 'a climate of disapproval grounds the belief that certain deeds are dangerous' (Douglas 1992: 27). Moreover, in the current political climate of Muslim/non-Muslim relations in contemporary Europe, the biological risk of cousin marriage provides 'scientific' grounds for disapproval of a marriage practice that singles out and blames a minority – Pakistanis, or, by erroneous extension, 'Asians' or 'Muslims' – for persisting in risky behaviour, resisting cultural conformity. The slippage between Pakistani, Asian and Muslim in much of the popular discourse on cousin marriage reflects contemporary political concerns about immigration and integration, which are, as I show below, played out in slightly different ways across Europe. In these political debates, cousin marriage has become a key marker of cultural difference, a marker, in Ann Cryer's view, of a 'sort of culture [that] is unacceptable in the twentieth century' (2005).

The imperative to do something about an identified risk has, in the U.K., resulted in various local public health and health education initiatives to address the issue through information about the genetic risks of consanguineous marriage, including the media and education campaign in Birmingham noted above. The leaflets, videos and press releases produced in such campaigns can exaggerate the risks of consanguineous marriage in their wording and presentation of statistics, and may fail to explain how cousin marriages increase the risk for recessive conditions (by making it more likely that a child will inherit two copies of an identical recessive mutation), instead creating an impression of cousin marriages as a cause of ill health (see Shaw and Ahmed 2004). The notion of a genetic condition is unfamiliar to many people in the general population, regardless of ethnicity (e.g. Lanie et al. 2004), and is not always explained in these materials. For example, the Birmingham campaign included an Urdu video drama in which a grief-stricken woman married to a cousin reports to her family, '*Mere bachche ka* genetic disorder *hai*' (My child has a genetic disorder), with 'genetic disorder' spoken in English and not explained in Urdu; the moment simply conveys the impression that something terrible has resulted from a cousin marriage.

National and local papers and television reports have at intervals discussed the risks of cousin marriages. The *Daily Jang, London,* an Urdu newspaper, published a report in Urdu entitled 'Dangers of marriage between blood relatives', which quite fully and accurately describes the findings of the Birmingham study (Iqbal 1997). The Birmingham genetics department also made a summary of their research findings available in Urdu. Usually the media reports highlight the dangers by presenting risks in relative rather than absolute terms, stressing, for instance, the doubled or sometimes tripled risks for consanguineous couples (especially where there is parental consanguinity in previous generations) compared with unrelated couples, and giving less space to genetic counselling issues. Thus, in March 2000, the Bradford *Asian Eye* carried a front-page feature with the title, 'We fear for the children: experts warn over genetic disorders in intermarriage':

> Interfamily marriages within the Bradford Asian community are contributing to the rising number of disabled children in the city, according to health experts. One doctor claims that babies born to married first cousins are at least three times more likely to suffer rare genetic defects which can lead to severe disability. And he today called for more education on the issue – in an effort to prevent heartbreak for families. (Asian Eye, March 2000)

The Bradford district, this report continues, 'Has more than twice the average number of deaf children in the country and higher incidents [*sic*] of youngsters of all sectors of the community suffering from cerebral palsy. And disabled children in Bradford account for about seven percent of young people in the U.K. who are diagnosed with progressive disorders which affect the brain' (*Asian Eye,* March 2000). The same article quotes a Leeds-based clinical geneticist in whose Bradford clinic for metabolic disorders three-quarters of the families are 'from an Asian background': 'Bradford has more metabolic disorders than anywhere else in the country … There's a condition which leads to smaller brains than normal and there are about five or six cases of this in the Caucasian population in Yorkshire compared to 30 from Asian families' (*Asian Eye* March 2000).

Later that year, a national paper, the *Independent,* printed an article entitled 'British Asians are warned over risks to children of inter-marriage', reporting that:

> Asians considering marrying within their own family are being asked to consider the genetic risks because of research that suggests the practice increases the chance of children being born with disabilities. The highly sensitive issue is being tackled for the first time by community leaders in Bradford, home to one of Britain's biggest Asian communities, where research has found that Asian children are 17.5 times more likely to be born with neuro-degenerative conditions than white children, three times more likely to suffer profound deafness and almost twice as likely to have cerebral palsy. Several studies have established a link between inter-family marriage and such disorders. (Herbert, 2000)

This article goes on to offer some absolute figures, quoting research by Bradford social services that deafness affects approximately five per 1,000 Asian children compared with one per 1,000 non-Asians in the city, cerebral palsy affects six per 1,000 Asians compared with three per 1,000 non-Asians children, and thirty-four Asians compared with six non-Asian children were listed as suffering from 'neurological damage'. However, it then reinforces its initial message by underlining the present and future scale of the problem: Bradford's Asian population is young and growing, the under-eighteen population being predicted to increase by 50 per cent by 2011. In fact, clinicians disagree on this point; some take the view that the problem may be short-term, as awareness of the risks increases and as the popularity of cousin marriage declines.

Marking Asians, Pakistanis and Muslims

In the reports just quoted, consanguinity is presented as a cause of a wide range of problems, particularly deafness, cerebral palsy, thalassaemia and learning difficulties, among British Asians. That this is an Asian issue is highly misleading, for there are very different marriage patterns, and, consequently, different risks, among the different South Asian populations in Britain. Ironically, in South Asia, marriage practices are critical markers of religious and ethnic difference. While some South Indian Hindus may favour marriages with maternal first cousins, for most Hindus and Sikhs first cousins are prohibited marriage partners.

Alternatively, the issue is often reported in a way that places Muslims rather than Asians under the spotlight. One *Guardian* report highlighting the dangers of cousin marriage draws from the original research relating to Birmingham Pakistanis, but begins by stressing the pathological aspects of what it implies is an outdated Islamic tradition: 'In Britain's Muslim community, wedding close relatives is normal. But a genetic backlash is hitting children … but now for the first time Birmingham health authority is challenging the centuries-old custom' (Haslam, 2001). The article implies that cousin marriage is an 'Islamic' practice, which it is not (Chapter 2) and exaggerates the figures on consanguineous marriages, particularly on uncle-to-niece marriage, which is actually prohibited by Islamic marriage rules: 'This practice of wedding close relatives ... is common among Muslims all over the world, and particularly so in Britain. In Birmingham, almost 80 per cent of arranged marriages in the 70,000–strong community are cousin-to-cousin or uncle-to-niece.' By combining several images of this 'Muslim' marriage practice, as 'centuries-old', 'arranged' and pathological, because it is now resulting in a 'genetic backlash ... hitting children', the article implies that the tradition is inappropriate in the modern world. In this way, religion, culture and morality are implicated in the discourse of genetic risk.

As we saw, the findings of the Birmingham birth study relate primarily to Pakistani Punjabis and to people from Azad Kashmir who comprise the majority of British Pakistani Muslims. Some British South Asian Muslims do not favour or do not often practise cousin marriage. Cousin marriages are less common among Bangladeshis than among Pakistanis and are disapproved of by such groups as the Khoja Shi'as, who are of Indian origin, came to Britain via East Africa and generally have more attenuated links with the Indian subcontinent than the Pakistanis.

Against the backdrop of professional debate and media publicity, some South Asian and Muslim associations have taken it upon themselves to publicise the risks of cousin marriages. These include the Asian Disability Action awareness (Bradford *Asian Eye*, March 2000) and a Bangladeshi community association initiative in Bradford (Herbert, 2000). The Khoja Shi'a website information on cousin marriages begins with statements by scholars of the Hadith (the traditions of recorded sayings of the Prophet Mohammad) that, in some of his sayings, the Prophet himself advised against cousin marriage. Providing a summary of recent medical evidence, the website advises that cousin marriages be strongly discouraged ('It is vital that our community is made aware of dangers of such marriages') and recommends that cousin couples wanting to marry have blood tests and genetic counselling first, and, if there is a family history of genetic disease or both partners have 'positive' test results, then 'such marriages must be stopped' (www.world-federation.org/MAB/Articles/cousin_marriages.asp).

The European context

To an extent, the medical discourse on consanguineous marriage and genetic risk is now global, although its local impact and political context vary. In contemporary Europe – in Britain, parts of France, Spain, Norway and Denmark – cousin marriage and the practice of arranged marriage with which it is usually linked distinguish 'old' settled Europeans from some post-war immigrant minority populations – mostly the Pakistanis (and often, by erroneous extension, other South Asians) but also people with Turkish and Middle Eastern origins as well as travelling populations. While some research has focused on long-standing consanguineous populations, such as Irish travellers, the adverse biological consequences of cousin marriages have been most hotly debated where they concern 'new' immigrants.

In Denmark, a government information campaign about the health risks of cousin marriage was launched just as a bill aiming to stop Pakistani immigration came before parliament. The Urdu version stated that 'research has proved that there is very great danger of inherited illness in the children of first cousins' (my translation). As in the U.K., Pakistani immigration to Denmark occurs mainly in the form of transnational marriages involving consanguineous kin (see Chapter 3). The bill that was eventually passed bans 'forced' marriages, but defines cousin marriages as 'forced' marriages on the grounds that marriages between people who 'share a close family relationship' are 'not voluntary'(www.udlst.dk/english/Family+Reunification/Spouses/forced_marriages). The publication of information on the health risks of cousin marriages seemed to be timed to deflect attention from potential criticism of the bill as denying a person's right to marry a cousin. In the U.K., in contrast, the issue of cousin marriage and birth defects has not been linked directly with immigration or with the issue of forced marriage, although significantly the MP Anne Cryer has previously campaigned against forced marriages. A similar debate is currently under way in Norway, where the focus is, again, on the links between cousin marriage, forced marriage and immigration, rather than on long-settled consanguineous populations such as gypsies.

The debates in Europe illustrate the moral and political power of a discourse of risk directed at a minority population. In many other parts of the world, consanguineous marriage is common: in the Middle East, for instance, it accounts for between 20 and 70 per cent of all marriages (Hoodfar and Teebi 1996, Teebi and Farangi 1997). Responses to the increasingly global medical discourse of genetic risk seem to be variable. In parts of Israel and Jordan, awareness of the potentially adverse effects of consanguineous marriage on birth outcomes seems to be related to a decline in the rate of consanguineous marriage, but this may also reflect changes in the socio-economic significance of consanguineous marriage (Zlotogora et al. 2002; Hamamy et al. 2005). In Lebanon, a law of 15 November 1994 requires a couple wishing to marry to undergo a 'medical fitness examination', as part of an attempt to reduce the incidence of genetic blood disorders and disabilities, a concern also shared, though not translated into law, in Jordan and Egypt (Kandela 1994). In contrast, some reports from Pakistan note a lack of public awareness of the role of consanguinity in adverse birth outcome and indicate a tendency for health discourse to focus on preventing cousin marriage rather than on developing genetic counselling facilities. The national newspaper *Dawn*, for instance, quotes a doctor in Islamabad saying that Pakistanis need to 'break away from the tradition of intermarriages ... to have a healthy new generation' (dawn.com/2001/11/15/nat32.htm). Another article reports from Karachi that marriages between cousins should be discouraged and the government should require couples to have blood tests before they marry, 'so that couples can be stopped from marrying and acquiring hereditary diseases' (dawn.com/2001/01/05/nat24.htm). As I show below, for the majority of the British Pakistanis in my study the discourse of genetic risk was new and one they associated specifically with the British environment, not with Pakistan.

Public and professional stereotypes

A comedy sketch in the popular BBC television series 'Goodness Gracious Me', written and produced by South Asian actors, featured a white English journalist, determined to get a story, interviewing a rather perplexed-looking Pakistani father about his arrangements for his daughter's marriage: 'You mean you are not forcing your daughter to marry her cousin from Pakistan who has only three fingers?' (BBC 2, 27 November 1998). While the comedy lies in the mocking of the journalist's assumption, for it takes some moments for the girl's parents to realise what the journalist expects and to act accordingly, the journalist's equation of a transnational Pakistani marriage with forced marriage, cousin marriage and biological defects reflects a popular stereotype of such marriages as socially and biologically problematic.

Given the extent of publicity given to the issue, it is perhaps not surprising that an image of cousin marriages as biologically dangerous has also filtered into other popular representations of Pakistani cousin marriage, as revealed, for instance, in Nadeem Aslam's novel:

> A girl in the audience ... is weeping to herself ... She is married to a first cousin brought over from Pakistan, and their first child was born with one lung smaller than the other, while the second child has no diaphragm in his torso, and, in the sixth month of her third pregnancy, she has recently learnt that the foetus has failed to develop ears; she has to have a scan every day. (Aslam 2004: 189)

In some medical and lay circles, consanguineous marriage seems to have become a popular general explanation for ill health among British Pakistanis, one that locates their poor health outcomes within their genetic and cultural background and obscures the role of poverty and problems in accessing services (Ahmad 1993, 1996). Waqar Ahmad (1996) notes that one consultant clinical oncologist believes that consanguineous marriage causes 'unusual tumours' in Asians. Genetic research indicates that consanguinity has some small effects on rates of rare recessive cancers and, moreover, may provide a tool for accessing the mutations involved (Sherridan 2005). Parental consanguinity may also have an effect on some common complex disorders (those caused by many genes in combination with environmental factors) (Rudan et al. 2003, 2006) though is unlikely to provide the overriding explanation for most common health problems. Nonetheless, concerns about its ill effects may be preventing some couples from having children at all. At one meeting where I presented some of my research, a young British Pakistani woman enquired afterwards about the effects of consanguinity on eczema. Her brother has eczema, is married to a first cousin and is apparently too afraid to have children for fear of a more severe form of eczema in their children. In this case, given that eczema is a complex condition and the contribution of parental consanguinity unclear, the young man would be best advised to see a genetic counsellor, who would take a family history and give more precise and probably reassuring advice.

Local responses: 'Islam knew this 1400 years ago'

As a public health discourse, the consanguinity thesis contains the potential for stigmatising difference or for creating a 'spoiled' self-identity (Goffman 1990), in this case at the level of a minority group, singled out as at risk on the basis of their marriage pattern, as well as for individuals. In subsequent chapters, I illustrate some of the ways in which the discourse of consanguinity and genetic risk affects people's personal experiences of genetic conditions, their understandings of genetic risk information and their views of marriage, particularly marriages within the family. In this section, I discuss aspects of local reactions to this risk discourse, in particular in relation to people's understandings of genetics.

Awareness of the possible biological ill effects of consanguineous marriage is not new. In Europe and America, medical concern can be traced back at least to the late eighteenth and early nineteenth century. It was partly informed by debates over the inbreeding of animals, but also reflected medical unease 'connected to hereditary diseases afflicting the European nobility' (Davidoff 2006: 33). In the mid-nineteenth century it was expressed by, among others, the prominent Victorian evolutionary scientist Charles Darwin, who was himself married to a first cousin. In the Islamic world, as I learnt from a local health-promotion video, awareness of the possible ill effects of marrying close relatives preceded modern genetic knowledge by about fourteen hundred years. In the video, a local *imām* (religious leader) was asked to comment on the research evidence that consanguineous marriage increases the risk of recessive disorders causing mental and physical disability. By claiming prior Islamic knowledge of risk, the intention was to deflect the stigma associated with the health education message of the video, and thus to make it less offensive to local viewers. The *imām* replied with the following story, which dates from about the sixth century AD , shortly after the death of the Prophet Mohammad:

> When we study Islamic history, we find that in the time of Hazrat Faruq-e-Azam [the second or third Caliph] a delegation from a tribe of Banu Saib came to Hazrat Faruq-e-Azam. Hazrat Faruq-e-Azam noticed that they all were physically weak, and asked them why. One of their elders replied, 'We

> have become weak from marrying continuously within the family.' Faruq-e-Azam's reply was, 'You should stop marrying close relatives and should marry unrelated people, so that your progeny will be both mentally and physically fit.' (Buckinghamshire Health authority, my translation)

Scepticism and lay epidemiology

Yet the video was not widely used locally; during my fieldwork I found boxes of the accompanying leaflets sitting, undistributed, at the local-health promotion centre. The video's message, I was told, proved too controversial, despite the *imām*'s cooperation. At a public meeting some senior, first-generation men from the local Pakistani population had apparently criticised the *imām* for siding with professionals in providing religious support for a discourse of risk they found offensive and alienating. It seemed, too, that the discussion had indeed alienated some users of genetic services. One father of several children with serious learning disabilities chose not to seek further genetic advice years later, when the time came to arrange his own children's marriages, and these marriages took place within the family, with kin from Pakistan.

For some of those in my study, genetics had become equated with the ill effects of cousin marriages. At the beginning of my home visit to Saleem Ullah, father of five children, whose two eldest children have learning difficulties, Saleem turned to his wife to explain the purpose of my visit; I had not previously met her as Saleem had brought their eldest child, an eighteen-year-old boy, to the genetics clinic. He and I had previously spoken in English. Speaking Panjabi, he told his wife that my research is 'about problems in the blood when people marry relatives'. This signalled an association between genetics, problems and marrying relatives. I then asked why their son had been referred to the genetics clinic. Saleem told me his son's problems had begun when he was a baby, after his first MMR injection took place while Saleem was in Pakistan. 'When I came back, after eight weeks, he was completely different,' he said. His son went on to attend special schools for children with learning difficulties, but was now of school leaving age:

> I wanted to make sure. I was thinking it was the MMR that caused the problem. Before that, he was very bubbly, very good, so it has to be to do with the injection. I was abroad. I don't know what they gave him at the GP surgery. I have wondered ever since. So I asked the paediatrician, 'What can we do to find out?' He wanted to check his brain in the scanner, but I did not think that my son would be able to do that. He would get claustrophobia – you have to put your head inside a tunnel. So the paediatrician said he would do the blood tests. That is why he referred to genetics. But I don't think it is to do with marrying in the family. I have seen some children, they are like my son, but their parents are not relatives.

> I don't see English people marrying in the family and I see plenty of English children like him. And I see less and less of this in Kashmir. I think it is the will of God. But I thought there is no harm in finding out.

For Saleem, then, genetics refers to the thesis that problems such as learning disability are caused by cousin marriage, a thesis of which he is sceptical on the basis of his observation that people who do not marry cousins may have children with similar problems. Later in our conversation, I asked him for a definition of genetics:

> AS: What do you understand by the word genetics?
> SU: Genetics? Yes, that's illnesses you get when you marry in the family.
> AS: What do you mean?
> SU: I had a couple of Asian interpreters come and say it is because you marry in the family that your child is like this. I did not say, English people have learning difficulties and don't marry cousins. I did not want to put them off so that they won't come, because my wife does not speak English and needs their help.
> AS: When did you first hear this?
> SU: I first heard it, oh, some years ago, when an Asian interpreter who came to the house with a health visitor was completing the form for disability living allowance. She said marrying in the family leads to learning disabilities. She said, 'because you marry in the family that is why you have got two children with learning disabilities. It's genetics.'

Since the consanguinity thesis did not make sense to him, Saleem was reluctant to pursue a genetic explanation for his son's problems (and, in this case, a genetic diagnosis proved inconclusive). The incident, as he narrates it, adds to the evidence of how medical professionals' views can alienate users of medical, including genetic services (Darr 1999). Miriam is married to a first cousin and has a niece and nephew who have a recessive condition. She told me that fear of professional disapproval of cousin marriages made her hesitate to seek a carrier test until after her first child was born, despite her niece urging her to do so earlier:

> We thought it was because we are married in the family that my niece is like that. When I came to the clinic where I met you, I felt, 'These people are going to think badly of me because I am married to my cousin.' Even when my niece said, 'Go for it. Go for the carrier test', I felt they would think badly of me. They shouldn't, though, because a lot of the time the girls have no choice about who they marry, and about 90 per cent of people who marry cousins do not have children with handicaps. But it is true, even the young girls in our community, they go round thinking we have abnormalities because we marry in the family. It makes you think twice about going to the genetics clinic, because you think you are going to be blamed.

Time and time again, study participants expressed scepticism of the thesis that cousin marriages cause disabilities, by making the accurate lay epidemiological observations that English people do not marry cousins but still have children with disabilities and the vast majority of Pakistanis marry cousins and have children who are perfectly healthy. Khalida's third child died suddenly and totally unexpectedly when he was nine months old. Khalida and her husband were then referred to clinical genetics because the post-mortem had indicated that their son had a genetic problem:

> KA: We were told at the clinic that it was a genetic problem. But there was nothing in my family, except my children's grandfather – my husband's father – who is also my Dad's brother – who died of a heart attack. That was thirteen years ago. But is there a genetic connection? I don't know. There are different kinds of heart problem. My Dad's Dad, he smoked a lot, he was over fifty – in those conditions, at that age, anything can bring it on. I just don't see the connection with my son.
> AS: Do you know why they said it is genetic?
> KA: Our Dads are brothers. Our Mums are sisters. You know how it's like in Pakistan. You have been there. The closer you are, the more likely you marry in the family. If they did not know we were cousins, or if we weren't cousins, they would not say it is genetic. In our culture, there are more people married in the family than out. But you don't see this going on with every family.

Husnain Ahmed, who is in his twenties, British-raised and university educated, attended a genetics appointment with his wife, a first cousin, because their infant daughter has a possibly genetic condition. Afterwards, he told me:

> HA: I don't agree with this cousin marriages and birth defects argument. There are many many people in our community who marry cousins, and in Pakistan too, but you don't see them all having children with medical problems. And English people don't marry cousins, and they sometimes have children with medical problems. How can this be to do with marrying a cousin? I disagree with that. I disagree that marrying a cousin causes a genetic problem. If something is going to happen, it is going to happen. There are millions of reasons why it might happen, especially if my gene is a strong gene, but still, it is not the only factor, it is not a main consideration.
> HA's wife: We might not marry her with a cousin.
> AS: Well, it is a question of an increased risk – not that marrying a cousin is a cause of birth defects, but that it is one of the factors that increased the chance of this happening.

HA: Well, yes, there is a risk, but there is a risk with everything. You sit and hear on television about the medical risks of cousin marriage, and you agree with it to an extent, while you are listening. Then, when the TV is finished, you go back to your old way of thinking. It goes in one ear and out the other. So that, even in six weeks' time, even when we are thinking about our daughter and about how this might explain her palate and spinal dip, it is not uppermost in our thinking. It is the media that brings it up into people's minds as an issue, and this is because it is strongly linked to Asians. If you break it down, they don't really mean Asian. Asian means Pakistani or Indian, and here they mean Pakistani – the media focus on one group, and they blow it all out of proportion. Because they have made it into an issue, we are more aware of it now than we would have been.

'There's more risk here than in Pakistan'

Alongside this general scepticism of the consanguinity thesis, families often had other explanations for a child's disorder, while also recognising that ultimately what happens is up to God. Their explanations included accidents, infections, fevers or, in a male infant, a circumcision operation that went wrong; alternatively problems may have arisen from an event in pregnancy such as a husband's violence or drug abuse, a mother's deficient intake of drinking liquids, or vulnerability to malicious spirits or an eclipse of the sun or moon. Some people also believed that many of the problems for which a child was referred to a genetics clinic could potentially be put right by treatments available in Pakistan, from religious specialists, through the use of Unani medicine (*hakīms*) or else because of the change of climate, air and diet. Saleem Ullah, who suspected that the MMR immunisation had caused his son's learning problems, thought such problems were less common in Kashmir because of the climate. 'In Pakistan's hot climate you sweat a lot, it's like being in a sauna, and everything bad comes out,' he said, but his responsibilities in the U.K. made it difficult to take his son to Pakistan.

Sometimes inter-generational differences with regard to the causality and management of a particular disorder produce conflict within the family. Sohrab Hussain is a three-year-old with obesity, learning difficulties and severe speech problems. His grandmother, anxious to understand the reasons for his condition (*bīmārī*) and whether it was simply the result of his 'fatness' (*motāpā*), reasoned (speaking in Panjabi) that if the British doctors can cure or treat him she would keep him in Britain, but, if they cannot, she would take him to Pakistan, where he would get 'smart' (using the English word that here means 'thin'). A few years earlier, she had taken an overweight younger son to Pakistan, and he became very smart (*bahut* smart *hogayā*), losing several stone in weight: 'It is cold in this country, and you get fat here. There, in the heat, you get smart. We had none of these illnesses in our family in Pakistan. Sohrab has not been to Pakistan. If there is no *ilāj* [cure/treatment] for him here, then I will take him to Pakistan.' She said she would also take Sohrab to a *pīr* (spiritual leader) and then he would start to talk. She had already obtained a *tāvīs* (amulet) for him, containing words of the Qur'an, from a *pīr* in Pakistan. The boy's father, in contrast, felt that it would be better to follow the advice of the doctors here. When the grandfather later joined our conversation, I asked him whether anyone in the family had Sohrab's problems of being overweight and not talking:

> Not in our family. Not in our family in the village in Pakistan. No, I have only seen it here. It is something to do with this country. It is a strange thing. In this country, my son's first child was born with this disability and the doctors told my son that this is a family problem, something to do with the blood. They also said that there is a danger that my son will have another child with this problem. In Pakistan, my three brothers and my wife's brothers and sister each have six or seven children, none of them disabled. There is more risk here than in Pakistan.

In a majority of cases, couples who were asked about their family history at a clinical referral would observe, 'We have never seen this thing before' or 'There is no one else in the family,' in this way implying that the disorder cannot be genetic if it's not in the family already. This observation is perfectly consistent with the incidence of rare recessively inherited disorders, which can be passed on by carriers without people necessarily being affected. Moreover, in many of the parts of rural northern Pakistan and Azad Kashmir that the study participants are from, fertility and perinatal infant mortality rates are high and facilities for establishing the cause of pregnancy loss, infant death and childhood illness are absent. It is therefore not surprising that illnesses or deaths that under modern medical surveillance can be attributed to genetic causes will be explained with reference to environmental causes or to the will of God. One young couple speculated about a possible family history among relatives in rural Pakistan, but had no way of confirming it; not only are causes of infant death not routinely investigated, knowledge of pregnancy loss or stillbirth may not be shared within the family.

Exposure to genetic risk is in these ways a feature of the new, British environment. Sohrab's grandfather's comment that 'there is more risk here than in Pakistan' reflects the prevalence of risk discourse in modern societies (Giddens 1991; Beck 1992). The names of the many rare genetic conditions identified, such as Roberts syndrome, Laurence–Moon–Bardet–Biedl syndrome, Fanconi's anaemia and so on, are in general unfamiliar, not just among British Pakistanis but to people of all social or ethnic backgrounds unless they have had family experience of one of these conditions or a training in clinical genetics. The exception, perhaps, is Down syndrome, at least for most British and Americans, for this seems to be widely known as a genetic condition involving learning difficulties, one that can be recognised by the characteristic 'moon face' of affected persons. Geneticists often mention Down syndrome when trying to explain what a genetic syndrome is, particularly one involving chromosomal abnormality. Rayna Rapp notes for America that Down syndrome has become emblematic of genetic syndromes in general, the 'iconic reason that medical professional explain and offer the [amniocentesis] test to pregnant women' over the age of thirty-five (2000: 264). However, I found that Down syndrome does not necessarily provide a cross-culturally valid model for learning disability among British Pakistanis (see also Shaw 2000b). Miriam, whose twenty-week scan showed problems with her third pregnancy, immediately thought 'Down syndrome' because this was in the family. Several other women had heard of Down syndrome in the context of special schooling and prenatal diagnosis but were unclear that it referred to a specific condition arising from having three copies of chromosome 21: rather, it was a generic term for different kinds of genetic condition. A city-educated woman, in the U.K. for six years following her marriage, who has two children with a recessive syndrome, told me she understood a 'Down syndrome test' is done in the U.K. 'to test if the baby has any disabilities, but there is no such test in Pakistan'. She had not understood why she had not been offered it: 'If they did Down syndromes for my children, they would have known about this condition. I don't know why they don't offer it. I have heard you can have it after the twenty-week scan but that you have to have it done privately.' Another woman thought it was a form of depression, as in being 'down'. As one mother told me:

> I have only heard of it here. It is not called Down syndrome in Pakistan.
> AS: Have you seen people who look like Down syndrome in Pakistan?
> Yes, it may be Down syndrome, but people have not heard about it in Pakistan. They don't know about it in Pakistan. My first cousin, my father's stepbrother's daughter (*abu ke step bhāī kī betī*) – she looks like Down's syndrome, but they don't know that is what it is. They accept that some babies are born like that – that God gives some babies like that.

Casting a further gloss on the idea of the novelty of genetic disorders in the U.K., one mother of three infants who died from an undiagnosed probably recessive condition that her doctors had linked to parental consanguinity told me she thought the contemporary discourse of genetic risk in consanguineous marriage is one component of the wider discourse of risk and danger to which the Qu'ran refers in association with *qiāmat* (the end of the world). The calamities of the modern world such as the increased risks of illness, terrorism, torture and the earthquake in Pakistan in 2005 are, she said, signs (*nishān*) of *qiāmat,* the Last Day, according to Qur'anic prophecy.

Conclusion

Media representations of the genetic risks of consanguineous marriage have had the effect of marking out a minority population by means of 'the neutral vocabulary of risk' (Douglas 1992: 28). Lay versions of the risk discourse are often also associated with some erroneous ideas about genetics, such as that genetic problems arise only if parents are cousins and that cousin marriage also causes complex disorders. At the local level, these representations are experienced, in effect, as a racialised theory of disability that marks out a particular ethnic group on the basis of its marriage pattern. While some research participants kept an open mind on the issue and others were deeply concerned, many of my informants regarded the crude form of the consanguinity thesis as quite simply wrong, on the basis of their own accurate lay observations, confidently challenging it with counter-examples of cousin marriages in which children are perfectly healthy.

Within public health discourse, the reduction of a complex social trend such as cousin marriage to a risky lifestyle issue, akin to having unprotected sex, drinking alcohol and smoking cigarettes, suggests a simple solution: 'Don't do it.' This strategy shifts the blame for adverse birth outcome on to the perpetrators of this risky behaviour. Yet, as Douglas has shown us, risk perception is socially and culturally shaped: we may choose to act in a particular way not on grounds of probability but because our choice of action matters to us for other reasons. As Douglas puts it, 'To invoke … probabilities of a particular dangerous event makes surprisingly little difference to the understanding of a choice. This is not because the public does not understand the sums, but because many other objectives which it cares about have been left out of the risk calculation' (Douglas 1992: 40). This central insight is frequently missing in risk analysis; the result is a deficient analysis. In Douglas's verdict, 'Risk analysis that only allows the cautious, risk-averse behaviour to be rational is convicted of crippling cultural bias' (ibid.: 44).

I encountered frequent examples of just such cultural bias in comments made by medical professionals such as family doctors, midwives, health visitors, clinical geneticists and paediatricians about British Pakistanis married to first cousins who have had children affected with serious recessive genetic conditions, yet who persisted in having more children and 'even' in arranging the marriages of their surviving children to first cousins; such genetically risky behaviour appeared to them to be irrational, beyond reasonable explanation. Are most British Pakistanis 'in denial' about the medical risks of parental consanguinity? I have argued here for a more nuanced understanding of British Pakistani reactions to the medical and public discourse of risk in cousin marriage and for situating this risk discourse in its social and cultural context. I develop this argument in the next two chapters, by examining the historical shaping of concern over cousin marriage (Chapter 2) and by analysing Pakistani cousin marriage as a complex and dynamic social trend in which genetic risk is just one of the elements to be weighed in the balance of risks involved in marriage choices (Chapter 3).

CHAPTER 2

CLOSE KIN MARRIAGES: SOME ANTHROPOLOGICAL THEORY AND EUROPEAN HISTORY

In Hosseini's novel about 1970s Afghanistan, when the narrator describes his household servant's marriage to a Shi'a Muslim ethnic Hazara woman, he adds that she is 'also his first cousin and therefore a natural choice for a spouse' (Hosseini 2003: 7). The use of the word 'natural' is telling, because, in many parts of the world besides Afghanistan, a first cousin is indeed considered a natural choice of marriage partner. Marriages between first cousins and other consanguineous kin account for between 20 and 55 per cent of marriages across the geographical region of the southern and eastern borders of the Mediterranean, including North Africa and the Middle East (see Figure 2.1). The North African countries in which consanguineous marriages are practiced include Morocco, Algeria, Tunisia, Libya, Egypt and Sudan, while the Middle Eastern countries include Syria, Jordan, Lebanon, Iraq, Saudi Arabia, Qatar, the United Arab Emirates, Yemen and Oman (Bittles 1990, 2001; Bittles et al. 1991). Although frequently associated with Muslims, who often prefer but do not prescribe it, cousin marriage is also practised within such groups as Christian Arabs and Hindu South Indians (Rao and Inbaraj 1979; Teebi and Farangi 1997). Consanguineous marriages also account for a proportion of marriages in Turkey and eastwards, in Iran, Afghanistan, Pakistan, parts of North and South India, Sri Lanka, and South America, where again they are often a preferred marital form (Jaber et al. 1998).

In contrast, in Western Europe and North America today, marriages between second cousins or closer relatives such as first cousins once removed, first cousins, double first cousins, uncles and nieces, and aunts and nephews are rare, except within particular minority populations. In mid-twentieth-century England, cousin marriages comprised less than 1 percent of all marriages, 'except in some fairly endogamous rural areas' (Fox, 1967: 223; see also Firth et al. 1970: 191; Coleman 1980); elsewhere in Europe too, rates of cousin marriage are generally low, one study from Hungary giving an estimate of 2.9 per cent (Czeizel et al. 1976). Moreover, marrying a first cousin tends to be regarded as unnatural and biologically risky, immoral and evocative of incest. It is also often regarded as illegal, as countering religious or civil law. And yet first cousins are not included in the Jewish,

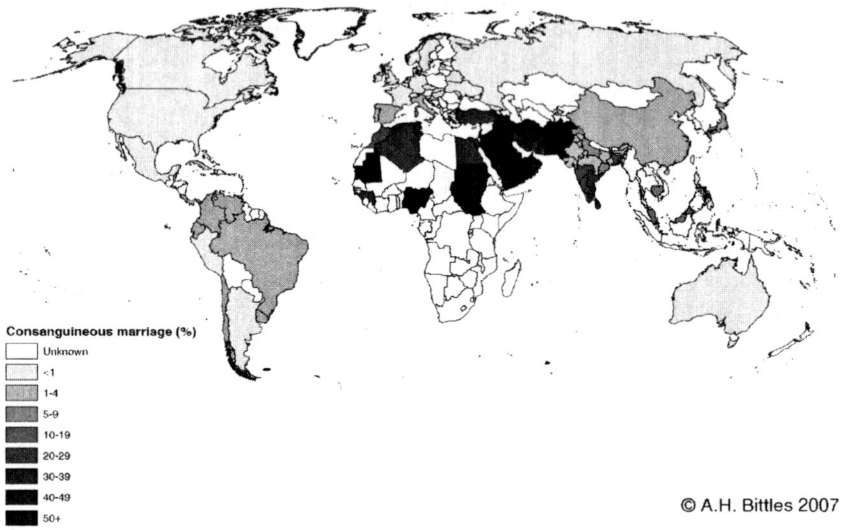

Figure 2.1The current global prevalence of consanguineous marriage: composite summary map (after Bittles 2001). Reproduced from www.consang.net with permission from Alan Bittles and Michael Black; see this website for original source data

Levitical (Old Testament) and Qur'anic lists of forbidden relatives (a fact sometimes cited in support of cousin marriage and sometimes against it) and prohibitions on cousin marriage were only introduced in the Roman Catholic Church from the fourth century AD. Within civil law, cousin marriage has been legal in England since 1540. In America, it is currently illegal in thirty-one out of fifty states, but there were no prohibitions before 1861 (Ottenheimer 1996: 37).

Why this apparent dichotomy between Western Europe (and North America) and the predominantly but not exclusively Muslim countries of the Mediterranean, North Africa and the Middle East, in attitudes towards and the practice of consanguineous marriage? More specifically, what light might anthropology, with its long-standing interest in human kinship and marriage, shed on this question? As I discuss in the first part of this chapter, anthropology has until recently been somewhat limited in its treatment of cousin marriage, particularly where it involves marriage within the descent group. Indeed, within the categories established by some prominent theorists, such marriage often 'appears as a sort of scandal' (Bourdieu 1977: 30). Part of the explanation for this, as I show, lies in the nineteenth-century evolutionary thinking that informed conventional alliance theory. Drawing on more recent anthropological and historical work, I then consider evidence for the popularity of close kin marriage (involving first cousin marriages and sibling exchange, whereby two brothers or a brother and sister from one family marry two sisters or a sister and brother in another) in early nineteenth century Europe, and ask how the far discourses of biological risk that circulated widely in the late nineteenth century in Western Europe and North America influenced the decline of the practice from the late nineteenth century onwards. Besides trying to answer the questions a general reader might ask about the origins of cousin marriage and reasons for its practice, historically and today, this chapter also aims to provide a backdrop for the analysis of British Pakistani marriages presented in Chapter 3. In so doing, it also seeks to highlight the cultural bias (documented in Chapter 1) within contemporary Western perceptions of British Pakistani cousin marriage and, through discussion of the popularity and subsequent decline of close kin marriage in Western Europe in the nineteenth century, to suggest continuities and discontinuities with the situation confronting Pakistani and other minorities in Europe and North America today.

Early origins: keeping the girls in the family for the boys in the family

According to the Old Testament, one of the wives of Abraham ('the holy prophet who engendered the Arabs and Jews') was his half-sister Sarah, of whom Abraham noted 'Indeed she is my sister; she is the daughter of my father, but not the daughter of my mother; and she became my wife' (Genesis 20: 12; Tillion 1983: 68). Other stories of close kin marriage in the Book of Genesis include marriages among Abraham's descendants. Abraham arranges his son Isaac's marriage to his second cousin, Rebecca, who is the granddaughter of Abraham's brother; Isaac and Rebecca's son Esau, after already marrying two foreign women, marries a paternal cousin, the daughter of one of Abraham's sons, in order to please his father, and Esau's brother Jacob also marries within his father's lineage – first Leah and then Rachel (for whom he waited fourteen years). Leah and Rachel are Rebecca's brother Laban's daughters; they are therefore related to Jacob as first cousins and also as second cousins in the paternal line, by descent from Abraham's brother (Tillion 1983: 68–70). Germain Tillion argues that in these passages from Genesis it is the fact of common paternity that made such unions lawful according to the social mores of ancient Israel: marriage within the patrilineage was the desired form of marriage.

Cousin marriage was apparently permitted and practised within ancient Israel, Greece and Palestine; one legend has it that Jesus Christ was born of a first cousin marriage (Goody 1983: 53). On the basis of scriptural reference, historical observation, and fieldwork, mainly in Africa among the peoples of the Maghreb, anthropologist Germain Tillion proposes in a small book called *The Republic of Cousins: Women's Oppression in Mediterranean Society*, first published in French in 1966, that the practice of cousin marriage and specifically of marrying a woman within the paternal lineage has very deep historical origins, pre-dating the rise of Islam. Not prohibited in the early Hebrew or Christian religion, it is 'infinitely more ancient than the revelation of the Koran' (Tillion 1983: 25).

Tillion offers an evolutionary explanation for the origin of the practice of cousin marriage, particularly the marriage of a man to his father's brother's daughter (FBD), and its continued popularity for centuries without being 'wiped out by the launderings of time', though not in a biological sense (ibid.: 35). She proposes that the 'Republic of Cousins' enabled a very lengthy transition from 'savage society', marked by the rule of exogamous marriage and zero population growth, to the 'Republic of Citizens', marked by respect for the individual, 'which thrives in [the] structured states' of the modern world (ibid.: 14). This transition is incomplete: many parts of the contemporary world, such as the Middle East, North Africa and the Mediterranean, can still be described in terms of features of the 'Republic of Cousins' and within European and American society the practices of endogamy and female seclusion have left a deep legacy.

Characteristic features of the 'Republic of Cousins' include the segregation of women and their exclusion from public places combined with a preference for marriage within the paternal lineage, between the children of brothers. These features, for Tillion, are key to understanding the beginnings of settled agriculture and thus of urban society, marking the transition from an increasingly precarious hunting and gathering existence to a lifestyle of agricultural production and stock-rearing during the Neolithic revolution. Along the European, Asian and African borders of the Mediterranean, cousin marriage emerged as a preferred means of promoting solidarity between kin holding land in common. Secluding women and denying them inheritance rights helped secure this new system by ensuring that no one outside the ancestral lineage acquired the family's land. Subsequently, inheritance rights for women, introduced in Islam (specified in the Qur'an), undermined this process; in consequence, systematically veiling daughters and marrying them to paternal relatives became even more important, indeed crucial, in protecting tribal or family interests in land (Tillion 1983: 30).

These processes, Tillion argues, ensured the high birth rates and dramatic population growth that marked the Neolithic revolution: endogamy, female seclusion and settled agriculture combined to promote production and reproduction and support this expansionist lifestyle. Throughout the entire ancient Mediterranean world, the most desirable marriage came to be defined as 'marriage with a very close relative belonging to your own lineage' (ibid.: 37). Rather than exchanging women, the ideal became 'to keep all the girls in the family for the boys in the family' (ibid.: 74). Besides creating a cultural ideal, these processes had emotional or psychological concomitants, chiefly with respect to gender roles and female dependency upon men.

Evolutionary theory

Archaeologists and historians might doubt that a single cultural logic united the entire ancient Mediterranean region; social anthropologists are likely to question the broad sweep of Tillion's evolutionary theory in, for instance, the extent to which 'respect for the individual' has replaced a more relational concept of person within so-called modern individualistic societies. Moreover, the analysis of gendered divisions of labour and use of social space as 'female oppression', historically and cross-culturally, is a matter of long-standing debate in anthropology (e.g. Strathern 1987). Most importantly, an origin theory for close kin marriage is not necessarily an explanation for contemporary practices, which may need to be understood in terms of other factors, which are likely to vary with locality and as circumstances change (Holy 1989: 12–14).

Even so, Tillion's hypothesis is striking in suggesting a common cultural origin for a practice permitted in the early Hebrew and Christian religions and pre-dating the rise of Islam, and for taking seriously a practice that had been either ignored or else redefined as a form of exogamy (marrying outside the descent group) within prominent anthropological scholarship. Nineteenth-century evolutionary theories had defined prohibitions against marrying close kin (such as those introduced in the early Roman Catholic Church) as characteristic of more fit and intelligent human groups (Lubbock 1870; Morgan 1871, 1877; Westermarck 1891), making cousin marriage problematic. Lewis Henry Morgan (an American lawyer and scholar), for instance, who viewed reproduction as the essential function of marriage, considered that prohibitions against cousin marriage were biologically protective evolutionary mechanisms that, under natural selection, would maximise physical and intellectual fitness and advance human civilisation (1877). In fact, Morgan considered not just physical characteristics but patterns of thought to be biologically inherited, 'handed down … through channels of blood' (1871: v; see also 4–13, quoted in Ottenheimer 1996: 112). His influential works described the evolution of human marriage in terms of a progression from primitive to complex societies and from promiscuity to monogamy: brother–sister exchange was an evolutionary advance on brother–sister incest, but if the rules governing this exchange did not involve marriage outside the descent group (exogamy) then this was a more primitive form of marriage (Morgan 1877).

The idea of primitive promiscuity was dropped in anthropological scholarship, but the idea that exogamy was more advanced than endogamy persisted; Morgan himself classified different societies on this basis (1877; Ottenheimer 1996: 110). But for Morgan exogamy referred not to genetic distance or, more loosely, to marrying 'outside' the group, but instead, following McLennan (1865), meant marriage outside the descent group (and endogamy meant marriage within it). His definition reflects the fact that human reckonings of kinship and descent rarely correspond to the understanding of consanguinity as genetic relatedness, and it also enabled him to exclude societies with specific prohibitions on marriage within the descent group (often combined with prescriptive marriage rules) from the accusation of being primitive. The North American Iroquois, for instance, prohibited marriage with the patrilineal clan, and, like another group, the Ojibwa

Indians, distinguished different kinds of cousin by specific terms (unlike the Europeans, for whom the term 'cousin' is generic). They forbade marriage with the father's brother's daughter (FBD), but prescribed marriages with the mother's brother's daughter (MBD) or father's sister's daughter (FZD) because these women belong to different descent groups. Morgan also noted that the Tamil and Telegu peoples of South India similarly distinguished different kinds of cousins and forbade marriage with a cousin on the father's side.

For Morgan, the important aspect of these marriage rules was not the focus on consanguineous kin, such as first cousins, as such, but the prohibition on marriage within the descent group. Like some other eminent Victorians, he had married (in 1851) a first cousin. Others included Charles Darwin, author of the *Origin of Species* (1859) and *The Descent of Man* (1871); the lawyer Henry Maine, who wrote on the origins of human marriage (1883) and Alfred Henry Huth, who reviewed the evidence on biological consequences of consanguinity (1887). As his wife was his mother's brother's daughter and therefore not of the same descent group, 'Morgan could view his marriage (Charles Darwin's marriage as well) to his cousin as ... neither endogamous not primitive' (Ottenheimer 1996: 111).

Morgan's theory therefore reflected nineteenth-century evolutionary concerns about inbreeding which, although unsupported by genetic science, were used to justify laws against cousin marriage in some American states. In the legal context his distinction between exogamy and endogamy was lost, but in mainstream anthropology the distinction persisted and took on a life of its own. Sir Edward Tylor (an English scholar) viewed exogamy as essential to socio-political survival because it enabled the formation of alliances (Maine 1883; Tylor 1889). Tylor's theoretical emphasis was less directly biological and more cultural. He stressed the socio-political functions of exogamy, famously writing, 'Again and again in the world's history, savage tribes must have had plainly before their minds the simple practical alternative between marrying-out and being killed-out' (Tylor 1889: 267). He distinguished parallel-cousin marriages (marriages of a man to his FBD or to his MZD) as endogamous, from cross-cousin marriages (MBD or FZD marriages) as exogamous, involving different descent groups. He considered that women played an important role in providing social cohesion in exogamous systems, because they would be motivated to resolve disputes between different descent groups as a result of their dual allegiances, to one group as sisters and to another as wives (ibid.: 268). The South Indian Dravidian kinship system became an exemplar of this system: within it, the preferred form of cousin marriage is marriage with the MBD, which is also the most common form of cross-cousin marriage. The links between cross-cousin marriage, exogamy and alliance were then most famously developed by Claude Lévi-Strauss (a French structural anthropologist) in his monumental *The Elementary Structures of Kinship* (1969), a work that is simultaneously evolutionary, structural and functional. It is premised on the centrality of the incest taboo: for survival human groups must exchange women –

the sisters of men in one group must become the wives of men in another – and the incest taboo and prescriptive cross-cousin marriage (MBD marriage) maintain the system. The theory, however, depends on a problematic characterisation of women's role in marriage: while Tylor stressed women's mediating role, Lévi-Strauss depicted women as objects of exchange by men, a characterisation that has persisted within much twentieth-century structuralist-functionalist analysis (Sacks 1979; Ottenheimer 1996: 141). And the model so famously depicted by Lévi-Strauss in fact relates only to a small number of societies worldwide (Parkin and Stone 2004: 16).

The dominant focus on cross-cousin marriage in anthropological theory had the effect of sidelining societies in which the preferred marriage is with a patrilateral cousin (FBD), or within the descent group (Ottenheimer 1986, 1996). From the perspective of conventional alliance theory, such marriage scandalously blurs lines of descent, since a person can be related to a paternal grandparent through both their father and their mother (Bourdieu 1977: 30). And yet, as we have seen, marriage with the FBD or within the descent group is significant in many parts of the world, including the contemporary Islamic world, and historically was of widespread importance across the Mediterranean region – according to Tillion, marriage between the children of brothers or within the descent group promoting solidarity between kin holding land in common (1983) – and even beyond it, in China and Japan for instance, until the mid-twentieth century (Imaizumi 1987; Bittles 1990; Bittles et al. 1991; Jaber et al. 1998). Yet anthropological discussion of it is noticeably absent in some key texts on marriage (e.g. Fox 1967; see Ottenheimer 1996: 142).

Cousin marriages: from economic or political functions to cultural transmission

In societies where FBD marriage or marriage within the descent group occurs, such marriages are preferential, not prescribed (Parkin 1997: 109), and occur alongside marriage of other types – with other cousins, more distant kin and outside the descent group (see, for example, Tapper 1981: 387; Ottenheimer 1996: 142). Indeed, in such countries as Pakistan, there is no marked preference for FBD marriage; the preference instead is for marriage within the kin group – as the Dhund of North-East Pakistan put it, 'It is better to marry a relative than someone you do not know' (Donnan 1985: 183) – but this preference is not followed in every case (Donnan 1985; Werbner 1990; Shaw 2001; Charsley 2003).

Explanations for preferential FBD marriage or marriage within the descent group have sought to account for the preference in terms of its positive functions for those who follow it or for the social system in which it occurs. The classic functional explanation for cousin marriage, especially for marriages between the children of two brothers, is that it keeps property, especially land, within the family

(Westermarck 1891). Pakistanis in Britain and in Pakistan often offer this explanation for cousin marriage, which also dominates in historical accounts of cousin marriages in Europe. Although it might seem that cousin marriage cannot create alliances because 'it unites people who are already connected' (Holy 1989: 1), many authors have noted how cousin marriages can strengthen existing links between kin. Preferential FBD marriage has been depicted in the Middle East as 'solidifying the minimal lineage as a corporate group in factional struggle' (Barth 1954: 171) or as a mechanism that confers strength and political flexibility in Arab society, since smaller lineage groups can break away from larger kindreds, or can regroup on the basis of shared descent, if necessary (Murphy and Kasdan 1959). Among Pakistanis, consanguineous marriage is viewed as a means of sustaining kinship links that would otherwise weaken. As one Panjabi proverb puts it, 'When the fence is old, it is your duty to put new wood into it' (Werbner 1990: 96); another has it that 'A new brick strengthens the wall' (Shaw 2000a: 155). For British Pakistanis, marriages with Pakistan-raised cousins are increasingly significant in maintaining links between transnationally divided kin (Shaw 2001; Charsley 2003).

Noting the lack of consensus in economic or political explanations for preferential marriage with the FBD or within the kin group, Ladislav Holy argues that the preference is best understood in symbolic terms – as a symbol of the cultural value of marriage with the closest possible kin (other than those prohibited as spouses by incest rules), which is related to other cultural notions such as the value of keeping property in the group and the importance of women's behaviour for male honour; for Holy, these notions (following Bourdieu) comprise the group's cultural resources or its 'symbolic capital' (Holy 1989: 113). These explanations for the existence of the preference, however, are inadequate as an explanation of the marriage choices people make in practice, since the marriage preference may have little bearing on actual marriage choices.

In an important contribution to the analysis of marriage choices, Hastings Donnan observes that the focus on a marriage preference in complex systems has meant that marriages not conforming to the preference are treated as exceptional (or as occurring only if a relative is unavailable e.g. Eglar 1960: 94), while the existence of the preference is assumed to be sufficient as an explanation of why people marry relatives. But, Donnan writes, identifying the function of a marriage preference, for individuals or for the society, may explain its existence as a cultural rule, but does not explain why in some cases people do marry kin and in other instances they do not. The reasons for a particular marriage choice are not necessarily – or simultaneously – the reasons why a marriage preference exists. He proposes a model for interpreting marriage choices that incorporates political and economic considerations (which anthropologists know are involved in marriage choices) 'on an equal footing' with cultural preferences expressed in terms of kinship (Donnan 1988: 209). Donnan argues that marriage choices and negotiations should be understood in strategic terms rather than in terms of a marriage preference: in this process, cultural preferences based on kinship (including the preference for marrying relatives and the obligation to consider spouses as kin) are important but not the only considerations. Also important are reputation, the balancing of a need for new contacts with that of strengthening existing connections, economic possibilities and personal preferences, the relative weight of each depending on the particular circumstances in each case. As Bourdieu has put it, 'Marriages which are identical as regards genealogy alone may thus have different, even opposite, meanings and functions, depending on the strategies in which they are involved. These can only be grasped by means of a reconstruction of the entire system of relationships between two associated groups and of the state of these relationships at a given point in time' (1977: 48).

This model has been useful in explaining the popularity of transnational cousin marriages among British Pakistanis (Shaw 2001), as well as in explaining why marriages may connect some relatives at the expense of others, effectively fracturing a wider network (e.g. Shaw 2000a: 144), and may take place with non-kin (Donnan 1988; see also Ahmad 1978; Jeffery 1996a: 98–99). For British Pakistanis, the additional strategic considerations involved in marriage include the benefits of opportunities for labour migration, particularly for Pakistan-based kin, although marriage migration introduces new risks associated with 'bogus' marriages (Shaw 2001; Charsley 2006).

The focus on strategy in the sense of maximising socio-economic resources may, however, overlook the significance of emotional connections between kin, which may be particularly heightened in transnational contexts (Charsley 2003; Shaw and Charsley 2006). Trust, too, is important within the motivations for close kin marriages, in diverse situations, including among urban Hindus in India (Jeffery and Jeffery 1996a: 98–9): marriages with relatives are seen as a means of reducing the risks associated with marrying outside the family, since the family provides 'referees in the form of mutual kin, who can advise on the character of the proposed spouse and their family' (Charsley 2003: 141). As we shall see in Chapter 3, among British Pakistanis, marriages involving spouses from Pakistan are also seen as important in the creation of a common religious culture in which to raise children in the U.K. Marriage with kin is thus not merely symbolic of the solidarity of the kin group but is associated with real pragmatic, social, cultural and emotional benefits, each of which needs to be identified in research.

Anthropological analysis has therefore moved from a focus on the function of marriage preferences to explaining actual marriage choices in terms of people's purposive strategies and motivations. Thus, in some situations, particular choices may be less a question of maximising resources or opportunities and more a reflection of affective ties between kin or concerns to manage the perceived socio-economic, emotional and cultural risks associated with marrying 'outsiders'. Nonetheless, marriage choices do have structural, socio-economic and cultural effects. Thus, Pnina Werbner notes that the flow of gifts and marriage partners between Pakistan and Britain is crucial to the creation and recreation of Pakistani ethnicity in the U.K. (Werbner 1990; see also Shaw 2000a). Martin Ottenheimer offers a more general theory: that cousin marriage is important for cultural continuity. He notes that, because they are the children of siblings, parents who are first cousins are more likely effectively to transmit a coherent set of cultural values to their children. Where one partner moves to their spouse's parental home on marriage, 'Both the husband and the wife will be living with members from the previous generation of their own unilineal descent group' (Ottenheimer 1996: 149); this will enhance cultural continuity, for instance, with respect to how the division of labour in a household is gendered. Cousin marriage is not the only way to achieve cultural continuity, however, and some cousin marriages do not have this effect; among British Pakistanis some cousin marriages flounder because of the discontinuities between spouses raised continents apart (Shaw 2001; Charsley 2005). Perhaps what is most important here is the perceived association between close kin, including cousin, marriage and cultural continuity, both in the motivations for such marriage and in attempts to prohibit it. Thus, Ottenheimer (1996) suggests that prohibitions against cousin marriage in the late nineteenth and early twentieth century in the U.S.A. effectively undermined the distinct identity of cultural and religious minorities. In contemporary Europe, debates over the potential biological risks of cousin marriage have become linked, in the popular imagination, with the non-assimilation or non-integration of mainly Pakistani Muslim cultural minorities (Chapter 1). As we shall see, various strands of these explanatory threads are present in historical and anthropological work on cousin marriages in Europe.

Cousin marriages in Europe

Establishing the historical popularity of cousin marriage in Europe (as elsewhere) requires reliable information on whether the parents of each partner in a couple are related as siblings, but this is not routinely recorded, in marriage records for instance. European historians have inferred the popularity of parallel-cousin marriages, at least, by analysing surname patterns – since these societies use a 'surname system' whereby a woman adopts her husband's second name on marriage, relinquishing her 'maiden' name. If both partners had the same surname before marriage, they might be the children of same-sex siblings; if the same sets of surnames occur among the parents and grandparents, this may indicate a continuing pattern of first cousin and sibling exchange marriage over the generations (Molloy 1986: 233). Shared surnames might not indicate consanguinity, of course, and the technique fails to identify cross-cousin marriages between children of different-sex siblings; it would also be of little value as a research tool in societies in which a surname system is not used. Nonetheless, this and other methods have offered some indication of the popularity of close kin marriage in nineteenth-century Europe and, later, in North America and the colonies.

There is some evidence that cousin marriage was a numerically significant minority marriage pattern in many parts of Europe well before the nineteenth century, from before opposition to it from the early Church in Europe and continuing despite such opposition and beyond, after the re-liberalisation of marriage rules during the Reformation (Goody 1983, Reid 1988). The Church's doctrine on incest (sexual intercourse between people forbidden by the Church to marry) was originally based on the rules set out in the Old Testament, which include certain close kin but do not include first cousins (Leviticus 18: 6–18) but a ban on cousin marriage was introduced into the early Church 'in the waning years of the Roman empire, towards the end of the fourth century' (Ottenheimer 1996: 63). However, the Catholic prohibitions did not necessarily prevent cousin marriage because cousin couples could be granted dispensations to marry. The Church benefited financially from the prohibitions, because the European peasantry routinely paid for dispensations (Goody 1983: 183–88). Indeed, the anthropologist Jack Goody speculates that the early Roman Catholic Church may have introduced the prohibitions precisely to gain lucre from the dispensations it expected cousin couples would pay for marriage licences, since cousin marriage was widespread in the regions served by the early Church at the time. Catholic definitions of prohibited unions actually fluctuated until the thirteenth century, when cousin marriages up to and including third cousins were prohibited except under dispensation. This remained the Catholic position up until the twentieth century. In 1917, a Papal decree reduced the range of prohibited kin, so that today only first and second cousins require dispensations to marry (Ottenheimer 1996: 63–68). Rates of consanguineous marriage within predominantly Catholic Mediterranean countries such as Italy fluctuated partly in relation to the ease with which the authorities granted dispensations (Ottenheimer 1996). Elsewhere, people living in remote communities may have been unaware of or able to disregard Church prohibitions (Molloy 1986: 240).

The Protestant Reformation in the sixteenth century brought strong opposition to the Catholic prohibitions on cousin marriage as well as to the system of church dispensations. Martin Luther, who led the Protestant revolt, called for a radical re-liberalisation of the marriage rules, accepting only the prohibitions listed in Leviticus. His supporter John Calvin reasoned that only relatives of the same degree or closer than those mentioned in Leviticus should be considered prohibited kin (Reid 1988; Ottenheimer 1996). Protestant reforms in marriage law were instituted first in continental Europe and soon afterwards in England, 'where they became embroiled in hotly debated political matters' (Ottenheimer 1996: 69).

In Henry VIII's England, Parliament legalised first cousin marriage in 1540 and denounced the Roman Catholic prohibitions, with the approval of many Protestant theologians. 'The immediate purpose of this law was to clear the way for the marriage of Henry VIII to Catherine Howard, who was the first cousin of a previous wife, Anne Boleyn' and was to become his fifth wife (Kuper 2002: 162). Henry had to legalise first cousin marriage in order to marry not his own cousin but his former wife's first cousin because of an argument based on the biblical description of a man and wife as being 'one flesh' (Genesis 2: 24, referred to also in Matthew 19: 6; Mark 10: 8 and Ephesians 5: 31). On the basis of this argument, the Catholic Church had extended the Levitical list of prohibited kin to include additional affines (kin by marriage). If a husband and wife are one body, the argument ran, then one spouse's close kin are also the close kin of the other spouse, and so are prohibited as marriage partners; 'for a man to have sexual relations with a wife's sister, for example, was equivalent to having sex with his own sister' (Kuper 2002: 161). The same reasoning applied to cousins, in that a rule forbidding first cousin marriage would thus also prohibit marriage to a spouse's first cousin. Henry VIII's reforms permitted first cousin marriage, making legal Henry's own marriage to a previous wife's cousin, but they did not challenge the logic of prohibiting marriage with affines, such as a deceased wife's sister or a deceased husband's brother; these prohibitions were to persist in England for almost another 400 years, being hotly debated in the nineteenth century and then lifted in the early twentieth century (Wolfram 1987; Kuper 2002; Simpson 2006).

Land, property and economic security: close kin marriage in the nineteenth century

The conventional wisdom is that industrialisation inevitably effects a transformation in kinship that involves the weakening of extended networks, in favour of smaller family units comprising couples and their unmarried children, and that this weakening of extended kinship is related, at least in part, to the decline in dependence on the land (Davidoff 2006). From this perspective, a decline in consanguineous marriage would also be expected, at least according to classic functional theory that first cousin marriage keeps property, especially land, within the family (Westermarck 1891). As we saw, preventing the alienation of family land is an important component of Tillion's explanation for prevalence of cousin marriage in the ancient world (Tillion 1983: 10). Goody's argument that the Roman Catholic Church prohibitions on cousin marriage 'broke the continuity of European family estates and maneuvered property into the church' is likewise essentially an economic argument relating to land and property (Goody 1983; Ottenheimer 1996: 68).

Functional explanations of this sort recur in historical accounts of cousin marriage in pre-industrial Europe. Historian Nancy Fix Anderson writes that in pre-industrial England, where investments in land were the principal source of income, 'marriages were often arranged by families, and among the propertied classes cousin marriages were a useful means of consolidating and expanding family land and capital' and that in this social class, 'cousin marriage was a common practice' (Anderson 1986: 285). Several studies show that cousin marriage was important in various farming districts of the Scottish Highlands in the late eighteenth century, and so may have been more widely practised across Scotland, England and Wales. Anthropologist Maureen Molloy reports for three Scottish kindreds that 'sixty percent of all couples [married in the early nineteenth century] for whom complete data is [*sic*] available had at least two parents with the same surname' (1986: 233). Marriages between the offspring of agnatic kin who held farms in joint tenure in the Scottish Highlands constituted 20.1 per cent of all marriages between 1775 and 1800, and 25.4 per cent between 1801 and 1825 (MacPherson 1968; see also Pryce 1993).

Recent research on marriage and family under early industrialisation suggests, however, that rather than heralding an immediate decline in close kin marriages, there were local increases in first cousin and sibling-exchange marriages in many parts of Europe, including some Catholic areas, where first cousin marriages were normally prohibited, and also in parts of North America and the colonies. The picture is far from complete, and the effects of industrialisation and urbanisation were extremely uneven, by region, locality and social class. However, historian Leonore Davidoff suggests that during this period of social change, there was a broad shift in patterns of significant kinship away from the wider network of the extended family towards a closer circle of kin, consisting of wife and husband, children, siblings, aunts, uncles, nieces, nephews and cousins, and it was from this closer circle of kin that marriage partners were often drawn (Davidoff 2006).

Perhaps the best-known illustration of a long-standing tradition of consanguineous marriage is that of the Protestant royal families in Europe, connected over the generations through transnational marriage. Over a period of 300 years following the crowning of King George I in 1714, close kin marriages accounted for one-third (29.9 per cent) of the marriages of rulers, defined as people who became or were expected to become reigning sovereigns (Fleming 1973). The fact that cousin marriage was traditional within the European royalty may well have added to its popularity in other parts of Europe in the nineteenth century. In England in 1840, Queen Victoria married her first cousin, her mother's brother's son Albert, who had been raised mainly in Germany. The match was first suggested four years earlier by Victoria's uncle, King Leopold of the Belgians; after her initial misgivings, Victoria decided in 1839 that she wanted this marriage, which lasted until Albert's death in 1861 (Lee 1997). George I and George IV also married first cousins, while Elizabeth II and George V married second cousins. The tradition can be traced back to the parents of James I, who were first cousins (Fleming 1973; Kuper 2002).

In the case of the Rothschild dynasty, anthropologist Adam Kuper suggests that cousin marriage may have been less a family tradition than a creative strategy to protect and promote economic interests, and that this strategy 'yielded them a competitive advantage that may have been decisive' (2001: 274). The conventional view is that family solidarity was the key to the success of the Rothschild bank, from the early nineteenth to the early twentieth century. Historian Niall Ferguson cites Disraeli as remarking that, in family unity, 'they were like an Arabian tribe' (Ferguson 1998: 105). The Jewish patriarch Mayer Rothschild, who had struggled to rise from the ghetto, founded a banking business in Frankfurt. Three of his five sons first joined the Frankfurt partnership, while two sons established branches in London and Paris; later, branches of the Frankfurt bank were established in Vienna and Naples. Cooperation between these five branches enabled the Rothschilds to become 'far and away the largest bank in the world' (Kuper 2001: 273).

Adam Kuper argues that the mechanism of this solidarity was not simply the fraternity among the five sons imposed by their father, which excluded women from the partnership. Links between the five branches of the bank were maintained by reciprocal visiting and by sending a partner's son for an apprenticeship in another branch of the bank (a practice also common in English middle-class family businesses; see below), but the strategic use of cousin marriages was more important in ensuring the structural continuity of the partnership. In the third generation (1824–77), cousin marriages were specifically arranged to sustain the links between the five branches, uniting the children of two partners. These, then, were marriages involving cousins whose fathers were brothers, or related in the male line, echoing the ancient Middle Eastern preference for marriage with the father's brother's daughter. Yet the Rothschild strategy, Adam Kuper argues, was unique in its time: the European Jewish elite usually arranged marriages outside the family with other wealthy Jews, while cousin marriages within the European royalty involved both maternal and paternal kin. By the 1870s, however, strategic cousin marriage no longer proved adaptive in a more nationalist and competitive economic environment (Kuper 2001).

In the mid- and late nineteenth century, increases in cousin marriages in some other parts of Europe where families still owned land seem to have been a response to laws abolishing primogeniture (the eldest son's right to inherit) and giving all children an equal right to inherit, since cousin marriages protected land from being overly divided (see Ottenheimer 1996: 91). Elsewhere, cousin marriages may have been a response to other economic transformations associated with industrialisation, such as, in Italy, the authorities' attempts to eliminate communal property from among the peasantry (Merzario 1990: 542). Consanguineous marriages had been common and dispensations from the Catholic prohibitions were granted fairly easily in many parts of rural Italy from the seventeenth to the nineteenth centuries (Merzario 1990). In one of many Italian examples, in the Mosso valley of northern Italy in the 1850s the proportion of cousin marriages increased significantly, to thirty per cent, during a 'decisive phase of transition for the community, with the weavers going to work in factories and no longer at home': consanguineous marriage 'was an obvious attempt to keep family patrimonies intact, avoiding dispersion' (Ramella 1984: 102, quoted in Merzario 1990: 540). After 1861 cousin marriages also increased because cousin couples had recourse to civil marriage without any need for dispensation (Ottenheimer 1996: 91).

In England in the late eighteenth and well into the nineteenth century as industrial capitalism developed, close kin marriages were also important among the middle classes, even without any direct links with the land. Leonore Davidoff argues that first cousin and sibling-exchange marriages provided families with, among other things, a flexible means of adapting to new economic conditions. English middle-class economic activities at this time were dominated by the ideals of family enterprise and family-based 'partnership'. These partnerships commonly consisted of a father and son (or sons), a father and brother or an uncle and nephew, and were often established after a younger male relative had received his training or apprenticeship from the older one. Marianne Kenrick, for instance, married her first cousin Samuel shortly after he had joined Marianne's father's buckle manufacturing business in 1812; in this case, Marianne was to experience deeply divided loyalties when Samuel subsequently quarrelled with Marianne's father and established a separate business (Davidoff and Hall 2002: 217, 219). In other instances, men sought business partners in their existing brothers-in-law, cementing a prior affinal link: 'sisters married their brothers' partners and sisters' husbands often became partners after marriage, thus binding two families into the fortunes of the enterprise' (ibid.: 217–18). There are some parallels here with British Pakistani marriages, where, for instance a man has married his business partner's sister, or where first cousin marriages involving British-based kin helped consolidate the joint businesses ventures of brothers or of brothers and a brother-in-law (Shaw 2000a: 129, 147).

Cultural, social and religious continuity

It would be misleading, however, to consider only the material aspects of cousin marriage, for religious and social continuity was often as important as protecting an agricultural livelihood or business interests as industrial capitalism developed. Even among people whose interests remained closely tied to the land, cousin marriages were more than simply instrumental to economic ends: they also represented a cultural ideal. Merzario notes that throughout pre-industrial Italy, where consanguineous marriage was closely linked with communal land ownership, the ideal marriage was always one made between kin. Consanguineous marriages, within the categories permitted by the church or contracted through fairly easily granted dispensations, were attempts to keep women 'within the same lineage', which reflected not just the desire to maintain landownership; rather, 'land and blood [had] become the fundamental values on which the community's social and economic system were based' (Merzario 1990: 544). In this we can discern parallels with studies of cousin marriage in the Mediterranean and the Middle East, which also emphasise its role in expressing the values given to the preservation of the agnatic lineage (Tillion 1983; Holy 1989: 112–13).

In such marriage arrangements, it is often difficult to disentangle family interests and personal choice and, in particular, to identify the role of spousal agency, an issue also present in contemporary debate over arranged and forced marriage in Europe. Adam Kuper (2001) reports for the Rothschild dynasty that senior kinswomen played an important role in arranging marriages between Mayer Rothschild's descendants and it was virtually unimaginable that a child would form emotional attachments outside the family. In 1839, Hannah Mayer shocked the family by marrying the son of an English aristocrat; this prompted her paternal uncle, Mayer's son James, to write to Hannah's brothers (his London nephews) to warn them of the threat to future marriages planned within the family of tolerating romantic attachments outside it. He reminded them that Rothschilds have been raised 'with the sense that love is to be confined to members of the family, that their attachment for one another would prevent them from getting any ideas of marrying anyone other than one of the family so that the fortune would stay inside the family' (Ferguson 1998: 321). As we shall see in Chapter 3, love and romance may also be present in British Pakistani transnational marriages involving cousins.

In many other European families, marriages were less formally arranged or were based chiefly or entirely on the personal choice of both partners, but this choice was exercised from within a person's economic, social and geographical circle and 'set in a carefully controlled context of mutual values and religious concerns' (Davidoff and Hall 2002: 219). Young people's opportunities for forging emotional attachments with the opposite sex tended to be found within their, usually local, close circles of family, friends and kin, in keeping with the social mores of the time.

Consanguineous marriage in England was not 'peculiar to any one religious, occupation or geographical area' (ibid.: 220–21) but was most likely to occur between people whose families were already connected socially, usually through common business or religious interests. The evidence for this comes mainly from the middle classes. A well-known example concerns the upper-middle-class Darwin and Wedgwood families. Erasmus Darwin, who would become Charles Darwin's grandfather, reached 'an understanding' with his friend Josiah Wedgwood I, founder of the Wedgwood pottery business near Stoke-on-Trent, that Josiah's daughter would marry Erasmus's son Robert. Susanna Wedgwood had 'been in and out of the Darwins' Derby house since childhood' and when she and Robert married in 1796, her inheritance from her father was 'an acceptable addition to the family fortune' (Desmond and Moore 1991: 11). In the next generation, two first cousin marriages helped maintain the link between the Darwin and Wedgwood families. In 1837, Robert and Susanna's daughter Caroline married her mother's brother's son, Josiah Wedgwood III. About a year later, Caroline's brother Charles married Emma Wedgwood, Josiah Wedgwood III's sister. From Charles's point of view, Emma was 'about the only eligible daughter left in his small circle of acceptable family acquaintances, and she came with a dowry' (ibid.: 258).

Sibling-exchange marriages involving siblings related as first cousins were quite common in middle- and upper-class business partnerships as well as in the marriages of European royalty (Fleming 1973; Davidoff and Hall 2002). Such marriages produce double first cousins in the next generation, for the children are related as cousins in two ways, through both their mothers and their fathers. These cousins, too, might marry one another: 'As in any such alliances, the connections were not only bound up in the two people involved but their parents, as in-laws, would be related to each other twice over and thus they would have a double interest in nieces, nephews and any grandchildren' (Davidoff and Hall 2002: 221).

The Wedgwood family provides an interesting instance of such complex consanguinity, as illustrated in Figure 2.2. Here, an earlier sibling-exchange marriage involving the Allen family had taken place in the previous generation of Wedgwood family marriages, when Josiah I's sons John and Josiah II married two Allen sisters. In the next generation, Henry Allen Wedgwood married Jessie Wedgwood; they were related as cousins through both their fathers and their mothers (see also Kuper 2002: 167). Such patterns also occur within some contemporary Pakistani kindreds: for instance, Khalida's father and her husband's father are brothers and her mother and her husband's mother are sisters; the same is true of her brother and his wife (Chapter 7).

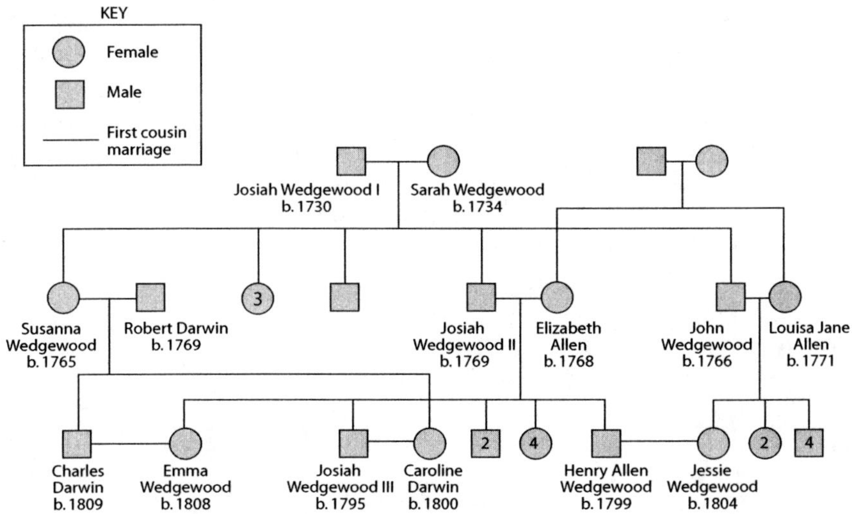

Figure 2.2 First Cousin Marriages in the Wedgwood, Allen and Darwin families in the eighteenth and nineteenth centuries. The figure is adapted from Wedgwood (1909: Chart XIIa). Among the first-generation descendants of Josiah and Sarah Wedgwood, there are sibling-exchange marriages (between the Wedgwood and Allen families); in the next generation, there are three first cousin marriages, two involving sibling exchange (between the Wedgwood and Darwin families) and one of double first cousins (Henry and Jessie Wedgwood)

Close kin marriage and cultural continuity: European immigrants in the New World

In the nineteenth and early twentieth century, first cousin and sibling-exchange marriages were also reportedly common within some European-origin emigrant communities in the New World (Canada, North America, New Zealand and Australia) with sometimes as many as 70 per cent of marriages taking place between cousins in some minority religious groups. Facilitating the effective transplantation of 'whole communities of kin', the marriage pattern produced close kinship ties that were central to the 'legendary success' of the migration and subsequent resettlement of these emigrant groups (Molloy 1986: 241). Close kin marriage in the colonial context was not simply a response to the circumstances of frontier settlement, because consanguineous marriage was already common at the time of migration. In fact, the assumed 'traditional' Highland Scots pattern of marriage within the line of descent through men (or clan) was already changing, in response to the political and social upheavals in Scotland at the time of emigration to the New World. The incursion of British rule and attempts by landlords to rationalise agriculture had resulted in an 'unprecedented exodus' of people from their traditional lands and was accompanied by increases in matrilateral first cousin and sibling-exchange marriages. It seems that the removal of clansmen from their hereditary lands decreased the impetus for clan-endogamous marriage, but increased matrilateral first cousin and sibling exchange marriages: 'In this period of social disruption, … families drew closer together emphasizing matri-lateral and affinal links as well as patrilateral ones. It is not that new marriage patterns were invented; it is simply that they were applied in different ways, sibling exchange marriage in particular ensuring that "strangers" who married in became "family" with strong multiple bonds' (Molloy 1986: 240).

Marriages were already largely endogamous within three large kinship groups of Highland Scots who migrated to Cape Breton in Nova Scotia in the early nineteenth century and on to Waipu in New Zealand in the mid nineteenth century. Spouses were frequently first and second cousins, or cousin's cousins, and no particular form of cousin marriage was preferred. There were also cross-generational cousin marriages and at least four widowers married their deceased wife's cousin, reflecting the ideal that a spouse be found from among affinal kin. Sibling-exchange marriages were also common, often also involving cousins. Marriages to people outside a particular kinship group were invariably followed by marriages with their siblings or cousins, so that 'in this sense the marriage alliances were between kin groups rather than individuals' (ibid.: 232).

In the process of migrating to and settling in the New World, this pattern of kinship and marriage was an asset. Kin groups tended to migrate on the same ships, take up adjacent plots of land and provide mutual support as the community established itself. In the next generation, in New Zealand, close kin marriages continued to be common, but there were fewer cross-generational marriages of close kin. There were also more marriages outside the kin group, and some outside the Nova Scotian community. Even so, by the end of the century, 'virtually any Nova Scotian descendant living in Waipu could trace a relationships to any other' (ibid.: 239).

In addition, their cultural and religious distinctiveness reinforced the Nova Scotian settlers' tendency to endogamy. They were dissenting Calvinists – dissenting from both the established Church of Scotland and the Roman Catholics. In Waipu, they felt themselves to be a community apart, religiously and linguistically, speaking only Gaelic at home. As pioneer shipowner John Munro put it, 'we have no inclination to mix with strangers' (quoted in Molloy 1986: 241). Similar patterns of close kin marriage have been noted for other groups of emigrant European religious minorities in the New World. A Presbyterian splinter group of Scottish-Irish immigrants to North America continued to marry consanguineously for more than 100 years from their arrival in the United States in the 1720s through to the mid-1800s (Reid 1988). For such groups, close kin marriages were important not just for economic survival but for enabling cultural and religious transmission over the generations. Yet, by 1861, cousin marriage was illegal in some states in America, and became so in others later. Martin Ottenheimer argues that prohibitions on cousin marriage in the United States were not based on any firm or convincing evidence of biological harm, but instead reflected the widespread acceptance of evolutionary thinking according to which cousin marriage was inimical to social progress: '[The laws] were enacted because of a belief that cousin marriage threatened the status of the United States as a civilized society, not because there was evidence of genetic risk to offspring' (1996: 113). Laws prohibiting cousin marriages can thus be seen as attempts to integrate relatively isolated minority communities rather than as measures to prevent genetic problems.

The decline of cousin marriage in Europe and America

The rate of cousin marriage declined quite dramatically, to its present-day low levels, from the middle of the nineteenth century in America and slightly later in Victorian England, except within some minority and relatively recent immigrant-origin groups. There is no evidence of any widespread disapproval of cousin marriage in England, despite periodic religious opposition and concern raised by some phrenologists, until the second half of the nineteenth century. By the end of the Victorian era, however, a definite change of opinion towards cousin marriage had occurred in at least in some social circles, where it was now seen as biologically harmful. A new scientific interest in biology and breeding had arisen with Charles Darwin's publications on evolution, particularly *On the Origin of Species* (1859) and *The Descent of Man* (1871). Darwin himself addressed the question of the biological consequences of inbreeding and of cross-fertilisation in a book called *On the Various Contrivances by which British and Foreign*

Orchids are Fertilised by Insects and on the Good Effects of Intercrossing (1862): from the observation that plants have evolved elaborate means of preventing self-fertilisation, he inferred that inbreeding in human populations is harmful and outbreeding beneficial. In *The Variation of Animals and Plants under Domestication* (1868) he proposed that by a 'law of nature' crossings between plants and animals not closely related are beneficial while prolonged inbreeding is 'highly injurious'. The extent to which this 'law of nature' applied to human populations, whether or to what extent parental consanguinity caused sterility, insanity, other forms of lowered fitness and, especially if prolonged, a general 'degeneration' of the human race, was then fiercely debated in scientific journals and in the popular press.

Dr Gilbert Child, a doctor at the Radcliffe Infirmary in Oxford, was sceptical that cousin marriage caused illness, observing that prejudice rather than careful scientific evidence had condemned inbreeding. From the observation that racehorses and domestic livestock are often inbred in order to produce very fine specimens through the intensification of traits, he inferred that consanguineous marriages cannot be intrinsically harmful. Since marriages of blood relatives 'have a tendency to strengthen and develope [*sic*] in the offspring, individual peculiarities of the parents, both mental and physical, whether morbid or otherwise', they would be problematic only if the parents had a characteristic or trait of disease, for in this case the disease characteristics would be intensified (Child 1862: 470–1). Whether a particular marriage is likely or not to be harmful to the children would depend on the presence of a harmful hereditary trait in both partners, which they might have inherited from one of their common grandparents. To ensure healthy children, he continued, it was probably more sensible to marry a consanguineous relative of known, healthy parentage than to marry a stranger whose family history is unknown. He advocated making case-by-case assessments of genetic risk instead of assuming 'that such marriages are in themselves contrary to some law of nature, and calculated to lead to degeneration of race' (ibid.: 469). In conclusion, he suggested that a physician who takes the trouble to enquire about his patient's family history would be able quite accurately to predict the likely health of the children of a consanguineously married couple, and that it is in fact the physician's duty to do this rather than, 'as some have asserted, to save himself all trouble by denouncing the match' (ibid.: 471).

Others took the opposite view: that there is intrinsic biological harm in marrying a cousin. In 1865, Arthur Mitchell, a doctor and deputy commissioner for lunacy in Scotland, examined the number of cases of consanguinity in the parents of 'idiots' and 'deaf mutes' and inferred that consanguinity was harmful. He also collected data from isolated Scottish island communities, where cousin marriage was reportedly common, but, instead of finding evidence of its harmful biological consequences, he found that, on St Kilda, where over one-third of couples were consanguineous, and on Lewis, the island was not 'peopled with idiots, madmen, cripples and mutes, [and that] not one such person is said to exist in it' (Mitchell, quoted in Kuper 2002: 169). Rather than discard his hypothesis, Mitchell suggested good living conditions might mitigate the ill effects of inbreeding and he thought the absence of any visible abnormalities in his data did not rule out the possibility of their appearance in subsequent generations or of the group's general deterioration over time (see George Darwin 1875: 175).

Sociological, legal and anthropological perspectives, viewing marriage to close relatives as threatening to the social order, were also added to the debate. In 1865, William Adam, a liberal parliamentarian, offered a sociological perspective on inbreeding that rejected Darwin's view of it as biologically harmful, but condemned it as socially undesirable, for its potential to confuse inheritance patterns and kinship categories, and to 'retard the formation of moral character and prevent real moral progress' (quoted in Anderson 1986: 293). Influenced by Darwin's insights about natural selection, the nineteenth century anthropologists who entered the debate in general agreed on the evolutionary advantages of exogamy or 'marrying out', but differed in the emphasis they gave to biological rather than social and political factors, some stressing the biological advantages of incest avoidance and exogamy (Lubbock 1870; Westermarck 1891; Morgan 1858 [1877]) others stressing its social and political advantages (Maine 1883; Tylor 1889).

Dr Mitchell's work prompted many further studies on both sides of the Atlantic, but, while it generated critical comment in England, it was uncritically accepted in the United States (Ottenheimer 1996: 85). Within the American Presbyterian Church, the revived theological debate about the propriety and moral consequences of marriages between affinal kin had shifted by the middle of the nineteenth century to a preoccupation with the fitness of consanguineous marriages, as reflected in Morgan's arguments that exogamy marked the passage from savagery to civilisation (Ottenheimer 1996). As noted, it was evolutionary thinking rather than conclusive empirical evidence of its harm that resulted in laws prohibiting cousin marriage being passed in a number of states in America in the nineteenth and early twentieth century (ibid.: 113).

The outcome of these debates in England was rather different. Charles Darwin worried about the potentially harmful biological and evolutionary consequences of inbreeding and the lack of evidence with which to decide the matter. In 1870, his friend Sir John Lubbock, a Member of Parliament, proposed including a question in the 1871 census about cousin marriage, to establish its effects on fertility and health. Parliament rejected the motion, 'on the ground that the idle curiosity of philosophers was not to be satisfied' (George Darwin 1875: 153); in one MP's view, the investigation would be 'purely inquisitorial; the only object could be to stigmatise certain marriages' (quoted in Huth 1887: 339).

Medical debate continued, however, with *The Lancet* stating in 1875 that an authoritative medical professional examination of the topic was necessary, because the question 'comes up at some time or another in almost every family' (quoted in Anderson 1986: 292), and, after Lubbock's motion was turned down, Charles

Darwin's son George undertook his own research. He investigated 18,528 marriage announcements in the *Pall Mall Gazette,* genealogical information given in *Burke's Peerage,* results of a questionnaire to 800 members of the upper middle and upper classes, and a sample of marriages from the register at Somerset House. Using a complicated method of surname analysis, he found that in 1873 the rate of first cousin marriage was highest, at 4.5 per cent, among the aristocracy and 3.5 per cent among the landed gentry and upper middle classes. This, he wrote, was 'in accordance with what might have been expected ... for the aristocracy hold together very much, the landed gentry slightly less' (George Darwin 1875: 164). His 'snapshot' may quite accurately reflect the prevalence of cousin marriage in England between 1873 and 1875 (Kuper 2002) but does not tell us whether cousin marriage was already, by then, in decline, as Anderson asserts (1986: 298).

To examine the biological consequences, George Darwin asked doctors working in lunatic asylums to collect data on parental consanguinity in the parents of inmates, and found that, in England and Wales, approximately 3.5 per cent of patients were the offspring of first cousin marriages. Since this percentage is almost the same as the percentage of cousin marriages in the general population, 'one can only draw the negative conclusion that as far as insanity and idiocy go, no evil has been shown to accrue from consanguineous marriages' (George Darwin 1875: 168), although, he added, 'it might still be shown by more accurate methods of research' (ibid.: 172). He drew the same general conclusion in relation to his data for blindness and the 'deaf and dumb'. George Darwin was aware that professional views on the topic ranged from the belief that a 'morbid constitutional tendency' is intensified when it is transferred through related parents to the opposite conviction that cousin marriage has 'no effect' in producing such traits (ibid.: 168–69). In his literature review, he concurred with Mitchell that 'favourable conditions of life' must mitigate the effects of parental consanguinity, an observation that, he wrote, was 'in striking accordance with some unpublished experiments of my father, Mr. Charles Darwin, on the in-and in-breeding of plants; for he has found that in-bred plants, when allowed enough space and good soil, frequently show little or no deterioration' (ibid.: 175).

In *The Effects of Cross and Self-Fertilisation in the Vegetable Kingdom,* Charles Darwin gave a qualified endorsement of his son's conclusions, commenting that, while cross-fertilisation was preferable, environmental conditions would tend to counter the effect of marriage between close relatives (1876: 461). In his revised second edition of *The Variation of Animals and Plants under Domestication,* he omitted the qualifier 'highly' injurious in his note on cousin marriages (1875: vol. 2, 177). In the revised edition of his book on the fertilisation of orchids by insects, he said nothing about the harm of close kin marriage, confining himself to stating the dangers of self-fertilisation (Darwin 1877: 297). As Alfred Henry Huth, a Victorian book-collector and writer, had demonstrated in his widely reviewed report, there was no conclusive evidence of serious biological harm (Huth 1887;

Anderson 1986: 295–96). As a result, 'the Darwinian establishment was no longer seriously concerned with the risk of inbreeding within prosperous families'; the eugenicist Francis Galton 'wrote enthusiastically to George Darwin that he had "exploded most effectually a popular scare"' (Kuper 2002: 173). Galton suggested that, if George Darwin (his cousin) wrote a book popularising his results, he would be guaranteed to sell at least 8,000 copies each year, since at least 2,000 cousin marriages occurred annually and all cousins intending to marry would buy it, as would their parents (Kuper 2002).

However, despite the reassurance offered by George Darwin's work, it seems the debate had already effectively stigmatised cousin marriages, for, by the late nineteenth century, medical opinion was 'almost unanimously against inbreeding' (Anderson 1986: 297). A tendency for consanguinity to 'intensify' parental characteristics, in both beneficial and deleterious ways, had indeed been observed; the problem was that doctors in the nineteenth century had no understanding of the mechanism of inheritance that would allow them to explain this observation. As Dr Gilbert Child had noted, 'no attempt has been made, so far as I am aware, to explain what this mysterious law of nature is, what are the limits within which it acts, or what is its *modus operandi*' (Child 1862: 461). This is because the nineteenth century debate pre-dated both the rediscovery, in 1900, of Mendel's work on the inheritance of recessive traits and the development of modern population genetics in the 1950s. In fact, according to modern population genetics, the genetic risks to the children of consanguineous marriage 'generally are within the limits of acceptability' for the children of first cousins 'appear to be in remarkably close agreement with the levels calculated by Darwin in 1875' (Bittles and Makov 1988: 164). However, the idea has persisted in many circles in Europe since the late nineteenth century that cousin marriages are inherently dangerous.

The literature of the late nineteenth century reflects this change in feeling towards cousin marriages. There are extensive examples of cousin marriages in early Victorian life: in the Darwin–Wedgwood family; in the lives of such literary figures as William Thackeray, Elizabeth Gaskell, Samuel Coleridge and Edward Barrett, who had children who married cousins; in the examples of John Ruskin and Lewis Carroll, who both had first cousin parents, and in the work of such prominent Victorian novelists as Charles Dickens, Anthony Trollope, William Thackeray and Emily Brontë (Anderson 1986). There are also accounts of love and marriage between cousins in many nineteenth-century novels, in Jane Austen's, for instance:

> In *Mansfield Park* (1814), Fanny married Edmund, her mother's sister's son. In *Persuasion* (1817), Charles Hayter similarly married his mother's sister's daughter, Henrietta Musgrave. In the same novel, Elizabeth Elliot dreams of a marriage with her cousin and her father's heir, William Elliot (apparently her second cousin in the male line), and he later woos her sister Anne. Any objections to these relationships had to do with such extraneous factors as

> the difference in status between Fanny and Edmund or Henrietta and Charles. There were similar marriages within Jane Austen's own family. Jane's brother Henry married his widowed cousin, Eliza de Feuillide, after Eliza had rejected his brother James. (Kuper 2002: 166; see also Tomalin 1997)

Adam Kuper notes that cousin marriages feature in novels and plays right up until the end of the nineteenth century, without being considered unusual or problematic. Oscar Wilde's *The Importance of Being Ernest* (1895) ends with the lovers discovering they are cousins: as the children of Lady Bracknell and her sister, Lady Bracknell could not possibly object to their marriage (Kuper 2002).

However, in the novels of the late Victorian period, the cousin marriages depicted are portrayed as foreboding the ill health of offspring (Anderson 1986). In Thomas Hardy's novel *Jude the Obscure* (1895) Sue Bridehead tells her cousin Jude that they should not marry because it is 'bad' for cousins to marry, in effect foretelling the tragedy to come. In John Galsworthy's *The Forsyte Saga* (1922) cousins Holly Forsyte and Val Dartie marry, but decide not to have children because of their consanguinity. In 1911, a biographer attributed John Ruskin's mental illness to parental consanguinity (see Anderson 1986: 297).

Cousin marriages did not decline everywhere in the late nineteenth century. In relatively isolated rural and emigrant communities there were strong social reasons for maintaining a tradition of close kin marriage, and these communities may also have been beyond the influence of the public disputes of the Victorian medical establishment or the disapproval of individual physicians who felt compelled 'to set their faces against such marriages' (Child 1862: 462). In fact, in some parts of Europe and the Mediterranean, cousin marriages increased, in response to changes in inheritance laws and the introduction of civil marriage laws, circumventing the requirement for first cousin couples to seek Church dispensations (Ottenheimer 1996: 90–91). Where it did occur, the decline in cousin marriage seems likely to have been influenced by a combination of changing attitudes and other forces of socio-economic change, such as an increase in commerce, a decreasing dependency on family land and the decline in family size. Probably the single most significant of these socio-economic factors was the dramatic decline in fertility that occurred in the late nineteenth century, beginning with the middle classes from about 1870 (Banks 1954). For cousin marriage to be a significant minority marriage pattern requires there to be enough eligible cousins and, therefore, a relatively high birth rate. A widespread reduction in family size would have meant that the next generation of adults would have had fewer aunts and uncles, and in consequence would have had fewer cousins from among whom they might find a spouse. Combined with this major demographic change, relationships between men and women in post-Victorian England were increasingly marked by greater social freedom than previously, making it more likely for individual men and women to find partners outside their immediate family circles. In particular, women's freedom from financial and emotional dependence on their close male kin, particularly fathers and brothers, would have assisted this process (Anderson 1986). In short, although the decline in cousin marriage is commonly understood to reflect a change in opinion about its desirability, by the late nineteenth century, the socio-economic factors that had supported and maintained this minority marriage pattern for hundreds of years previously had also altered.

Conclusion

Under early industrialisation, it seems there were increases in several types of close kin marriage, including the marriages of first cousins, even though the socio-economic significance of links with a wider circle of kin was decreasing. Close kin marriage has been noted among people as diverse as the royalty, the aristocracy, the middle classes and sections of the peasantry. While this practice does not lend itself easily to historical analysis, it appears in many cases to have been important as a means of conserving resources during economic expansion and uncertainly, within the constraints imposed by legal or religious laws. For the middle classes and within the lower reaches of the gentry in urban and rural England, close kin marriage seems to have been important in securing business interests in an uncertain and competitive environment, in which the economic and legal apparatus of modern business had not yet evolved. For the Rothschild European banking network, patrilateral parallel-cousin marriage represented a specific strategy suited to the economic environment of the early nineteenth century.

The examples discussed in this chapter lend some support to the strategic analyses of marriage strategies presented in the work of Bourdieu (1977) and Donnan (1988), that cousin marriages represent a means of protecting socio-economic and, sometimes, cultural and religious interests – or a strategy to contain or reduce risks in an uncertain environment; they also support aspects of Ottenheimer's (1996) general argument that cousin marriages facilitate social and cultural continuity. As we shall see in the next chapter, an increase in the rate of cousin marriage has also been noted in relation to the marriages of second- and third-generation British Pakistanis, marriages that mostly involve cousins from Pakistan. Such marriages may be viewed by the participants themselves as a means of reducing the risks associated with marrying 'strangers', risks perceived as particularly acute in a new or uncertain cultural and religious environment.

Yet there are also some significant differences. On the one hand, the contemporary increase in consanguineous marriage among British Pakistanis coincides with a quite widespread discourse of cousin marriage as genetically risky and morally problematic, which has a potentially global reach, through the education system and modern communications media; it may thus feature directly in particular negotiations of cousin marriage, as I show in the next chapter. On the other hand, the demographic and social factors that facilitated a decline in cousin marriage in the nineteenth century, such as smaller family size and new patterns of gendered social interaction, may have variable influences on British Pakistani family networks which extend to South Asia. Moreover, the availability of modern genetic services in the U.K. means that avoiding consanguineous marriage is not the only way of preventing the birth of a child with a recessive genetic disorder. As the remaining chapters of this book show, individuals and couples, including those in consanguineous marriages, may negotiate reproductive risk in a variety of different ways. So, although, in the current situation, the discourse of disapproval has the potential to be more complete in its social reach, any decline in cousin marriage might be less complete or consistent than in the late nineteenth century.

CHAPTER 3
BRITISH PAKISTANI COUSIN MARRIAGES: BALANCING MARITAL RISKS

Husnain is a twenty-six-year-old British law graduate who describes himself as a 'second-generation Pakistani'. He has lived in England since he was four years old. Commenting on his marriage to a first cousin from Pakistan, he told me: 'Marrying within the family is the normal thing to do. It's a cultural issue. I don't think the medical issue even crosses our people's minds. It certainly didn't concern me. You just assume you will marry a cousin. That's what I did. It is the natural thing to do.' Yet, like many other young adults, he was also acutely aware that this is not the view of many non-Pakistanis in Britain:

> [White] people ask you, 'Are you married to a cousin?' They can't take it in, a lot of white people. I am using the term 'white' in a general way, please don't be offended. They can't understand it, for them, marrying a cousin is beyond their imagination. People say, 'How can you do that, she's your cousin!' It's a no-win situation, because if you say, 'It was a love marriage'; they [white people] will say, 'Really, how come, were you allowed? How did you get to marry out of the family? How did your parents allow you to do that?' And then your own community will say, how did your parents allow you to do that? If I say it's an arranged marriage they [white people] would ask loads of questions, so now I say it's a love marriage with parents' consent. That stops the questions.

This chapter offers a framework for understanding British Pakistanis' continued preference for marriage with cousins or other close kin, particularly cousins from Pakistan. Indeed, there is some evidence that, rather than declining, the popularity of consanguineous marriage has increased among British Pakistanis (Darr and Modell 1988; Modood et al. 1997: 319; Shaw 2001). Significantly, many of these marriages are transnational, involving a partner from Pakistan or elsewhere in the Pakistani diaspora who then applies to join a spouse in the U.K. (Shaw 2001). The apparent increase in consanguineous marriage more accurately and specifically represents the current popularity of transnational kin marriages among British Pakistanis. While marriage migrants are typically South Asians, there are more incoming spouses from Pakistan than from India and Bangladesh combined (Home Office 2001). This trend counters my earlier expectation that British Pakistani marriages might increasingly be arranged within the U.K., on the basis of common interests, as evidenced by marriages between children of brothers who are business partners, and the compatibility of spouses (see Shaw 2000a: 147, 159 note 10). It also counters the Home Office's (2002) more recent hopes with respect to integration. The numbers of incoming spouses are substantial. In 2000, just over 10,000 Pakistani partners – 4,720 men and 5,560 women – obtained U.K. entry clearance (Home Office 2001). These figures represent a sustained rise in male in comparison with female marriage migrants since the abolition in 1997 of the Primary Purpose Rule, which required incoming men to prove that immigration was not the main motive for their marriages (ibid.), with numbers fluctuating somewhat since. How can this significant and apparently enduring trend be understood?

Previous research has tended to view the popularity of transnational consanguineous marriage in socio-economic terms as a means of circumventing increasingly restrictive immigration regulations, as part of a family-driven strategy for socio-economic advantage, in keeping with pioneer migrants' and their families' original intention that migration should benefit relatives 'at home' in Pakistan. Roger Ballard notes the intense pressure exerted by siblings in Pakistan upon pioneer-generation British Mirpuri parents to accept offers of marriage on behalf of their children (1987: 27). In Pakistan, the obligations of kinship underpin a family's financial and social security in the absence of state social and health provision, and as such are important in motivating international labour migration. Although the British Pakistani population now comprises united families of several generations' depth, many British Pakistanis still remit some money to support relatives in Pakistan and for charitable purposes. Legal remittances (through banks) from the U.K. (and elsewhere) to Pakistan continue to be important to the Pakistan economy. Within transnationally divided families, marriage plans for children can become entwined with the possibility of emigration, not just as a strategy to enable male wage-earners to enter Britain, but more broadly as a means of sharing the benefits of migration – earning potential, educational opportunities, British citizenship – with other members of the family.

The image of the Pakistani *birādarī* or extended family as a corporate group with a shared interest in the marriage of its members can, however, obscure the fact that marriage is also a matter of individual calculation, a balance of sometimes conflicting and competing interests (Ballard 1987; Shaw 2000a, 2001; and, for a study in Pakistan, see Donnan 1988). From this perspective, the individual motivations of different family members interact with social and cultural conventions (such as a sense of obligation to kin in Pakistan and the approval that accrues from making a culturally appropriate marriage choice) in the negotiations that determine which, for instance, of the available spouses in a family are chosen for a particular son or daughter, or even if a particular marriage takes place within the family at all. Individual choices thus cannot be reduced to statements about culturally preferred marital forms (Donnan 1985). Whether a boy is married to his father's sibling's or his mother's sibling's daughter, for example, involves such considerations as which other marriages have already taken place or may in the future take place between the households in question and the relative strengths of each parent's interests in a particular marriage arrangement (which in turn reflect the strength of personal connections with particular siblings), as well as the preferences of the boy and girl in question (Shaw 2000a, 2001). As Bourdieu has put it, 'matrimonial strategies are often the outcome of power relationships within the domestic group and the relationships can be understood only by appealing to the history of this group and in particular to the history of previous marriages' (Bourdieu 1990: 69).

Recent research augments our understanding of the motivations for arranging transnational cousin marriages by considering the role of emotional ties of kinship. These are evident in parents' desires to maintain connections with kin such as brothers and sisters overseas and in their concerns to secure their children's future happiness, security and well-being. From this perspective, an arranged transnational kin marriage can be regarded as a strategy to reduce the emotional and social risks for children of marrying outside the family, even though transnational marriage introduces new marital risks (Charsley 2003, 2006). Moreover, affective ties among transnationally separated kin may also motivate marriages between the children of pioneer-generation migrants and their Pakistani cousins. Indeed, the main impetus for at least some transnational Pakistani marriages comes from the young people themselves, who may speak about their experiences of engagement and marriage in quite strongly romantic terms (Charsley 2003; Shaw and Charsley 2006). In what follows, I incorporate perspectives from this more recent research in exploring the considerations involved in British Pakistani marriages with spouses from Pakistan. I draw mainly from the research with couples attending the genetics clinic but also from ongoing contacts with families from earlier research, and I begin with a discussion of the cultural rationale for arranging marriages within the family.

A good *rishta*: prior knowledge and risk reduction

For South Asian parents, arranging children's marriages is, generally, a central concern; securing children's marriages constitutes perhaps the most fundamental parental responsibility. The insecurities that surround marriage arrangements are usually regarded as greater with regard to daughters, who are viewed as the dependents of men and for whom premarital courtship is discouraged; indeed, the matter of a daughter's marriage can become a matter of family honour (see Donnan 1988; Holy 1989). These insecurities are also connected with the fear of a bride's mistreatment by her husband or in-laws after marriage. For Pakistanis, this responsibility informs the expectation that a match (*rishta*) will be found within the family. Sometimes grandparents or other elders attempt to settle the issue of finding good *rishta*s by making informal, unspoken betrothals between their grandchildren; in some families, children grow up aware of these expected matches, sometimes teasing each other about them as they approach adolescence (Charsley 2003). Given these fears, and the expectation that a *rishta* will be found within the family, it can be difficult for parents to contemplate matches outside the family (See Shaw 2000a: 126–34; 151–58; 2001: 326). Since kin, especially siblings, expect to have 'first refusal' in the matter of the marriages of their relatives' children, refusals must be handled delicately, usually through a trusted relative as go-between, to avoid major disruptions to ongoing relationships within the extended family.

Ideally, in a 'good' *rishta*, the partners are well matched for social background and education. Indeed, marriage between equals is a central principle of marriage choice, recommended, according to one Hadith, by the Prophet Mohammad (Ahmad 1978: 14), and assumed to facilitate a happy and stable marriage (Hussain 1999: 456; Fischer and Lyon 2000: 298; Shaw 2000a: 132; see also Samad and Eade 2002). Pakistanis often say they prefer cousin marriages because prior knowledge about the suitability of a potential spouse and their immediate kin will be more accurate within the family than outside, where there is greater uncertainty and risk of false information. The couple should also be well matched for personality and disposition, and in this respect the behaviour of older close kin, particularly the same-sex close kin of each prospective spouse, is considered to provide useful predictors of the young person's future behaviour (Fischer and Lyon 2000). A couple's physical characteristics, such as skin colour, height and build, should be similar or complementary, although physical appearance may be given less emphasis than personality, education or other considerations, including the need for care, where marriages are arranged within the family; in particular, a woman's beauty is less harshly judged than in marriages with outsiders. In contrast, advertisements for 'proposals' or 'matches' placed in the matrimonial columns of Urdu and English Pakistani newspapers in Pakistan typically specify that the man be of a good family, be educated and have a secure job, whereas a bride must be beautiful and educated (Charsley 2003). Even so, the lesser emphasis on physical characteristics in arranging *rishta*s in the family can sometimes cause concern: in some of the letters to the problem pages of an Urdu weekly published in the U.K., brides-to-be worry that their cousin's short stature or dark complexion is incompatible with their good looks: it 'does not look right' (*jorā achchā nahīn lagtā*) – in such cases, the paper's agony aunt typically advises that beauty is only skin deep and the complainant should be glad of her prospective spouse's other good qualities (Shaw n.d.).

Family-based insider knowledge of prospective *rishta*s is also regarded as a means of minimising the risks of being given false information about potential spouses

(Donnan 1988). People tend to assume that if parents are seeking a spouse from outside the family for a son or daughter there is something 'wrong' with that child, such as a disability, long-term illness, undesirable character trait or tainted past, for otherwise they would be pursuing a *rishta* within the family. One such arrangement, made by intermediaries, involved a British man and a woman from a 'good' wealthy and educated family in Pakistan. Soon after her arrival in England, the British family discovered that the young woman had a terminal illness and concluded that they had been deliberately deceived by the woman's parents, who were presumably anxious to secure their daughter's medical treatment abroad. The British family returned the woman to Pakistan and arranged for their son to marry a first cousin from their home village instead.

Such incidents reinforce the view that marriages arranged within the family are 'safer' than marriages arranged with 'outsiders', because mutual kin can provide information about prospective *rishtas*, including about any possible chronic illness and disability that might detract from an otherwise attractive match – for this is more difficult to conceal from relatives. Health problems, illnesses or disabilities introduce additional insecurities into arranging marriages within the family, such that the affected person or their parents may strive to conceal the details of the problem from kin (see Chapter 7), because the perception of an illness running 'in the family' can sometimes affect the marriage prospects not just of the affected person but of other, unaffected, kin. On the other hand, arranged marriages may also provide an important source of support for people with a long-term illness or disability, especially where the person's special needs are known or made clear in advance. Riaz's wife, who is his cousin, is deaf, as are three of their children. Riaz told me that, for a girl with a problem like deafness, a marriage within the family means she is less likely to be ill-treated, because her husband and in-laws already know her and her limitations, so will make allowances for her: 'They won't shout at her, because they know she can't hear.' Indeed, the expectation of care for a spouse who has a permanent disability or a chronic illness can sometimes inform transnational marriage arrangements, made both within the family and with non-kin, in which the disadvantages of a *rishta* that involves providing additional care may be balanced against the perceived advantages offered by such marriages (see Chapter 8).

Some young British-born Pakistanis use Web-based marriage introduction services aimed at South Asians resident in Europe and North America (such as shadi.com) or the relatively few Pakistani matchmaking organisations such as Rabta ('Contact'), but intermediaries, matchmaking services and newspaper matrimonial columns seem to constitute minority routes for securing *rishtas* and to be generally viewed as strategies of last resort. As a British Pakistani woman who had joined a U.K. matchmaking organisation to help her brother find a partner after a failed love affair commented, 'This is not for the majority, it is only for the desperate.'

In finding a good *rishta*, it is also important to assess the personalities of the prospective parents-in-law, especially the mother-in-law; traditionally, a bride joins her husband in his parents' household after marriage. If a woman's future mother-in-law is her mother's sister, father's sister or another close relative, the new bride is considered more likely to be treated well in her new home than if she is 'from outside' (*bāhir se*). This, as noted above, is an especially important consideration where there is chronic illness or disability. As a natural consequence of the informal and formal activities of extended family life, the bride's parents and the bride herself are also likely to know and be able to assess the character and personality of the prospective mother-in-law and of other close kin, such as any married brothers' wives already living in the in-laws' household, who can also significantly shape a daughter-in-law's future happiness. The other side of this is that dual loyalties can also mean that relatives withhold critical information about a prospective spouse and their family (see Charsley 2003).

When she received a marriage proposal for her eldest daughter from her favourite cousin Usma, in Pakistan, Shamim was particularly pleased because Usma's son was an only child: 'Usma will treat my daughter like her own daughter, not a daughter-in-law, and the boy does not have any brothers, so my daughter will have no sisters-in-law to order her about and treat her harshly.' Similarly, the marriage of another daughter into a household where one daughter has already married is sometimes favoured, because the relationship between sisters-in-law is predicted to be smooth if they are already sisters: they are more likely to be allies than rivals. In fact, 'one response to the hazards of marriage arrangements is to take someone from a family ... which has already been proven; where one marriage has [already] been seen to be successful' (Charsley 2003: 153). Another quite common arrangement effectively entails the exchange of opposite-sex siblings; it is called *watta-satta* marriage. It is recognised as more problematic than same-sex sibling exchange because, while drawing upon a reliable prior connection, it introduces the additional risk that a difficulty in one marriage will cause a problem in the other – specifically, there is the risk of 'direct revenge being taken out on your daughter should your son's marriage run into difficulty' (Charsley 2003: 155).

A wife's brother is expected to support his sister in any marital difficulty, but a man in a *watta-satta* marriage may upset his own wife (who may side with her brother) by supporting his sister; however, if he supports his wife and his brother-in-law rather than his sister, he risks incurring the resentment of his own siblings and parents. Shamim's husband's brother is married to a first cousin, his mother's brother's daughter, and has a sister married to his wife's brother – a man who later deserted and divorced his wife. Shamim's brother-in-law was both criticised and praised, by different relatives and outsiders, for staying with his wife when this happened – criticised for implicitly condoning his wife's brother's behaviour and for being 'under his wife's thumb' and praised for being loyal to his wife. Marriages within the family are considered generally conducive to marital stability because relatives are likely to offer a couple support in times of difficulty; they also contain the risk of serious rifts between kin when marriages fail. As one young father put it, 'And then there are worse consequences if the marriage goes wrong. It's much worse to stop talking to your brother than to stop talking to a stranger.'

How far does a proposal that fulfils most or all parental criteria for a 'good' match also reflect their son or daughter's feelings? Whether British Pakistani arranged marriages are, in many cases, 'forced' by parents upon unwilling participants acting in their own interests has been a topic of recent public concern (Samad and Eade 2002). Typical normative statements about Pakistani arranged marriages, such as that *larkīyān inkār nahīn kartīn* (girls do not refuse), may easily be taken to imply that such marriages are necessarily 'forced' (*zabardastī se*), but the distinction between acting in someone else's interest and inflicting harm or duress is not always clear-cut, particularly in cross-cultural contexts, since concepts such as autonomy are themselves culturally shaped. Further, so-called forced marriages may themselves be motivated by parents' desires to act in their child's best interests. As a British Pakistani woman married at sixteen against her wishes to a man she had not met before told Charsley, 'I was lucky, I was forced to marry a really nice bloke' (Charsley 2003: 142).

The young adults in my fieldwork were aware of these debates around arranged marriage. In many cases, children agree with their parents' judgement of what is a good *rishta,* while at the same time parents' assessments of particular proposals are also influenced by their understandings of their child's personal preferences. When she was sixteen, Zareena's father, a man of Mirpuri background, received a proposal from a sister, also in the U.K. However, Zareena – herself born and raised in Britain and now a mother of teenagers – knew immediately that she did not want to marry this particular local cousin, in whose house she had stayed as a child:

> It was not the cousin himself, the man is good. It was something about my auntie. When I was about twelve, I went there for a weekend, my Dad took me over. For some reason, my auntie went out and left me with the baby to look after. The baby screamed and I did not know what to do. The whole situation just did not feel right to me. So I phoned my Dad and asked him to bring me home. He didn't ask why, he just fetched me back. Some years later, when my Dad suggested a *rishta* with them, I knew I did not want to marry that cousin. My Dad respected my feelings. In the end, my sister married him. It is okay, because they live separately from his parents now, but I was not wrong about my feelings about my auntie.

Unlike her sister, Zareena later married transnationally and outside the family, having met her future husband through family contacts while visiting Pakistan. Her father was initially upset by this *rishta* because it was outside the family and would make it harder for Zareena's family to intervene on her behalf should the marriage run into difficulties. Twenty years on, though, Zareena's father regards this son-in-law as a part of the family, a family that 'does not give daughters to outsiders'.

Transnational marriages: negotiating new risks

At first glance, we might expect that for young British Pakistanis, being raised in a developed Western country introduces a fundamental inequality into a transnational *rishta*, compromising the presumption of equality and compatibility between kin. We might also expect that young adults, influenced by the Western discourses of autonomy, love and free choice will increasingly disagree with parents' plans for their marriages. In earlier research in the 1980s, I speculated that we might see more marriages between British-raised Pakistanis (kin and non-kin) and fewer transnational *rishtas*, on the basis of my informants' emphasis on equivalence of status in a 'good' *rishta*. In one Oxford Arain *birādarī* in particular, a pattern of marriages between British-raised cousins, as well as outside the *birādarī*, had helped consolidate local family businesses, and a mother in this kindred and her children concluded from a return visit to Pakistan that the cousins there were too 'wild' and 'uncultivated' to be appropriate spouses. In this way, it seemed that, as in Pakistan, smaller inter-marrying groups might splinter off, on the basis of common socio-economic status, from a wider transnational *birādarī* network (Fischer and Lyon 2000; Shaw 2000a).

Transnational cousin marriages clearly introduce some new risks, particularly for brides. In my first fieldwork, several marriages of British women to Pakistani cousins or other kin were, in retrospect, a means of male immigration that had resulted in wives being abandoned by their husbands. Within a few weeks of arriving in Britain and after having a registry office marriage, Alim's cousin, a father's sister's son, had departed for London, where he became involved in various criminal activities (Shaw 2000a). By the time of my subsequent research in Oxford with the same families, marital instability had become a topic of major local concern. Several incidents of unsuccessful or deceitful transnational marriages had occurred, and some elopements involving British-raised South Asians 'escaping' arranged marriages had been reported in the local press. After Alim's sister experienced a similarly unsuccessful marriage to another Pakistani cousin, the younger sisters in this family refused every subsequent proposal that their father received from kin in Pakistan. Charsley reports similar cases from Bristol, noting that sometimes husbands contract second marriages in Pakistan once their position in Britain is secure, but she cautions that it is often hard to tell if this was the husband's original intention, or a later decision resulting from an unhappy marriage. For those involved, these experiences show how shared kinship is in itself no guarantee of compatibility or commitment, despite the widespread assumption that a *rishta* within the family is 'safer', for women especially, than marriage outside the family (Charsley 2003: 188).

The new risks of arranged transnational marriage vary by gender and social and cultural circumstances. For British Pakistani women, the most serious risks include being used as 'passports' to enable male immigration or becoming 'immigration widows' via marriages to Pakistani husbands who are then refused entry visas (Menski 2002; Werbner 2002). Parents have responded to the risks for

British-raised daughters by, for instance, separating out elements of the marriage ceremony, so that a daughter whose husband is refused a visa will not be left effectively single but no longer a virgin (Charsley 2003). A woman in Pakistan whose marriage is arranged to a British Pakistani man risks the shame of a broken *rishta* if the man proves unwilling to bring his wife to Britain. Husbands from Pakistan can experience a range of social, cultural and economic difficulties following marriage to British Pakistani women, particularly in connection with the fact that they often live, initially at least, as dependents within their wives' parents' households in Britain, a position comparable to the traditionally undesirable status of the *ghar dāmād* or 'house son-in-law' (Charsley 2005). More generally, there has been public concern for British spouses of both sexes over marital incompatibility, particularly with respect to language use and education; this issue, in turn, is linked with both national and local debates over arranged and forced marriage.

Transnational connections and continuities

Despite these new hazards and concerns, transnational cousin marriage remains the dominant marriage pattern among U.K. Pakistanis, suggesting that, for most families, the reasons for arranging such marriages seem, on balance, to override the risks (Shaw 2001; Charsley 2003). The assumption of inevitable socio-economic inequality between transnationally divided kin clearly underestimates the transcontinentality of British Pakistani families, who maintain active links with kin in Pakistan and elsewhere abroad (Kelly 1990). It also does not follow that British-based Pakistanis will necessarily have unreliable knowledge of close kin in Pakistan. In contrast to when Pakistani migration to Britain began fifty years ago, Internet and telephone connections now link once quite remote villages with British cities. For many British Pakistanis, Pakistan seems closer today than it has ever been, relatively cheap air travel enabling many families to visit kin in Pakistan fairly regularly. Khalida's Pakistan-born husband returns to his ancestral village near Jhelum for a few weeks every year for his father's death anniversary, to visit his mother and unmarried sister; Shamim's British-raised husband has telephoned his mother every week since she returned to live in Pakistan after her husband died.

Many children have experienced at least one extended school holiday spent in Pakistan, family finances permitting (see also Cressey 2006), while others travel 'back home', as British Pakistanis often describe Pakistan, much more frequently. Tahir's three-year old nephew has already been to Pakistan three times, most recently accompanying his grandmother, Tahir's mother, to the family's ancestral village in Jhelum and to Karachi to attend the wedding of a young kinswoman. While there may be interpersonal cultural differences between young people raised in Pakistan and those raised in Britain, there are also significant social continuities, facilitated by global communication and travel, enabling individuals to maintain transnational connections in various different ways. Kinship, for many British Pakistanis, is still experienced transnationally.

Many rural-origin British Pakistani families now have contacts far beyond their original villages, with kin who have moved to nearby towns or more distant cities. As Tahir's mother told me, 'We have our own people (*apne bande*) in every city in Pakistan.' As in Bristol, where middle-class families talked disapprovingly of British Pakistani parents who arranged their children's marriage with uneducated village cousins (Charsley 2003), so for families in Oxford and in High Wycombe the children of city-based or city-educated Pakistani relatives are regarded as of approximately equivalent status to those raised in British cities. Since a transnational marriage contains the possibility of the Pakistani spouse's migration abroad, most British families are now in a strong position to find a 'good' match from among city-based or city-educated relatives, a process also evident in the 1980s (see, for example, Shaw 2001: 329).

In the transnational context, the preference for arranging *rishta*s within the family is experienced through the obligations of kinship within a framework of global economics. The marriage of at least one child to a relative from Pakistan, such as a sibling's son or daughter or a spouse's sibling's son or daughter, is a means of reinvigorating, through the reciprocities of visiting and participating in life-course rituals, ties of kinship that might otherwise become weakened through living continents apart. As one pioneer-generation migrant told Charsley, 'I wanted to keep a link with Pakistan. If I have [had] found all my three kids *rishta*s here [in the U.K.], my link to Pakistan would have been broken' (Charsley 2003: 113). For other couples, a husband and wife's desires to maintain links with kin in Pakistan may result in several transnational marriages, and thus in multiple links with kin overseas. Hanif, who came to Britain in the 1960s, arranged his elder son's marriage to his sister's daughter Shamim, wishing to strengthen his connection with his sister, who had moved upon marriage to Kuwait. His wife Hamida's wishes prevailed when they arranged their younger son's marriage to Hamida's favourite brother's daughter in Pakistan. A few years later, they made a *watta satta* (brother-sister exchange) marriage by marrying their daughter into Hamida's brother's household.

Pioneer-generation migrants in the U.K. may be particularly aware of the centrality of marriage, more than any other life-course event, in strengthening connections between people, and its possible practical consequences in offering options for retirement or more long-term residence in Pakistan. After her husband died, Hamida returned to her village in Attock district and then to the nearby town, where her favourite brother and her British-based younger son live with their families. Her younger son has a degree in engineering from a British university and was joined in Britain by his wife (his mother's brother's daughter) on marriage, but, after his children were born, he and his wife returned to Pakistan, in order to raise their children in an Islamic society.

Nevertheless, younger adults, particularly those who have themselves had transnational marriages, are also aware of the significance of marriage in strengthening relationships between kin in disparate locations. While marriage migration reconnects kin, it creates distance between the new migrant and the kin they leave behind; new migrants in turn, may seek to reduce this distance through the marriages of their children. For Hanif and Hamida, their eldest son's marriage strengthened Hanif's relationship with his sister, but for their daughter-in-law Shamim, marriage migration meant separation from her only sister, her brothers and her parents. Now, with her own children's marriages, Shamim wants to reduce this distance:

> I have seen my sister very little since my marriage. I came to England in 1980, she went to Kuwait. I said to her on the phone the other day, wouldn't it be nice if we make a *rishta* between your daughter and my son ... My sister has no son; if we make a *rishta* there, it will be for our son. For one daughter, we are thinking of Usma's son, in Pakistan. For our younger daughter, we are thinking of the son of my brother who lives in Kuwait. They have asked us, and we are talking to him about it. It is making us brothers and sisters closer.

Shamim's husband supports these arrangements, since he does not wish his more problematic relationship with his only brother to become complicated by *rishtas*.

Young adults' views: individual responsibility

So far, I have emphasised the desires of pioneer- and second-generation parents to renew connections with kin overseas, but what of the motivations of the young British adults in transnational marriages? Are they frequently coerced to consent to a *rishta*, agreeing for fear of upsetting their parents? How far are these *rishtas* their own choice or the result of coercion or fear of upsetting their parents? Assuming that her marriage had been arranged by her parents, I asked Neha, who is twenty-three and married to a cousin from Pakistan, if her mother felt in any way responsible for the baby's problems – since her baby had just been diagnosed with a rare recessive condition. She replied:

> No, she does not feel guilty or responsible at all. How could she? It was my choice to get married to him! He came here with his family for a visit – it was nothing to do with thinking about getting married – and he got on with my brother very well. And we got to know each other as well. This was after I had spent two years in Pakistan. Of course I knew him then, but we never thought it would happen that we would get married. But then we got to know each other over here, and my brother and my husband were good friends, and my husband wanted to come over here, so we decided to get married.

Neha, whose parents are from Lahore, stressed that this marriage was her choice – her own decision – in fact, she added, first cousin marriages are not particularly common in her family. Shamim's younger daughter, Iram, who is twenty-two years old and studying for a degree in fashion, also emphasised how her recent marriage to twenty-four-year old Ikhlaq, her mother's brother's son, was largely her own decision, even though cousin marriages are common in her family:

> I met him at my sister's wedding in Pakistan, four years ago – he was there from Kuwait and I was there from England – and we have been in touch even since. I liked him as soon as I met him. We spoke to each other first, and he told me he liked me. Then I let my parents know and he let his parents know, and our parents they got on with it then. So I couldn't say it was totally an arranged marriage. Actually, it was just him and me to start with. I have had it easy, compared with other girls. I consider myself very lucky. It was my decision at the end of the day. Living in this day and age, I wanted to marry someone who I would be comfortable with. It's a coincidence that it's him, my cousin. It could have been someone out of the family. He is educated – he is studying, in Pakistan, for a master's degree in business and finance – and we don't have any major differences. We decided to get married this summer, to just get it done, since our families were both back in Pakistan, and my husband's Dad wasn't well. He's studying until January and then he is going to come over here, because I have two years of my degree left. I think he wants to move to Dubai, so I'll have some options of things to do.

There is a common stereotype among Punjabis that Mirpuris are particularly likely to force their daughters into early marriages with kin from Pakistan, in contrast with city-based or better educated Punjabis or Pakistanis, who allow young people to take the initiative or responsibility for marital choices. In practice, this perceived difference may be less a matter of coercion than of differing and changing expectations. Zareena's father, originally from rural Mirpur, respected his British born and raised daughter's feelings when she said she did not want to marry a local cousin and subsequently accepted her decision to marry out of the family. In contrast, Rukhsana, who is the same age as Zarina but born and raised in rural Mirpur, told me that she would not have thought to question her parents' choice of a husband for her – in this case, her father's sister's son, whom she had not met and who was living in England at the time. For her, it was enough to respect her parents' judgement, but, she continued: 'It is different now, because sometimes children's ideas and experiences are very different from their parents. Children should not agree just to keep parents happy, if they are not prepared to take responsibility themselves.'

The theme of individual responsibility recurred in younger adults' accounts of their own recent marriages and in their views on marriage generally. Hamid Ullah, also British-born, with family origins in Azad Kashmir, is thirty years old and married to a first cousin. He referred directly to the issue of forced marriage in his emphasis on the importance of individual responsibility:

> You can marry a relative if you want, but both have to agree. In Islam, it is quite clear that you should not marry in the family if it is not your decision, if you have not taken responsibility for it. Even if your fathers were brothers and they forced our marriage, we would have to take responsibility for it. But in Qur'anic terms, the people who will get punished are the fathers.

Rashida, who is twenty-two, with paternal grandparents in Rawalpindi city and maternal grandparents in a village in Jhelum district, also referred to the issue of forced marriage when telling me how she envisaged her own marriage:

> There was an article from Bradford I think about parents taking girls back to Pakistan saying they are just going for a holiday, then doing *nikah* [Islamic marriage contract] and leaving the girls there. That is forced marriage. That is against Islam. I have read a lot about Islam, and I don't agree with forced marriages. My parents agree that it is not in Islam. They will wait until I tell them I want to get married. First I will talk to my Mum, and she will talk to my Dad. My Mum wanted to do *haj* [pilgrimage to Mecca] last year, but it was my sister's wedding. So I think they will do it next year. When that is out of the way, then I will tell them. I have decided that I will go with my parents' decision, with who they choose, and I will tell them when I am ready. I don't want much, but I want someone kind, who will look after me. My parents will be a good judge of that. I will be happy with someone from Pakistan. All I will say is that if I discover there is something in what I hear about him that I don't like, then they must listen to me. They will listen, they won't force me.

If a child is unwilling to accept a particular proposal, the rejection needs to be handled very carefully, especially if it is in the family and particularly if it is expressed at a relatively late stage in marriage negotiations, for it may otherwise reflect badly on the parents. Tahir's parents, originally from rural Jhelum (bordering Mirpur), cited their son's desire to continue his studies in their explanation to relatives in Pakistan for their son's last-minute change of heart over a long-expected marriage to a kinswoman in Pakistan. This was also one of Tahir's reasons for rejecting the proposal. In his justification of his decision he also distances himself from the stereotypical Mirpuri:

> I don't agree with these Mirpuri people who marry their sons and daughters at a young age, as soon as they finish school. I am twenty-one, and I don't want now to be burdened with supporting a wife and kids. I have been working for a couple of years, saving the money for university. I want to study for a couple of years. Besides, I have found someone else.

Tahir knew the *rishta* was important to his parents so had consented when the engagement was first suggested two years previously, but felt increasingly unwilling to go through with the marriage as the date approached, particularly since he now had a girlfriend. Eventually his mother and aunts insisted he make a final decision, and so he firmly refused. Although the decision did not really surprise her, his mother was very upset, and his father was so angry that he turned him out of the house, blaming his wife for putting 'too much pressure on the boy. If they had let the matter drop, he would have agreed eventually.'

Yet, despite the pain of this experience, Tahir's parents accepted his right to disagree. Tahir's mother's brother, who had played an important mediating role when emotions were running high, explained this as an Islamic principle: 'If you ask your son, and he says no, you can ask him again, and you can ask him one more time. But if after three times he still refuses, then you should leave it [let the matter drop]. That is what Islam says.' Tahir's sister's husband added that it was better for the girl in Pakistan, who is, after all, a relative towards whom they also have some responsibility, that the engagement be broken now when another *rishta* can be found for her from within the family. For Tahir too, the experience was also extremely painful, not least because of his awareness of how it would affect his parents, particularly his mother:

> My Mum is suffering, I know. I really felt for her when she had to go to Pakistan to my cousin's wedding – the cousin I was supposed to marry. Luckily the family there found someone else for her. My Mum, she had to go, because she is that girl's auntie and has to give something at the wedding, so she had to face all those people. She felt ashamed, embarrassed, about what had happened, and that is my fault. The thing is, whatever I do, my mother will suffer people's criticisms, they'll say she did not bring me up right and stuff. The thing is, I don't want to marry in the family because there's always so much trouble. There is too much history, history that goes back for generations, and you get embroiled in it although it's all about things that mean nothing to you. And there's this thing about blood.
> AS: Blood, what do you mean?
> TH: That there can be problems with marriages between people who have the same blood. Well, I have heard it. It makes you want to avoid it.

For Tahir, the shared kinship on which this marriage would have been built and the fact that the marriage has implications for connections between a wide range of other relatives in England and in Pakistan were experienced as negative features of this proposal, to which he added the issue of biological risk. However, for other young adults, the prior connection of kinship gives marriage within the family a particular appeal, reconnecting a couple within a wider family network (see also Donnan 1988: 316). The security that such *rishtas* offer can be as important for young people as it is for the parents making these proposals: 'I think it's quite a bonus ... because if you marry in the family, you know, they know you. You've got that strong bond before you even start ... And you've got the family support as well' (Charsley 2003). While 'family support' is sometimes experienced as interference, it is also recognised as a strength, entailing a commitment to make the marriage work. Saima, too, now twenty-eight, whose parents are from Rawalpindi, could have married an English boyfriend, but finally decided to accept the *rishta* her father had proposed with his brother's son, who was then living in Saudi Arabia, because, she said, 'I suddenly realised what I would be throwing away.' She was referring to the social and emotional support of her own family and of her husband's family, as well as her own cultural heritage, all of which was packaged into this culturally acceptable proposal.

Transnational *rishtas*: identity and cultural reproduction

In the pioneer generation, one of the effects of, if not the motivation for, 'family reunion' (women and children joining men in Britain) from the 1970s onwards was to ensure that the men did not lose their cultural and religious roots. Occasionally this was an explicit reason for arranging a marriage. Hamid Ullah told me that his father was married to a woman in Pakistan for just this reason:

> My father was getting very Westernised [he had been living with an Englishwoman]. He had been over here a long time. Someone who knew my father and who knew my mother's family, they got the two families in touch with each other. My father's friend and his family, they thought it was time my father got married, so he did not forget his culture.

Some British Pakistanis are wary of *rishtas* with other British Pakistanis for fear that they will have been 'contaminated by the amoral climate of the West' (Charsley 2003). This fear comes to the fore in the context of marriage and childbearing, because these processes most centrally concern cultural and religious reproduction.

British Pakistani men may say they would prefer a Pakistani wife over a British-raised one, because women raised in Pakistan are more dutiful and less independent, assertive, argumentative or likely to 'do fashion', besides also being better able to impart Pakistani ways and Islamic values to their children, thus compensating for British-raised men's own perceived lack of religious practice and knowledge (Charsley 2003). Husnain stressed the importance of a 'common religious culture' in which to raise children, by commenting on the cultural differences he assumed would be present in interfaith marriages, implying here that marrying a British-raised Pakistani woman would be like marrying outside the ethnic group:

> The problems will arise when you have children. Imagine if I had married a Christian or a Jew. I would want my children to attend the mosque on Friday and be brought up as Muslim, while my wife would want to the child to go to church on Sunday and be brought up as a Christian. In the long term, what helps marriages work is a common religious culture and common family culture.

A match between two British-raised people is viewed as potentially unstable, because both partners will be 'too Westernised', whereas marriage involving a spouse from Pakistan is more likely to endure because of the more committed approach to marriage that a person raised in a Muslim country will bring. Arranged South Asian marriages appear to be more stable than among the majority British population because, despite evidence of rising divorce rates, divorce remains less common and the number of single-parent households is fewer (Berrington 1994). In part, this may reflect the cultural expectations associated with arranged marriage. As Husnain put it:

> With an arranged marriage, you start with the expectation that this is a marriage, that you will be a husband and a wife to each other. It is a totally different thing from a love marriage; where you have been girlfriend and boyfriend, how do you convert to husband and wife? You can't always be thinking of yourself if you want your marriage to work.

Nonetheless, during the recent fieldwork, marital stability was an issue of local concern. To date, there has been little research on disjunctions in practice between marital expectations and outcome in Pakistani Muslim marriages, with the exception of Charsley's (2005) work on the difficulties experienced by Pakistan-raised husbands. The gendered dimensions of marital success or instability reflect the fact that Pakistan-raised women are generally perceived to have been brought up to expect to adapt to their husband's family after marriage, to respect their husband's and elders' -particularly their in-laws' – wishes and dress and behave modestly, whereas confrontation may be more likely with a British-raised woman. Khalid, now forty-five years old, who has family origins in Mirpur, described himself with some pride as having been 'the first to marry out of the family' in his local community, but he added that the failure of this marriage to a British-raised Pakistani woman made him re-evaluate the security of 'traditional' inter-family marriages and the value of marrying a woman raised in Pakistan. He is now married to a twenty-one-year-old cousin (who is also his sister-in-law, his sister's husband's sister).

It is not just men, however, who may actively prefer a spouse from 'back home'. It is worth recalling Rashida's sentiment, quoted above, that 'I will be happy with someone from Pakistan.' British women sometimes consider British-raised men unsuitable as husbands, for reasons that include the view that local men are deficient in their work ethic, religious practice and values or, alternatively, too materialistic, as well as more likely to be unfaithful (Shaw and Charsley 2006). Farhat, who is twenty-four and waiting for her Pakistani husband to receive entry clearance, explained:

> I had a few proposals from men here too. They would come round. But their proposals were mainly financial; they all talked about the money they would earn. They said I could continue working; 'You work, and I will work.' It seemed it wasn't really a commitment to a life together. I was not happy with them. A man from Pakistan is different. He knows his culture, he is more religious, less obsessed with money. Men from here, they are too forward, too confident in talking to women. A man from Pakistan, I don't think he would cheat on me.

Transnational cousinhood: introducing distance

Young British Pakistanis usually have some British-born and raised cousins whom they could marry, and such marriages sometimes take place, but there are several reasons why young adults and their parents may consider these matches 'too close'. One has already been mentioned: such a couple will be 'too Westernised', whereas a partner from Pakistan would redress any imbalance in cultural and religious values. Another is the concern with balancing distance from and closeness to in-laws. Insufficient physical distance from a woman's natal kin can be problematic, because excessive close contact between a woman and her close kin can cause conflicts between her parents and her in-laws (Jeffery and Jeffery 1996a: 216–17). Ghazalla's mother disapproved of her daughter's wish to marry her father's brother's son, who lives locally, because the prospective father-in-law was known to be domineering; Ghazalla thought that, if this marriage went ahead, she would find it hard not to interfere, out of a desire to protect her daughter; she would prefer her daughter to marry a man from Pakistan, who would be more independent of his parents' control. The other side of this is that immigrant husbands can experience difficulties in being dependents upon their wives' parents' households (Charsley 2005).

The dominant discourse of disapproval of cousin marriages, as being akin to incest or as illegal (even though cousin marriage has been legal in England since the sixteenth century; see Chapter 2) also informs young British Pakistani ideas of cousin marriages, particularly marriages to British cousins, as 'too close'. Several parents reported that quite young Pakistani children are taunted by white children in the school playground about marrying cousins; they then return home from school asserting that they will not marry a cousin. Husnain told me:

> Our youngsters here – my nieces and nephews – they are saying, 'We are not going to marry cousins.' It's a peer group influence, it is brainwashing, even at the age of thirteen or so, even as young as seven. Their white friends, they say to them, 'You're going to get married to your cousin,' and the kids, they are trying to defend themselves, so they come home and say, 'I am not going to marry a cousin.' One of my nieces is seven. Her friends say it to her at school, 'You'll definitely marry your cousin.'

Rubina, who has two daughters and a twelve-year-old son, said that, when he is contemplating marriage, she will show her son her nieces, but:

> I think he won't want to marry them. He thinks of his cousins as his sisters. When he was ten, he came to me and said, 'Are you allowed to marry a cousin?' I said, 'Yes.' He said, 'I don't want to marry one of my auntie's girls.' I asked him, 'What about your uncle's daughters?' He said, 'No, they are like sisters.'

The discourse of disapproval (Chapter 1) has reached many young people via the media and in schools, including in the GCSE and A-level syllabus on genetic science. Khalid said his sons would not marry cousins for this reason:

> My sons [one studying for A levels, the other at university] know there is a problem marrying cousins. My kids say to me, Dad, we would not do that – we have learnt about it at school. But some kids would not be able to say that to their parents. It is a matter of understanding and culture. There are people who are my age whose children just would not mention it to them, just as I would not mention it to my parents.

Husnain, Rubina and Khalid, all of whom had attended a genetics clinic in connection with a family history of a genetic (or possibly genetic) condition, paid particular attention to such comments from their children, nephews and nieces because of the family experience. Tahir, too, who referred to the discourse of genetic risk when justifying his rejection of a *rishta* with a Pakistani cousin, was perhaps particularly aware of 'this thing about blood' because his sister has a child with a recessive genetic condition. Yet I have also heard these concerns expressed by people in other families unaffected by genetic conditions or not connected with this study involving referrals to a genetics clinic. For instance, one mother told me her thirty-year-old son mentioned the genetic risks of consanguineous marriage among his reasons for turning down a *rishta* in the family. In these cases, children's views reflect the effects of the wider discourse of disapproval of such marriages discussed in the previous chapter.

Pakistani kinship terminology contains some ambiguity with regard to cousins, for in Urdu and Panjabi the full kinship terms for cousin mean, literally, the brother or sister born to a maternal or paternal aunt or uncle. British Pakistanis often adapt this terminology by using the English words brother or sister in statements about cousins, saying he's my 'brother', or he's my 'cousin-brother' or she's my 'cousin-sister.' Katharine Charsley suggests that young Bristol Pakistanis utilise this ambiguity 'to negotiate the category of potential spouses', for within Pakistani kinship – and according to Islamic marriage rules – siblings are not permissible spouses while first cousins are. By referring to a local cousin as a brother or a sister, they may be indicating to their parents that a local cousin, whom they know well and who might otherwise be considered a potential match, is in fact 'too close' to marry: 'A certain distance, then, is necessary to make space for affinity within bonds of kinship and locality' (Charsley 2003: 151). In contrast, British Pakistanis 'do not have these uncomfortable feelings about cousins in Pakistan whom they may only have seen occasionally' (ibid.: 151). 'The possibility of transnational marriage introduces potential spouses who are equally close in terms of kinship, but distant enough in other ways to be acceptable partners, whilst fulfilling the criteria of connection needed to be confident of social approval and the reduction of risk involved in such arrangements' (Charsley 2003: 152). This combination of closeness and distance – in a relationship with someone with whom you did not grow up but to whom you feel closely connected – may contribute to the romance of some transnational *rishtas*. As we saw in the Introduction, Yasmin fell in love with a cousin while on holiday in India. Among British Pakistanis, attractions between transnationally distant cousins sometimes develop on visits to Pakistan. 'It was love at first sight,' one man said of the cousin he met at his brother's wedding in Pakistan. Iram met her future husband Ikhlaq at her sister's wedding in Pakistan: 'I liked him as soon as I saw him.' Such attractions can lead to rapid changes of parental plans where parents had a different cousin in mind, and yet the criterion of connection is maintained. Thus, the emotion of love is not necessarily incompatible with 'playing the game' but may provide important insights into its process; as Bourdieu writes, 'To love is always to some extent … another way of fulfilling one's own social destiny' (1990: 71).

Although 'arranged' and 'love' marriages are usually viewed as polar opposites, some *rishtas* begin as an attraction between two young people who then ask their families to arrange the marriage (Fischer and Lyon 2000: 309; Shaw 2001: 324). Indeed, the stereotypical distinction between 'love' and 'arranged' marriage obscures the role of love and romance even within conventionally arranged marriages, for, in a purdah society like Pakistan, romantic attraction and love marriages are more likely to occur between cousins, who, as 'family', have opportunities to meet (Fischer 1991: 102). Even in more conventionally arranged marriages, there may be romance in long-distance phone conversations with fiancés and in chaperoned visits. Farhat (introduced above) said she insisted on having a 'romantic' month in Pakistan before her wedding in which to go out with her fiancé, accompanied by a sister and brother-in-law. Indeed, the cultural conventions surrounding arranged marriages, including the expectation of love after marriage rather than through premarital intimacy, may intensify the attraction of a transnational *rishta*.

Conclusion

For Husnain, the twenty-six-year-old graduate quoted at the beginning of this chapter, as for most of the young couples in my research, 'Marrying within the family is the normal thing to do.' Countering the dominant media images of transnational marriages forced upon unwilling participants in response to cultural and psychological pressures exerted by their parents, these young people often indicate a preference for a spouse from Pakistan rather than from the U.K., for reasons that indicate a desire for cultural and religious continuity as well as social and emotional security in a multicultural world.

From both the parents' perspectives and, in rather different ways, the perspectives of the young adults themselves, the continuing popularity of consanguineous Pakistani transnational marriages can be understood as a means of balancing the social and emotional risks entailed in marriage as an inherently insecure process. Marriages involving close and trusted kin are thought to minimise the risks of deception and marital insecurity that are perceived to be greater with marriages arranged outside the family. Transnational marriage arrangements do, however, bring a variety of new risks, such as the possibility that an entry visa will be refused and the danger that marriage is being used as a route to immigration and U.K. citizenship. The dominant public discourse in the U.K. and elsewhere in Europe that links consanguineous marriage with the risk of genetic problems – sometimes to the extent that, for some, genetics has become equated with 'what happens when you marry within the family' – can provide grounds for the rejection of particular proposals. Yet bringing into focus the social and cultural objectives and emotional motivations in choices of a transnational spouse helps explain why such marriages may still be regarded as 'safer' than marrying out of the family.

This discussion raises a number of issues relevant to considering the likely continuity of this complex social trend. Transnational marriage sets in place a structure for maintaining transcontinental links in the next generation, through the incoming spouse. The extent to which young British-raised Pakistanis' decisions about work and marriage will continue to be shaped by relationships with parents and other kin, locally, nationally and in transnational networks, will depend, in part, on global political and socio-economic processes. Within these processes, local, national and increasingly global awareness of the issue of genetic risk in consanguineous marriage – of which even children as young as seven years are aware through their interactions with other children in school playgrounds – will play an as yet unknown part. Relevant, too, will be the experiences of children and young adults with personal experience of genetic conditions, either from being affected themselves or having close affected relatives. However, it is important to emphasise also that contemporary genetic services in the U.K. offer a means of avoiding the births of further affected children in at least some of the families in which a recessive condition has been diagnosed without the need to avoid consanguineous marriage. This is because, for at least some conditions, the risks for other members of the family can be managed by offering individuals carrier tests, and, for carrier couples, by appropriate prenatal diagnosis with the option of ending an affected pregnancy. The following chapters explore some of the ways in which individuals and couples at risk of having an affected child negotiate these options, beginning with the question of establishing a genetic diagnosis.

CHAPTER 4
MEDICAL SURVEILLANCE AND DIAGNOSTIC UNCERTAINTY

Sofia: four unsuccessful pregnancies

Sofia Ali, twenty-six years old and raised in Azad Kashmir, has been living in England for seven years since joining her British-born and raised husband. As is typical in families in which intermarriage has been practised for generations, her husband is related to her in several ways: as her mother's brother's son (first cousin), as her father's brother's daughter's son, and as her father's sister's son's son (her husband's parents are first cousins). For Sofia, the U.K. provisions of antenatal care and hospitalised births contrasted with the limited services available in rural Pakistan and Azad Kashmir (and their availability only to the wealthy in urban areas) and had, at first, held out the promise of successful childbirth when she became pregnant for the first time:

> I was very happy. I went for my first scan – twelve weeks I think – and they said everything was fine, the baby was okay, and I was very happy, very grateful. In Pakistan, they don't have these facilities, no check-ups before. There is only a midwife [*dāī*] in the village. When my son was born and they said he had a problem, it was a shock, not at all what I expected ... The doctors told me they had noticed a problem at birth. They said he had one kidney bigger than the other and both were not working properly. They said he would be on these machines for two weeks and then he would come home, but after some hours his breathing stopped. When my husband got back to the hospital [he had gone home to inform his family about his son's birth] the baby was dead. Here, I have a photograph of him in his father's arms [shows a photograph of the dead baby].

After that, Sofia had two miscarriages and although she then carried a fourth pregnancy to term, this baby was diagnosed from prenatal scans as having the same fatal kidney problems as the first baby. The couple decided to continue the pregnancy, but the baby died within a few hours of its birth.

> Women come to the house – neighbours, friends of my mother-in-law, people I don't know well. They say, 'It happened to me two or three times, then I have this child and this child and they are okay.' But it is no comfort. It is as if you are really really hungry. You have cooked a meal. It is right in front of you. And then someone puts it to one side and you are told, 'It's no good, you have to cook it all over again.' I can't think of a better way of explaining. You are so hungry, so very very hungry, you want the food now, you don't want to wait.

Over three years of four unsuccessful pregnancies, Sofia and her husband made several visits to the genetics clinic, to which they were initially referred for investigation of the reasons for the miscarriage. At the original appointment, Sofia recalled being asked if any tissue from the miscarried baby had been stored, but, she told me, 'I was on my own when it happened. It was like a heavy period and I flushed it away. I did not know that the doctors would have liked to look at it.' The couple returned to the genetics clinic after the second miscarriage and this time received a full medical explanation for the first infant death, which they had initially understood to have been caused by 'something to do with the kidney or something to do with the lungs'. They learnt that the immediate cause of death was a developmental problem with the lungs, as a result of a problem with the formation of the kidneys, which were full of holes, like sacs, and therefore unable to make urine. The lack of urine had meant the pressure of amniotic fluid around the baby in the womb was insufficient for the lungs to develop properly. This kidney condition is a recognised recessively inherited condition, with a recurrence risk of one in four. The doctor also raised the possibility that a prenatal test might be available in another pregnancy:

> Sometimes one gene carries a fault but there is usually a backup copy to compensate. In this case, your child, by chance, got two copies of the gene with the fault, one from each of you. This has caused the condition. The chance of this happening is one in four. We could take blood from you to see if we can do a genetic test in your next pregnancy, to see if another baby has a double dose of the faulty gene.

Sofia's husband's response indicates a willingness to consent to genetic investigations that might permit a prenatal test and give information about a future pregnancy, but not necessarily for the purpose of ending an affected pregnancy: 'I'd rather have a healthy baby than not; I would like to know if it is healthy. I don't think she [indicating his wife] would want you to do anything that might harm the pregnancy. I won't think she would terminate, or that our religion would allow it.' Although the possibility of mutation research involving a laboratory in Birmingham, U.K., was discussed, the doctor considered it unlikely to provide a result in time to be useful in the next pregnancy. Instead, the couple gave blood and signed papers consenting to its storage and use for a clinical test to investigate the cause of miscarriage. The doctor also promised to investigate whether any tissue from the dead baby had been stored and could be used in research. Three months later, the couple learnt that the test to investigate the cause of miscarriage was negative.

Eight months later, Sofia was pregnant again, but her twenty-four-week scan showed the same fatal recessive condition. The couple requested another genetics appointment, as they were considering whether or not to terminate this pregnancy and thought some test results might be outstanding. The doctor mentioned a possible new clinical test at a U.K. laboratory, because a gene causing the kidney condition had been recently discovered in America. There was also a new research possibility involving a laboratory in America, but this would require DNA from the next baby: should the parents continue with the pregnancy, a note would be written into Sofia's prenatal records to alert the obstetricians and paediatricians to the need for DNA from the baby to be taken at birth. The nurse counsellor remarked after the consultation, 'It is imperative that we get a DNA sample from this baby. We need to get the DNA stored, from the cord blood if the baby goes to term, because we might be able to do a molecular diagnosis.'

Sofia and her husband decided to continue the pregnancy. It was already quite advanced, and termination would have involved feticide, as Sofia learnt by listening to her husband and sister-in-law talking in English in the car on the way home after the hospital appointment at which this was discussed. Immediately after the birth, the baby was whisked off by medical staff. Sofia's later recollection of this raises questions to which I return in Chapter 6 about the management of childbirth in the case of known fatal abnormalities:

> This time, I was fully conscious, I had not had any painkillers or injections, only the cut that they put stitches in afterwards to get the baby out, so I could see everything. I wanted to see her and I said can you give her to me, but they took her to one side and put her on a machine like a thing you weigh someone on, and after that they took her out to another room, and they told me, 'Be patient' [*sābar karo*]. Then they came back and said there is nothing more that they can do and they brought me a photograph of her. I did not get to hold her. I think now that they knew she was going to die, why did they not just give her to me? When they said, when I was pregnant, that she would die and I should think about having the injection, I thought about it and knew that I did not want to kill her. Then she was born and they took her away. Now I think perhaps they killed her. I know the doctors try, but, in the end, they cannot solve anything, they cannot change anything, there is nothing they can do for me. Though there are one or two methods . . .

As this indicates, Sofia's attitude to the clinical genetics service was, by now, decidedly ambivalent. On the one hand, she comments, 'I know the doctors try, but, in the end, they cannot solve anything, they cannot change anything, there is nothing they can do for me.' On the other hand, she adds, 'there are one or two methods . . .'. She had, in fact, returned with her husband to the genetics clinic after this second infant death, and the couple had agreed to their own and their dead baby's DNA being sent for mutation research to America. As Sofia explained:

> The doctor told my husband that there is something, some test they can do in pregnancy, take some fluid or something, and from that they may be able to tell if the baby has the same problem or not . . . But I would not end the pregnancy, that is illegitimate [*nājāiz*] in our religion. But I am thinking, if I get pregnant again, I won't tell the doctors at all.

Three years on, then, after two infant deaths and two miscarriages, this couple and their second dead baby had been enrolled, via their blood samples, in mutation research.

Enrolment, resistance and the challenges of genetic diagnosis

These extracts relating to Sofia's case over three years of engagement with genetic services introduce the central concerns of this chapter: the enrolment of men, women and children in genetic diagnostic processes and the challenges confronting doctors and patients in endeavours to 'find the gene' for rare conditions. As I shall show, two slightly different sets of interests govern doctors' and patients' participation in genetic diagnostic processes, although a degree of cooperation and co-participation is necessary for their pursuit. That patients like Sofia attend genetics clinics and give blood samples indicates that, 'at least to some extent', they share with their doctors a common interest in solving the problems of unsuccessful reproduction and of a range of different forms of ill health (Lock 1998: 206). Sofia's husband had told the clinical geneticists, 'I'd rather have a healthy baby than not; I would like to know if it is healthy.' However, Sofia's later ambivalence (desire for research results but resistance to early prenatal investigations) indicates that the degree of or limits to patients' engagement in genetic diagnostic processes remain open to exploration and may change over time.

Clinically, a genetic diagnosis means that a cure, in the form of correcting the changes or errors the DNA sequence in an affected person, is unlikely, even though therapies can reduce the ill effects of certain conditions (depending on the bodily system they affect); the causes of changes in chromosome or genetic structure are currently beyond human control (regardless of whether they arise anew, as 'mistakes' occurring at conception, or originate in the structure of parental DNA). A genetic diagnosis in a baby or child also means the parents may be at risk of having another similarly affected pregnancy and (unless the identified mutation or chromosomal rearrangement has arisen anew in the child) diagnostic accuracy is thus crucial to risk assessment, since different inheritance patterns (dominant, recessive, etc.) imply different reproductive risks (Introduction), with implications for risk management in subsequent pregnancies. The genetic change may also be shared by and have health and reproductive implications for other close blood relatives, because biological relatives share some of their DNA. A chromosome rearrangement or alteration in DNA sequence could also be passed on to subsequent generations. Work in clinical genetics thus entails making diagnoses and establishing and communicating to patients the associated health and reproductive risks for individuals, couples and the wider family and the options for risk management via, of instance, genetic prenatal and carrier testing (Chapters 5 and 7). Genetics doctors also provide information about the condition's prognosis, management and therapeutic possibilities; these aspects of work overlap, to some extent, with that of paediatricians and specialists in other medical disciplines, where discussion focuses on management rather than on the genetic aspects.

However, achieving a genetic diagnosis is not always straightforward but may be slow and uncertain and pose significant challenges for clinicians, especially in relation to rare conditions such as those affecting Sofia's children. A genetic diagnosis itself is not a foregone conclusion and, while some conditions may be established as genetic on the basis of their presenting features (phenotype), the underlying change in gene sequence (genotype) may not yet be established, precluding genetic prenatal or carrier tests. The underlying genetic causes of many known and unknown conditions remain unidentified, limiting the possibilities for genetic prenatal diagnosis and carrier testing, despite often inflated popular and scientific claims that molecular science is transforming clinical medicine. Nearly a third of the cases in this study had an uncertain diagnosis, while the category of certain diagnoses included many in which the diagnosis was made from clinical observation and test results rather than by molecular means.

Of the sixty-nine different conditions observed in the study sample (Introduction), fifty-seven were considered genetic, nine remained unknown and three had non-genetic causes, such as a trauma of pregnancy or birth (Hurst 2005). Diagnosis was certain for more than half (46/57) of the conditions including for thirty-three of the forty-four recessive conditions (one being the fatal renal problem that affected Sofia's two infants). But diagnosis was probable or possible (rather than certain) for a quarter (11/44) of the recessive conditions, of which many are rare and some are considered 'orphan' conditions because they have not been previously recorded in other families. Overall, although most conditions could be categorised as genetic or non-genetic (rather than unknown) in most cases (60/69), and although diagnosis was certain (dominant, chromosomal, recessive or non-genetic) rather than unknown for nearly two-thirds of the sample (49/60), it remained unknown or uncertain (as possibly or probably recessive) for over a third of cases (20/69). The precise genetic change was identified for about half

(16/33) of the certain recessives but not for the other recessive conditions, and so in these cases a genetic prenatal or carrier test was not available and the genotypic characterisation was deferred to a point in the future (Latimer et al. 2006), even where a firm diagnosis had been made on the basis of the phenotypic features (Shaw 2003b).

Achieving a genetic diagnosis thus presents various challenges for patients and their doctors. For doctors in genetics, as I shall show, these include negotiation of the rather grey area that delineates clinical practice from research, especially with respect to rare disorders. For patients, these include such things as understanding genetic terminology and the rationale behind particular tests, the need for consent to clinical tests or for research enrolment and why doctors may ask about parental consanguinity. In what follows, I present extracts from cases chosen not so much because they represent different diagnostic categories (a possible non-genetic condition, a recessive condition, etc.) but because they illustrate some of these challenges: I could equally have illustrated these with cases representing other diagnostic categories (dominant, X-linked, etc.). The order of presentation, does, however reflect to some extent the clinical process of differential diagnosis that governs genetic diagnostic work. Differential diagnosis first involves defining as genetic rather than non-genetic in origin problems such as infertility, infant death or long-term difficulties with physical or mental health. These problems may present as single conditions without any other associated features (deafness, for instance, often involves only deafness) or else they may present as syndromes involving more than one unusual clinical feature, including characteristics – such as an unusually small head, low-set ears or extra fingers and toes – that fall outside the range of normal variation and are not characteristics of the family in which they appear (Shaw 2003b). Doctors then seek to establish the underlying genetic cause (genotype) within the person's DNA, distinguishing chromosomal conditions (involving changes in chromosome structure) from single-gene conditions, and then, for the latter, to identify the causative mutation (change in gene sequence).

Various theorists have described the processes of assigning an underlying genetic cause to problems with reproduction and health as geneticisation or genetic essentialism and then asserted that, in these processes, genetic explanations are being prioritised over other understandings of health and illness (Lippman 1992; Nelkin and Lindee 1995). Geneticisation in the sense of assigning a genetic cause can be understood as a form of what Ivan Illich calls the medicalisation of life (Illich 1992: 230), referring to the rise of Western biomedical knowledge, practice and control by means of surveys and investigations of the physical body (Foucault 1973, 1979; Atkinson 1981; Armstrong 1983). Research and clinical work in genetics are undoubtedly a part of this process, involving genetic epidemiology (population-wide assessments of genetic risk, etc.) and clinic-based scrutiny of the external body (its skeleton and organs, via scans, X-rays, etc.) and its internal structure or 'building plan' as set out in cellular DNA. But, as I hope to show here, it does not necessarily follow from this that geneticisation in the sense of reducing a diagnosis to an underlying DNA sequence is either inevitable or straightforward in the diagnostic process or within patients' understandings.

Are Zobeen's birth abnormalities non-genetic, chromosomal or genetic?

Husnain and Humaira's first child, Zobeen, was born after Humaira had previously suffered a miscarriage. The parents were referred to clinical genetics when a prenatal scan had shown a slightly unusual curve in the baby's spine. At birth Zobeen was noted to have a small head, low-set ears, mild club feet, a heart murmur and a cleft palate as well as a slight spinal curvature (scoliosis). Zobeen's parents were shocked to learn about these problems, but reassured to hear that the cleft palate could be repaired, and did not consider the small head particularly problematic. 'I look at Husnain', Humaira said, 'and he has a narrow head, long and narrow. I think that a small head is normal in Asian families.' Nevertheless, they returned to the genetics clinic for a review of Zobeen's progress and to find out if there was now a diagnosis. However, as the clinician explained:

> Dr A: Zobeen has not got something that jumps out to us as X syndrome. We are going to do tests [including scans to check the structure of spine and heart] over the next few weeks or months to give an assessment of whether it is genetic or not … If there is more than one problem, we see if it fits into a syndrome – a named condition; if it does fit one, we would look for a cause. Her chromosome test is normal. That does not mean nothing is wrong in the genes or chromosomes, but on the current sophistication of routine testing of chromosomes there is nothing missing or extra. A chromosomal condition would have been high on our list, but it isn't obvious from this. If there is a chromosomal problem, it's too small to pick up.
> Husnain: What else could it be?
> Dr A: There were no problems in pregnancy. The mother did not take any medication. Something like interruption of the blood supply to the baby through the placenta, which we have no knowledge of, could have caused it – and that would have nothing to do with genetics. Or it could be a genetic thing. That's the problem.
> Husnain: I don't know the difference between the chromosomes and the genes.
> Dr A: The chromosomes are the structures that carry the genes. The chromosomes come in parts, half from the mother, half from the father. Along the chromosome there are many hundreds of thousands of genes which give individual genetic messages. When we look at the chromosomes, we can't see single genetic changes.

Having noted that the chromosome test is 'normal', the clinician first considers non-genetic causes of Zobeen's problems in answer to Husnain's first question as to 'what else' the problem could be, if it is not chromosomal. She rules out environmental causes (problems in pregnancy, taking medicine in pregnancy, interrupted blood supply to the baby, etc.) for lack of evidence and returns to the possibility of a genetic explanation, using the term genetic generally, to refer to either chromosomes or genes. Husnain's next question picks up on this frequent ambiguity in clinicians' use of the word genetic: on the one hand, they use it to distinguish environmental from chromosomal or submiscroscopic changes in DNA sequence, and, on the other hand, they use it to distinguish a chromosomal from submicroscopic molecular causes. Husnain asks for clarification of the difference between chromosomes and genes, and the clinician's answer focuses on submicroscopic changes detectable by molecular techniques.

The logic of differential diagnosis usually involves ruling out first non-genetic conditions and then chromosomal causes before proceeding to mutation analysis, but sometimes clinical investigations do not happen in this order and sometimes a genetic diagnosis may be made in the absence of a confirmatory molecular test.

Sohrab: why do they need more blood if there is no blood test?

Sohrab Hussain is the eldest son of first cousin parents and lives with his parents, his paternal grandparents and his father's unmarried siblings. He was referred by a paediatrician for genetic investigations just before his third birthday. His clinical features include severe obesity, learning difficulties and an extra toe on each foot. Six months previously, a paediatrician aware that a rare disorder of fat metabolism had recently been identified in another consanguineous Pakistani family in High Wycombe had arranged for a blood test to be sent to a particular research group, but the result had been negative. At the genetics clinic, the doctor explained the need to take more blood, because Sohrab's chromosomes had not yet been checked:

> It is curious they did a mutation test without checking the chromosomes. It's like doing the fancy stuff without doing the basics first. If you are doing chromosomes you put the blood into a tube with an orange stopper – if you are doing some other test, you put the blood in a different tube – and the blood gets prepared differently according to what test you are doing. So it is likely that when they took the blood before, it was stored in such a way, or, rather, prepared in such a way, that makes it unusable for any other test such as doing the chromosomes.

Obtaining another blood sample was very difficult. Sohrab was very frightened and resisted violently, the doctor had trouble inserting the needle into a blood vessel, Sohrab's blood flowed very slowly into the tubes, and the doctor thought the amount obtained might be insufficient.

Dr B: I am sorry we had to do that ... We need to take his blood to check his chromosomes. We may need to take more blood for that, if this is not enough.
Do you know what chromosomes are?
Father: No.
Dr B: They are long strings which contain genetic material. I think that these chromosomes will be normal. What I think is that because he has more than one problem – his weight, his lack of speech, a few other problems, and extra toes – this may be a genetic condition. I do not know yet what the condition is. We need his blood to check the chromosomes. My suspicion is that he has a particular condition characterised by developmental delay; if it is this, he may have kidney problems in the future, so he will need a kidney examination, and he may have eye problems. Children with this condition sometimes have extra toes.
Father: What is the condition?
Dr B: It is called [she names a syndrome]. But there is no test to confirm it that we can do, at this stage. There is no blood test for this syndrome. Instead, we will look in his body, his heart, his kidneys, to see if there are other things that are described in the syndrome that he has.

Sohrab's father asked about the implications of this diagnosis for Sohrab's health, but the doctor cautioned that she must first rule out a chromosomal disorder – hence the blood test.

At home, some weeks later, the family learnt that the blood obtained at the clinic was indeed insufficient and the clinicians suggested another sample be taken under anaesthetic in the paediatric outpatient's ward at the local hospital, having double-checked that the blood taken for the earlier mutation test was unsuitable for chromosome analysis. Sohrab's mother was worried by this prospect 'because he is not like normal children, I am afraid he will not wake up like normal children, that making him unconscious will have some bad effect'. His grandmother was worried by the idea of taking more blood, believing that Sohrab's condition may have been caused by losing an unusually large amount of blood when he was circumcised as an infant. Despite a home visit from a genetic counsellor and interpreter, the family remained puzzled that more blood needed to be taken, because the consultant had said there is 'no blood test' to confirm the diagnosis. Why, then, was this new blood test necessary? If its result was negative, surely it would show that Sohrab did not have the condition? However, Sohrab's father felt the clinicians should complete their investigations, and eventually more blood was taken, under anaesthetic, with, fortunately, no difficulties, and the family waited anxiously for a result. Sohrab's grandparents found it particularly difficult to appreciate that a negative blood test result would not necessarily mean that Sohrab did not have a genetic condition; indeed, his grandmother seemed to view the test as if it would be definitive. 'I want the blood test result quickly,' she told me tearfully, 'I want him not to have any illness.'

Some six months later, at the genetics clinic, the clinicians confirmed that Sohrab has most of the features of the condition they had in mind. The blood test had helped them rule out a chromosomal condition, and the clinical tests – kidney scans, eye tests, etc. – had helped them establish the diagnosis, since, as the clinician explained:

> There isn't a blood test yet. There are five or six different types of this condition In only one of these types can you do a blood test to identify the problem, and this one type has been identified in an Amish population in the United States. We would have to send blood to the U.S. to get an answer on just this one variant. But it is unlikely to be the same variant.

In this extract, the clinician considers the option of sending Sohrab's blood to the United States and then rejects it as unlikely to assist the clinical diagnosis, because the mutation identified in the U.S. is unlikely to be the same as the one underlying Sohrab's condition.

In this case, therefore, as with more than half of the certain recessives in this study, a genetic condition was diagnosed on the basis of clinical features and a negative chromosome test result, rather than on the basis of a confirmatory molecular genetic test. There is currently no genetic (molecular) test for many certain recessive conditions, although, for one of them (Roberts syndrome), a chromosome test produces a characteristic result in which the chromosomes have a 'puffy' appearance. For several certain recessives, the underlying mutation was discovered and genetic (mutation) tests became available during the course of my study, but not at the time of the initial diagnosis being made. In other words, clinicians do not rely on molecular tests alone but draw on a range of different kinds of clinical evidence to diagnose rare recessive disorders (Shaw 2003b; Shaw et al. 2003).

Consanguinity in differential diagnosis: 'I can't ignore the fact that Zobeen's parents are cousins'

In the process of first considering and then, if there is no evidence for them, ruling out non-genetic or chromosomal conditions, clinicians must also note any parental consanguinity, as this increases the likelihood of recessive conditions (as discussed in Chapter 1). Zobeen's and Sohrab's parents are first cousins, as are Sofia and her husband, and, in each case, this fact was relevant to the differential diagnosis. In Zobeen's case, although the doctor seemed to be ruling out molecular causes in favour of a chromosomal explanation, there was another factor she could not overlook:

> Dr A: Often the underlying cause is not genetic [i.e. is chromosomal]. We have to note that you lost a baby in your first pregnancy [because this would

> indicate a chromosomal problem]. [However] Being cousins increases the risk of having a child with certain genetic diseases, but I don't know if this is one of them. I can't ignore the fact that Zobeen's parents are cousins, and [I] factor this in. This is a plus in favour of a genetic [i.e. molecular] explanation. There does not have to be a family history. These are very rare conditions, and may be individual to a family.

Her comments that 'there does not have to be a family history' and 'these are very rare conditions and may be individual to a family' refer to the fact that rare recessive conditions can arise for the first time in a family and can be virtually unique. Clinicians sometimes describe these as 'orphan' conditions: since no other cases are known to exist, such conditions lack 'kinship' with any other affected individuals in any other families.[1] The doctor continues: 'We have to look through the literature, and see if there are any other cases like her. If you weren't related, I would think it is most likely a chromosomal problem, rather than a hereditary problem, but I think it is too early to say.' In this case the doctor's inclination, based on her experience of observing other similarly affected children, is towards a chromosomal rather than a genetic (molecular) diagnosis; the fact that Zobeen's chromosome test had not shown a chromosome change did not conclusively rule one out. She therefore arranged for further clinical investigations, including a check of the parents' chromosomes, because 'sometimes an imbalance in one of the parents' chromosomes but no imbalance in the child's can explain the problems'. However, her advice to the couple about the recurrence risks – that 'the highest risk is a one in four risk' – allowed for the possibility that Zobeen's condition may be recessive; a chromosomal diagnosis usually gives a lower recurrence risk.

After Zobeen and her parents left the clinic, the doctor remarked, 'If she was born to non-consanguineous U.K. parents, it doesn't shout recessive; it could be chromosomal,' implying she would not be considering a recessive diagnosis if there had been no parental consanguinity. The child's features combined with her parents' consanguinity mean that a possible recessive diagnosis must be seriously considered, even if the clinician's diagnostic intuition might be towards a chromosomal condition. Zobeen's parents, too, remarked after the consultation on the clinical interest in their consanguinity. For Husnain, as for many Pakistani couples, the public focus on consanguinity, genetic risk and British Pakistanis (discussed in Chapter 1) suggests a racialised prejudice that a consanguineous couple's child's problems must be to do with their consanguinity. As Husnain put it, at home after the clinical appointment, 'I think there is an automatic assumption that it is because you are cousins. Is it the first question they would have asked a white family? No, they ask Asians.' As we have seen, doctors must consider the possible significance of parental consanguinity when looking for an explanation for a child's problems, since this increases the risk of recessive conditions, but they cannot assume that a condition is recessive because the parents are consanguineous. Nonetheless, parents may experience the question as implying a prejudged diagnosis. As Khalida, who is married to a double first cousin (their mothers are sisters and their fathers are brothers), remarked sceptically after the genetics clinic appointment at which she and her husband learnt they are carriers of two different recessive genetic disorders: 'I don't believe in this. I don't believe in this stuff that it's genetic. They try to say that it's your fault because you are married to a cousin. If they did not know we were cousins or if we weren't cousins they would not say it's genetic.'

Negotiating research enrolment

For rare conditions, a routine clinical test may be unavailable because the underlying mutations have not been identified, but doctors may be able to offer genetic tests on a research basis. This potentially extends clinical options (to include prenatal genetic and carrier tests) available to patients to whom a full clinical service cannot yet be offered, either because the causative mutation for their condition has not been found, or because it has been identified by a research group but a clinical test is not yet available. Much of the genetic research into rare conditions only proceeds because clinicians are willing to identify potential research participants. The potential benefits are mutual. Mutation research is central to the expansion of the clinical diagnostic repertoire, but cannot proceed without the recruitment of patients, via their DNA. Typically, a published paper identifying a causative mutation for a particular syndrome acknowledges the doctors and genetic counsellors who identified the patients whose blood samples were analysed. Indeed, some clinicians view research as an extension of the clinical service – as one clinician put it, 'The families want a result; they would give the blood for a clinical test, it's just that the clinical test is not available right away' – and some clinical geneticists are also actively engaged in genetic mutation research. One research resource stores blood samples and accompanying phenotypic data from consanguineous families affected by rare syndromes so that these samples can be made available to research groups as and when interest in particular rare conditions develops (Chapter 1). Doctors seek to keep up to date with developments in genetic research, not just because research results can quickly become transformed into clinically available tests, but because they may find that an interested and willing research group can offer tests on a research basis that are, nonetheless, likely to offer particular patients a clinically-useful result.

However, a number of challenges for doctors and patients emerge at this somewhat blurred boundary between mutation research and clinical practice. Although the 'substance' required for clinical genetic tests and genetic research is the same (usually a sample of blood or bodily tissue containing DNA), a clinical test entails patients consenting to an established procedure that will yield a positive or negative result within a predictable timescale, whereas mutation research cannot guarantee results and often operates to an indefinite timescale. Often likened to a fishing trip because of its uncertain outcomes, genetic research requires more complex consent procedures than clinical tests (Parker et al. 2004); for instance, two types of research consent may be required: one for samples to be stored, another detailing use of research results should research go ahead. Doctors may sometimes be unwilling to embark on complex research consent procedures if, in their view, a clinically useful result seems unlikely, especially where documents must be translated or interpreted, and so may decide to withhold research enrolment.

When Sofia and her husband had blood samples taken in the clinic, the doctor mentioned, considered and rejected a research possibility:

> We will need blood from both of you to send to a laboratory in Birmingham, to see if you both have the match [the same faulty gene]. To do this test will take time, it may take more than six months, so it is unlikely to tell you anything useful for the next pregnancy. Instead, we can check a future pregnancy with scans. In any case, with an amnio[centesis] you would risk losing the baby, and, given the problems with falling pregnant, it would not be worth the risk.

This research possibility, in the doctor's view, is unlikely to produce a result in time to enable a prenatal test in another pregnancy; besides this, the couple are ambivalent about prenatal diagnosis and the problem for which another pregnancy is at risk can be detected by ultrasound. The doctor also does not know, at this point, if any tissue from the affected baby was stored and could be used for research. As the consultation proceeds, she also establishes that Sofia's husband is unwilling to agree to the part of the research consent that required results with implications for other family members to be made available to relatives.

For patients, the distinctions between consenting to blood samples being taken for a clinical test, for storage or for research may be not at all obvious. Patients may expect results in each case to be equally likely, and so be puzzled when, having given blood, a result is not forthcoming. Khalida and her husband lost two newborn babies to a fatal kidney problem and a third baby in infancy to a rare metabolic condition for which the mutation was discovered during my fieldwork. At their first genetics clinic appointment, the clinician confirmed both diagnoses, explained the reproductive risks, and mentioned that a researcher in Scotland could look for the mutation involved in the metabolic problem:

> We would send the bloods [blood samples] for storage; he [the researcher] will send the forms, and you will have to consent to the research. If he finds it [the mutation], you will have to decide how the information should be used, for example for prenatal testing, or just to do a test on a newborn baby. I have already asked him and he is willing to try. What do you think, shall we take the bloods?

The couple consented immediately. Khalida's husband's response was, 'Do it, take the blood.' The clinician proceeded to take blood samples from them both and said she would see them again in a year, to discuss how genetic tests might be used in another pregnancy and to chase up the research – unless the couple were thinking of starting a pregnancy sooner and wanted an earlier appointment. Four months later, Khalida was pregnant again and seemed caught between wanting genetic test results and not wanting prenatal testing. 'I think that in future I won't go for any tests or anything, particularly not amniocentesis,' she said. She was annoyed that there were no results from the tests done in clinic: 'They should have had results by now.' In fact, there was no research result to wait for, because they had only consented to blood being stored and not, yet, to research.

A rather similar confusion arose in Sofia's case, after she and her husband had given blood samples in the clinic and consented to a clinical test – a chromosome test to investigate the reason for miscarriage. They had been informed of a negative chromosome test result by letter. After this, at the consultant's request, I telephoned Sofia to follow this up by raising, again, the issue of the couple's consent to mutation research. Sofia's reaction was frustration: for her, the act of giving blood seemed to constitute an effective consent to research; besides this, they had signed some consent forms in the clinic. To add to the confusion, she had not seen the consultant's letter:

AS: Dr A wanted me to ask you about the genetic research.
SA: Is there a result?
AS: No, not yet because they need your consent for the research.
SA: Do they need more blood?
AS: No they just need consent.
SA: Why?
AS: Because the test might find information that they might want to tell to other members of the family.
SA: But they said there would be a result in six weeks. I have had nothing. There has been no letter since, but we gave blood in the clinic.
AS: You are right that they said in the clinic that they would have a result from the blood test in six weeks. That test was a chromosome test, to find a reason for the miscarriage. They got a result, but not after six weeks – after eleven weeks, and they sent you a letter. The date on it is ...
SA: I have not had that letter. No letter has come at all.
AS: This letter, it also said that there is a research group ... that would take the blood that is stored ...
SA: Is this the test for my son?
AS: Yes, there is a research group in Birmingham, and they will take the stored blood, and in the future they will do a test to find the reason for your son's illness.

> SA: When will they do that?
> AS: They can't say, because it is a very rare illness, and usually people do research on common disorders. But they are asking you now for your permission so that as soon as there is someone who wants to do research on this illness they can give them the blood samples immediately. The consent form is very long, and you and your husband will have to read it and to sign it.
> SA: Yes, I want them to do that; yes, I give my permission.

A week after receiving the forms, Sofia and her husband remain undecided about the research. They wanted a healthy baby but were concerned about the implications that any results might have within the family. The clinicians also seemed reluctant to push for recruitment into genetic mutation research, partly because of the complexity of the consent required, which would have to be discussed via an interpreter, and also because of the uncertain outcome of enrolment in this particular project, which would not guarantee a result that could be used to test a future pregnancy or provide carrier tests for other family members. So it was left that the family should contact the clinic should they want to pursue the research. As this shows, 'finding the gene' can be a very lengthy process, taking months or years, and clinicians sometimes withhold research enrolment in the hope of a more specific research opportunity or that a clinical test will become available. In Sofia's case, when the couple returned to the clinic during their fourth pregnancy, it emerged that a clinical test was not available. The doctors also mentioned a new research possibility, involving a group in America working directly on the genetics of the kidney condition. But it was only after the clinical test proved negative (indicating, in this case, that the same condition can be caused by different mutations) and Sofia and her husband had lost a second newborn baby that this couple and their second dead baby were enrolled, via their DNA, in international mutation research.

For patients, this long-term engagement with diagnostic processes may increase familiarity with genetics but does not necessary dispel uncertainties about genetic research. Like Sofia and her husband, Khalida and her husband are enrolled in mutation research for the kidney problem, which, the clinicians hope, might permit early prenatal or, more speculatively, preimplantation genetic diagnosis (a technique enabling embryos fertilised in vitro to be checked for the presence of the genetic condition and implanted in the woman's uterus if they are free of the condition). As yet, it has not produced a result. Like Sofia, Khalida is ambivalent about it: 'The trouble is, once you have got into it, this high technology medicine, and into thinking about risk and the options, it is hard to get out of it. My husband says I should just put it out of my mind. I might go to Pakistan, at least for a rest.'

Bilaal: 'they can't find the faulty gene – that's the biggest problem'

Nighat Sadiq and Nasir Ahmed are second cousins whose second son, Bilaal, twelve years old when I first met him, has learning difficulties and a metabolic problem diagnosed in infancy. A month before his birth, the only indication of a problem was that prenatal staff considered him 'small for dates'. At birth, he weighed only four pounds and the clinicians noted that he had a very small head. At first his parents were not unduly worried. As Nighat said, she herself is slightly built and Nasir's sister had given birth to a baby weighing only one-and-a-half pounds who had 'caught up', but the medical staff:

> kept an eye on him, and the health visitor used to come more often ... like normally they might come like every other week or so and then stop coming, but for him they had to keep coming. From the start, we didn't know what the problem is. He was underweight, I mean he used to make up an ounce or so in a week, and then when he was 5 months old he stopped gaining weight altogether. The health visitors told us, you had better see the doctor in the hospital. After that, they had a lot of tests taken, blood tests and sweat tests and they did the biopsy test; Bilaal was in hospital [in London] for some weeks – and after that they were trying to see what sort of diet he was going to need. When they found out they told us he won't have ordinary milk, he has to have a special formula.

Bilaal has been on a special diet and vitamins ever since and has grown well and made progress at school despite his slight build and learning problems. Fortunately, when he was seven months old, a London-based consultant diagnosed, from biochemical tests, a specific disorder of protein metabolism that could be managed by a special diet. This diagnosis did not account for Bilaal's small head and developmental delay, but nonetheless Bilaal's parents are very grateful, because it indicated a therapy: 'We have to thank him [the consultant] that Bilaal's problems are not worse than they are.' The diagnosis also suggested a recessive single-gene disorder. 'We were told he has a damaged gene ... it is a gene to do with how the body uses protein,' Nasir told me at our first meeting. His wife added, 'For Bilaal's problem, they can't find the faulty gene – that's the biggest problem.'

Pinpointing the mutation has indeed proved elusive. When Bilaal was five years old, a research group had found a mutation causing the same metabolic problems in other children. Genetics doctors promptly arranged to test stored blood samples from Bilaal and his brother, thinking Bilaal would share the mutation and his brother would not. Surprisingly, the result was negative, for both boys. The doctor concluded that Bilaal's biochemical condition must be caused by something other than the gene that usually causes it. Seven years later, a different genetics doctor reviewing the case wondered if Bilaal's three different symptoms – learning difficulties, small head (microcephaly) and metabolic problems – might be linked as a syndrome caused by a different gene altogether. The family consented to stored blood samples being sent to a research group in London to investigate this possibility.

Later, at a routine genetics clinic review when Bilaal was approaching school leaving age, the doctors asked about the metabolic condition:

> Dr A: How is the treatment going?
> Nasir: Last time, they mentioned the genetics. They were going to see if any repair therapy for the faulty gene has been developed, because they were doing some research on the genes. We thought this appointment might have resulted from that conversation.
> Dr A: We sent your bloods [blood samples] to Professor S and he replied last week that so far he hasn't been able to find anything. He looked for the main gene and can't find the genetic change. Most people with this problem have that change ... this does not mean there isn't something, just that they couldn't find it. Now they are looking at a different gene. You wouldn't normally see learning difficulties, a small head and small ears with this metabolic problem.
> Nasir: Is it not connected?
> Dr A: Maybe it is, but it might be a rare form, perhaps caused by a change in a different gene. The balance of opinion is that this is typical for the metabolic problem but unusual in that he has not found the genetic change yet but they may find it at some stage.
> Dr B: We thought another genetic cause might connect all three problems – but it doesn't. None of these tests are 100 per cent, so there is always a catch.

Nevertheless, the doctors held out the hope of future research: 'Professor S has currently come to a standstill but we have the samples stored in the lab, if anyone has any bright ideas ... and we will see Bilaal again in clinical genetics in two years' time.' Reflecting on the appointment afterwards, Nighat understood that 'they had nearly found the faulty gene; that is why we came to the clinic last time. They said they were getting close, but don't raise your hopes too high.' In Bilaal's case, seventeen years have elapsed since his metabolic condition was first diagnosed, yet a firm genetic characterisation of Bilaal's particular problems remains elusive. Such cases are not closed but deferred to a point in the future when there will be new knowledge or when a doctor has a 'bright idea'. The possibility that, one day, a research group will find the relevant mutation means that such cases are not closed but held indefinitely within the clinical system (Latimer et al. 2006).

Why does 'finding the gene' matter?

Bilaal's metabolic and learning problems, Sohrab's obesity and learning difficulties and the kidney condition affecting Sofia's and Khalida's infants are all clinically considered certain recessives, but ones for which the relevant causative mutations are not yet identified. In Nighat's view, this is 'the biggest problem'. Both patients and doctors may set great store by the possibility of 'finding the gene', but this can motivate their engagements in diagnostic processes in rather different ways.

From a clinical genetics perspective, 'finding the gene' in principle extends clinical options for patients, via genetic prenatal and carrier testing. It is important, though, to note that diagnosing a genetic syndrome with a known inheritance pattern, even when the causative mutation has not been identified, usually enables doctors to offer patients information about the condition's likely progression (or 'natural history') on the basis of what is already known, to give recurrence risks for another pregnancy (e.g. one in 4 four or 25 per cent, with recessive conditions) and perhaps to offer some prenatal investigations. Certain features of some conditions are observable by ultrasound scan, and prenatal staff can be advised to look for these: polycystic kidney disease may be indicated by areas of greater or lesser density in the lung, for example, and the major limb abnormalities associated with Roberts syndrome may be visible (although small features, such as extra digits, may not). Some metabolic conditions can be diagnosed by biochemical tests on amniotic fluid, in the absence of a molecular test.

The limitation of a prenatal confirmation of a genetic condition by scans or amniocentesis is that it may be considered 'too late' for termination of pregnancy to be a realistic option; an early termination is often considered more acceptable (Chapters 5 and 6). An early prenatal mutation test (via CVS), if available, includes the possibility of an early termination. Clinicians sometimes suggest patients contact them before they start another pregnancy, to allow time for checking the latest research and clinical possibilities. After her first genetics clinic appointment, Khalida said:

> We were told that if we decided to have another child we should let them know if we were thinking of it, rather than turning up and saying you are pregnant, you should tell us. It was like asking their permission. My husband was very upset at losing two children in one year and we wanted another baby, so I phoned to say that we were thinking of having another baby … and she said, get in touch when you are pregnant! I did not understand why she said let us know if you are thinking of having another baby if all they say is get in touch when you are pregnant.

Clinicians expect women with known risks to register a pregnancy as soon as possible, to allow time for early prenatal scans and testing, and may feel frustrated when women do the opposite. Sofia did not attend the prenatal clinic until twenty-four weeks with her fourth pregnancy, missing a twenty-two week anomaly scan. 'Why did she come in so late?' a genetics nurse-counsellor exclaimed. As the couple said later, they were feeling positive about this pregnancy so saw no need for early surveillance. These acts of resistance, in the form of 'at risk' women's late registrations of pregnancy, seem to represent a desire to avoid or delay confronting the possibility of foetal abnormality.

Another clinical advantage of a molecular characterisation of a rare genetic disorder is that, rather than being restricted to describing theoretical risks for other family members, doctors can inform patients that a carrier test is available (raising issues concerning risk communication in the family, discussed in Chapter 7). These, then, are the clinical advantages of molecular research into rare disorders, which, as later chapters discuss, raise issues and suggest outcomes and actions about which clients may feel ambivalent or be resistant. But what motivates patient engagement in genetic mutation research?

Hopes for treatment and cure: 'We are willing to go to any lengths to make sure the baby is fine'

To an extent, the NHS referral system means that patient engagement in clinical genetics processes in unavoidable. Some patients initially have very little knowledge of what distinguishes 'genetics' from any other medical referral. A few couples in this study requested a genetics appointment to establish their carrier status because of a known risk in the family (Chapter 7) and occasionally a referral was motivated by the desire to prevent a particular pregnancy on genetic grounds (Chapter 5). Usually, though, patients were more concerned with seeking a treatment or a cure – concepts described in Urdu and Panjabi by a single term, *ilāj* – for a problem than with risk assessment and management. Time and time again, individuals and couples referred to genetics clinics would ask, 'Is there a treatment/cure for this? [*is kā koi ilāj hai?*]' Sofia's desire to participate in research was motivated more by her desperation for a healthy baby and her willingness to avail herself of techniques that might assist this aim, than by the desire to control the possibility of adverse birth outcome via testing or termination. For Khalida and her husband, carriers of two recessive conditions, the discovery of the mutation for one of them (a metabolic problem) resulted not in their requesting a prenatal genetic test but in their choosing to have the next baby checked at birth, via a biochemical test followed by a confirmatory molecular test (ultrasound scans had already ruled out the kidney condition in this pregnancy). The parents felt that even if this baby's life would be curtailed by the metabolic condition it was more important to preserve it than to risk harm by prenatal genetic testing (CVS or amniocentesis carrying small risks of miscarriage). To ensure that the parents' decision was fully 'informed',[2] doctors emphasised the seriousness of the rare metabolic condition:

there are only sixteen cases in the world, lifelong dietary treatment to reduce the effects has had dubious success and affected children are vulnerable to infection and heart problems and need regular specialist medical surveillance. Humaira and her husband felt sure it would be wrong to risk harming the baby via prenatal genetic tests and said that, in the absence of no-risk prenatal therapy to reduce the likelihood of the condition (such as modifying the mother's diet), they would do everything possible for an affected child after its birth. 'We are willing to go to any lengths to make sure the baby's fine,' Humaira told the clinicians.

Parents of children with known and unknown, genetic and other congenital problems often become involved in long-term, complex collaborations with clinicians, usually across more than one medical discipline, to manage and where possible ameliorate the conditions' worst effects. Having a diagnosis, in the form, for example, of a named condition, is useful in facilitating appropriate clinical management and learning support for the child as well as social support for carers, but a precise genetic or molecular diagnosis is not necessarily crucial to these processes. Nonetheless, as Carlos Novas notes for patient associations in the United States, parents of children with named genetic conditions may become active supporters of molecular genetic research in the hope that discovering the gene will enable more accurate therapies to be developed that will be specifically tailored to work on the metabolic, neurological or other pathway that the 'faulty gene' in effect disrupts (2006: 289). The parents in this study were not 'activists' in the ways Novas describes (for further discussion, see Chapter 8). Nonetheless, the hope that mutation research will one day lead to a cure for genetic conditions was a striking feature of some personal and family experiences.

At our first meeting, after telling me that Bilaal 'has a damaged gene … a gene to do with how the body uses protein', Nasir asked me, 'Have they any cure? Do you know if they can repair damaged genes?' The answer is no – at least, not in the body of an already grown child or adult – because the 'damaged gene' is contained within every cell of the body and replacing every cell's 'damaged gene' with an unaltered copy would be impossible. Research is exploring the possibilities of gene therapy at conception, combined with the use of preimplantation genetic diagnosis: a 'faulty' gene would be replaced by an unchanged copy before the embryo (formed from parental gametes) begins to develop into a baby, but this technical possibility would not help the quest to 'cure' Bilaal's problems.

Nighat and Nasir have a good grasp of what medical science currently offers for Bilaal's problems – namely, treatments via medication and dietary supplements, to counter the effects of the metabolic problem, but not a cure: 'Some things can be cured with medicines and all, [but] he has not got any disease like that, which he needs medicine to get rid of … He is only taking medicines like vitamin supplements and for energy and because he can't produce fat.' Nonetheless, they continue to pin their hopes on gene therapy. As Nighat put it:

> They can't find the faulty gene – that's the biggest problem. If they can find a faulty gene, then they can probably operate on him as well. They can get rid of this problem. I am really hoping for it. Every time when we go somewhere, people ask, 'When will he grow out of this? Will this problem be finished?' I say, 'I hope so.' It is very difficult to say, 'No', so I say, 'I hope so.' These days the technology can change overnight. That is why I told the paediatrician last time that there might be some new research, something might have come up. That is what I am hoping that some day ... It is possible with new research they will know, they will find something that might be able to cure him. That is all I want, that he can be cured.

This extract suggests that Nighat's hopes for gene therapy include the possibility of a surgical cure to remove the 'faulty gene'. She also mentioned another local Pakistani family with a metabolic condition for which the mutation has been identified and for which there is now a treatment, if not a cure:

> They have found a gene for obesity. I know someone who is being treated with American medicine ... The mother takes her daughter to Oxford for treatment. The condition runs in the family – her brother has a son like that too. The treatment is in the form of injections. The medicine is new, from America. I don't know how often she goes to America.

Talk of genetic research prompted one of Nighat's relatives in the United States to put Bilaal's case on the Internet to seek a research group that might be able to locate the gene and, perhaps, find a cure. 'We would pay whatever is necessary, if the funds could be found, if someone, somewhere, is interested in doing more tests on Bilaal to find out what the gene is,' Nighat told me.

Illness causality and faith

Gene discovery may thus be associated with the possibility of treatment and cure. Moreover, for some patients, the idea of a cure may entail the idea of 'removing' the gene from the body – for which the gene must first be identified. This concept of cure may take its form from other ideas patients have about what causes illness in general, and these ideas may in turn suggest treatment strategies that patients may pursue while also enrolling in genetic research, sometimes despite reassurance from clinicians that the condition in question was not caused by environmental factors.

Spiritual and other treatments and potential cures for genetic problems sometimes make more sense to the older generation in particular, as well as to some younger Pakistan-raised adults, than the investigative strategies and technologies of Western medicine and clinical genetics. Indeed, for many people in the general population in Western Europe and America, the concept of a 'genetic' disorder as something originating in an altered (and virtually immutable) instruction in the DNA in every cell of the body is very unfamiliar (see, for example, Lanie et al. 2004). To accept a genetic theory of causality can, in effect, require a leap of faith. For some of the participants in this study there was comfort in considering more familiar methods of illness management, such as consulting *hakīms* (practitioners of Unani medicine) or religious specialists. Almost all of my research participants had, or had considered, alternative explanations for genetic conditions, even as they engaged – sometimes fully and sometimes with scepticism of the consanguinity thesis (Chapter 1) – with the terminology and techniques of medical science. Their alternative explanations include environmental factors (accidents in pregnancy, infancy or early childhood, birth trauma, a childhood immunisation, a childhood or adult infection, a loss of blood at circumcision and a sense of heightened risk in the U.K. environment) as well as spiritual causes.

Sohrab's grandfather used the word gene synonymously with the Urdu/Panjabi word *jerasīm*, which means germ (and is also sometimes used for sperm or semen), implying that a gene is an infective agent. His grandmother thought Sohrab's problems originated with his losing blood at his circumcision and thought changing his environment by taking him to Pakistan would cure his obesity. Khalida's husband asked if a snake bite in childhood might have caused at least one of the two mutations he carries. Rukhsana, who knows she carries a recessive mutation and has a 25 per cent chance of having another affected child, asked if the genetics doctor would retest the parents' blood because 'the gene might no longer be there', since her husband had stopped using drugs. Sofia's in-laws blamed Sofia's miscarriages and infant deaths on her going out at night in pregnancy, which, they thought, had made her vulnerable to the effects of malicious spirits, and Sofia herself worried about these possible effects on the healthy baby she eventually gave birth to:

> My mother-in-law said there is no fear of ghosts there [in the hospital special care baby unit], because there is so much metal and so many machines. The baby's bed is his metal and has high sides; this protects him. In the years I have been in this country, I have not heard of ghosts harming a baby. In Pakistan, ghosts lurk behind bushes and you do not leave a baby alone in the first few weeks.

Nadia had heard from an elderly neighbour and from female relatives in Pakistan that her baby's limb abnormality, involving foreshortened arms folded inwards, results from a pregnant woman sleeping with her arms curled up during an eclipse of the moon or sun (*chānd garīn, yā sūraj garīn*). Nadia checked her dates, noted there had been no eclipse during her pregnancy and was advised by another neighbour to think no more of it. Birth defects such as cleft lip may be attributed to pregnant women holding sharp objects, such as knives, in their hands during an eclipse – the object's image is then imprinted on the baby. Zobeen's mother did not tell her relatives in Pakistan about Zobeen's curved spine and cleft lip: 'They would be on at me, you did this, you did that; I wanted to avoid it.'

Such theories may imply alternative treatments or cures that may be seriously considered, especially if Western medical treatment is ineffective or unavailable (or if its cost is prohibitive, as it may be in Pakistan). Beliefs in the curative power of *pīrs* (religious specialists) can offer the hope of a cure for conditions such as deafness, lack of speech or other forms of developmental delay (Shaw 2000a: 204–12). Besides believing that the change of environment would cure Sohrab's obesity, Sohrab's grandmother believed that taking Sohrab to a *pīr* in Pakistan would help him start to talk – she had already obtained an amulet (*tāvīs*) for him containing words of the Qur'an from a *pīr* in Pakistan – but her son, Sohrab's father, wanted to keep the boy in the U.K. until medical investigations were complete.

Other parents contemplate such treatments as homoeopathy. Sabrina's husband, a lawyer, and her in-laws, who are from Lahore in Pakistan, were pursuing homoeopathic treatment with help from relatives settled in Germany, for Sabrina's child's probably genetic condition. Nighat, educated in the United States, was cautious about the use of alternative therapies such as those prescribed by *hakīms* (practitioners of Unani medicine) in Pakistan, but, she added, there is 'only one I might try'. On a visit to Pakistan, a family friend with no prior knowledge of Bilaal's problems but renowned for his intuitive diagnostic ability had observed that Bilaal has a 'bad digestive system' and recommended that he take ground almonds and black pepper in the early morning for several days. Nighat had not tried this yet, wanting first to seek the U.K. dietitian's advice, since he had advised against oily foods and, as Nighat said, 'Almonds have oil.'

Nighat accepted the medical genetic account of her son's condition and told me that her relatives in Pakistan had not suggested any alternative theories:

> [Just] like me and you and the doctor [here], they don't know why it has happened, what caused this problem. We tell them whatever we know – what they know is what we tell them – they don't have their own views, because it is all medical, you see. And in a way, you can pray to God, that one day he will be better.
>
> AS: And your parents?
>
> NS: No, I think they understand all the genetic problems, because we explain to them, that he has not got any disease like that which he needs medicines to get rid of ... They never ask ... why is that, what is the reason. I mean, we have not got the answer, and they understand that as well. They still ask us, 'Will he every get rid of this problem?' That is the only thing which everybody asks. Apart from that, I think they accept it. This is it. I mean, there is nothing they can do.

However, she acknowledged that, if she felt medical science offered no hope, or if she did not understand what the doctors were trying to do, then:

> I might, you know, you might try some religious ritual. There is an *aiyat* (a verse) you can read … but … it never came into our mind, because we know it is a medical condition. We are happy with the treatment we get here. We know that people are doing all they can. But I do wish he would get cured. I do pray for that. I think that maybe if I was in Pakistan, I would not have the same feeling or the same views … If I was in Pakistan, I don't think we would have ever been able to find out what the problem is, to be honest.

She therefore recognises the power of prayer, that 'you can pray to God, that one day he will be better', and of reading particular Qur'anic verses. A belief shared by most of my research participants is that ultimately these matters are in the hands of God. However, I was told about one father who abandoned his faith following the birth of a child with a serious metabolic condition, because 'he was no longer able to believe in a God who could do this to him'. Nonetheless, for many Pakistani Muslim parents, the emotions associated with having a child with serious disabilities – the shock, fear, pain, sadness, anger, guilt, blame, shame and sustained grief for the child that might have been – may coexist with, and sometimes be tempered by, the belief that the quality of a person's life and the timing of their death are processes under God's control and for which God has a purpose. In this context, prayer is perfectly compatible with making use of Western medicine and, for some, may also open the door to as yet unknown treatments and cures.

Akhtar's brothers: 'The faulty gene will repair by itself, through massage and the warmth of the jacuzzi'

Akhtar is married with five children and came to England from rural Azad Kashmir as a small boy. He has five now-adult brothers who have a known recessive neurological condition that affects their physical coordination and balance, the signs of which appeared in their late teens and early adulthood. I first met them when I accompanied a clinical geneticist who wished to inform them about the progress of mutation research:

> There is good news. We think we have identified the chromosome the mutation is on. It is on chromosome 9, near the end of chromosome 9. But it is one of, say, 200 genes. If we can get some more blood samples from people with the disorder, we may be able to find the gene more quickly – it just takes time.

She went on to discuss whether they knew of other affected relatives or families from which she could obtain blood samples for research.

The family were clearly pinning their hopes on genetic research as a route to a cure. 'I always thought in the future it would get better, not that it would get worse,' one of the brothers told me. He had learned the Qur'an by heart as a teenager, but now, if he goes outside, the police think he is a drunkard, his gait is so wobbly. 'I would like to have my time again. If I had known, I would have done things differently.' On the other hand, another brother said, 'Our mother says its all right, this disability, because we are at home, not outside, not getting into trouble, doing drugs, doing bad things.' Their father, clearly associating me with the mutation research, chipped in, 'If you and [the doctor] can cure these boys, I will have a big party and I will buy you a car.' Referring to his brothers, Akhtar said, 'All they are interested in is a cure.' The clinician stressed that possibilities for a cure are remote, even if finding the gene might illuminate the neurological pathway involved.

Several years later, Akbar talked about how he understands the cause of his brothers' condition and the purpose of the mutation research, which would, in principle, provide a carrier test and diagnostic or predictive tests:

> In Pakistan, there would not even be any research. There you have to pay 200 rupees for a test, to be told there is no cure – what's the point of that? Here, this genetic research for my brothers, it has been going on for years. It did not begin with Dr X. There was a Dr Y … he was quite young then … I thought he only wanted the blood, and I think when he could not find anything he went on to something else. Dr X, she said she will not give up. She said she might want to take more blood, to send to New Zealand … A few years ago, she wrote saying that the gene is on chromosome 9, and later she said she will be sending the blood samples to France. My hope for the research is to get the balance controlled, that would be enough. I thought that with the technology being advanced with genetics nowadays there would be a cure.

He acknowledged that genetic research might not lead to a cure, but thought that knowing where the faulty gene is could lead to treatments by other means:

> Last year, I took him [one of his brothers] to a *hakīm* [in Pakistan] and he found this gene in his spine. He uses a drill to numb the spine and puts the medication in. After an hour, the medication brings something out of the spine. But the *hakīm* said there is a risk it goes wrong, and I am not going to do it.
>
> AS: How do you know the gene is on the spine?
>
> Akhtar: Dr X said it's on the ninth or the tenth line. There are three genes and the middle one is missing from the twelfth line.

He dismissed this potential treatment, involving the removal of the gene from the spine (apparently equating vertebra number nine with chromosome number nine), as too dangerous. Nevertheless, he continued to be hopeful of the possibilities for gene repair:

> All'ah says there is a cure for every disease, whether the doctor finds it or whether the spiritualist guide finds it. So you must try all routes. We have found one, but it only works for a month. It involves the new spiritualist, warm water and jacuzzi. Someone massages them on the spine, and the spiritualist guide locates the point on the spine. We are massaging from the toes to the spine, along the neck line. That faulty gene will repair by itself, through the massage and the warmth of the jacuzzi.

The 'new spiritualist' to whom he refers has reputedly cured psychiatric and medical conditions 'through the spirituality of All'ah'. One of Akhtar's brothers has recently benefited considerably from prayer (*namāz*), having consulted a *pīr* in Pakistan: 'The *pīr* said reading *namāz* was exercising, and, by doing it, [my brother] might be able to cure himself from within. It might send signals that the gene might disappear. We believe in the *pīr*s and in spirituality.'

Conclusion

This chapter has detailed some extents and limitations of patients' and doctors' commitments to finding genetic solutions to reproductive and health problems. Genetic categorisation could not proceed without patients' participation, from the initial taking of a family history and observation of the proband (affected infant, child or adult) and the enrolment of patients, via their blood samples, in genetic mutation research to discussing the implications of test results. As Margaret Lock writes, 'Without the desire of "consumers" to cooperate, reproductive technologies and genetic testing would remain confined to the research laboratory' (1998: 206).

Aspiring parents, parents of children with medical problems and adults with genetic conditions who provide DNA samples for genetic diagnosis and research (or consent to some aspects of these processes but not others) are neither simply passive conduits through which the power of the medical establishment is exerted nor necessarily fully committed to a genetic theory of illness (or, as discussed in the following chapters, to prenatal genetic diagnosis, ending an affected pregnancy or carrier testing). Identifying the mutation underlying a particular condition may motivate their pursuit of genetic counselling or may become a motivation over time, but patients' reasons for attending genetics consultations vary and a desire for a 'normal' pregnancy and birth or for a treatment or cure for an existing problem may be more important than avoiding the birth of an affected child. Patients' participation in clinical diagnostic processes involves varying degrees of compliance, may include selective resistance and may change over time. For families, clinical diagnostic uncertainty is often mediated by the hope of future research, gene discovery, therapy and cure, but the fact that therapeutic possibilities are currently limited also constitutes grounds for scepticism and ambivalence about the value of genetic research and may, in effect, support patients' alternative theories of causality and use of alternative treatments. All of the families enrolled via their DNA samples in genetic research had considered and sometimes actively pursued other explanations and treatments, although individuals differed in their views of the reliability of genetic science versus other systems of knowledge. Client participation in genetic diagnostic processes is thus neither passive nor necessarily indicative of fully embracing the values of the modern management of genetic risk but represents a form of 'ambivalence coupled with pragmatism' that often represents women's responses to medicalisation (Lock and Kaufert 1998: 2).

Even within clinical genetics, processes of geneticisation (as identifying underlying genetic causes for problems with reproduction and health) may be incomplete and uncertain, especially regarding rare recessive conditions diagnosable as such from their presenting features but for which molecular testing is currently unavailable. Clinical geneticists may utilise possibilities for genetic research to advance a clinical diagnosis but mediate this use by considering the clinical value of research and the need for patients' informed consent. U.K. health policy defines patient participation in clinical processes as based upon the individual's right to utilise services and to exercise an 'undirected' choice through informed consent. This definition of doctors and patients as co-participants might be viewed as a form of biological citizenship that is changing citizens' understandings of illness causality, risk and responsibility to others (Rose and Novas 2005). However, these processes may operate for doctors and patients in different ways and be incomplete.

As regards informed consent in clinical genetics, doctors are required to provide information and discuss options so that patients' consent is informed, but how much information or understanding is necessary for a client's choice to be informed, particularly in relation to mutation research with uncertain outcomes? Can or should clinicians ensure that their clients fully understand clinical information, particularly where their initial understanding of genetics may be limited and their communication with medical personnel may have to be mediated by interpreters or other family members? Despite the principle of non-directiveness, providing genetic information to enable choice requires patients to consider a theory of illness they may not have previously encountered, and consider possibilities they would not have contemplated (such as prenatal genetic testing, termination of pregnancy and carrier testing in the family) had a foetal abnormality not been detected, a genetic diagnosis not been made or a causative mutation not been identified. The next three chapters explore patients' negotiation of these issues, first considering couples' responses to receiving information about reproductive risks in future pregnancies.

Notes

1. This kinship with affected individuals in other families, which Paul Rabinow (1992) calls biosociality, usually provides the basis for the formation of patient support groups. There is also a support group called Unique for people with very rare or 'orphan' conditions.
2. The principles of informed consent and non-directiveness in genetic counselling represent attempts to distinguish contemporary clinical genetics from its origins in late nineteenth- and early twentieth-century eugenics and policies of racial purity (Kessler 1979, Kevles 1985; see also Clarke 1994). In the U.K., these principles sometimes sit uneasily alongside clinical and government demands for cost-effective services and concerns to reduce the socio-economic burden of genetic conditions. In a free-market economy such as the U.S.A, choice is not necessarily freer but may be biased in favour of the wealthy or motivated by a sense of a right to have a normal child, while commercial interests may drive the use of prenatal technology (Ratcliff 1989; Wertz and Fletcher 1989; Keller 1992).

CHAPTER 5
RESPONDING TO REPRODUCTIVE RISK

Providing information about reproductive risk is one aspect of the diagnostic work performed in clinical genetics. Couples attending genetics clinics because their baby or child has a problem presumed to be genetic, or because of a family history of a genetic condition, usually receive an assessment of the chances that any future children they have will also have the condition, an assessment that will vary according to the inheritance pattern of the condition and the level of certainty attached to the clinical diagnosis. Doctors giving reproductive risk assessments usually also discuss with patients the implications for the management of another pregnancy and, if prenatal genetic testing is available, will inform couples about the comparative risks of the available procedures. In this way, patients receiving reproductive risk information are also invited to consider routes into more complex risk management. Clinical geneticists will strive to give numerical risks that are as accurate as possible, and for this, making as accurate a diagnosis as possible is therefore crucial. Where diagnosis is uncertain, clinicians may 'hedge their bets', for instance by offering a risk 'in the region of between 25 per cent and 50 per cent' for a condition that is possibly recessive, but also possibly dominant.

The clinical assumption is that reproductive risk information will inform patients' decisions about whether or not and how – that is, using which tests or techniques – to proceed with a new pregnancy. Thus, risk assessments are more than statements about the probability of a future event occurring, for they imply that the identified risk must be avoided, or at least managed. A new pregnancy, from this perspective, requires conscious decision-making. Making such a decision, in the light of clinically identified risk, thus becomes 'a burden of being at risk and not just a dependent variable' (Lippman-Hand and Fraser 1979: 333). The expectation of such decision-making and the processes involved reflect the preoccupation with risk identification and management characteristic of modern society and the value accorded to individual choice (Giddens 1991; Beck 1992). At an individual level, it may have positive psychological effects, as a means by which individuals gain control over uncertainty (Miller 1983), or negative effects, by increasing anxiety and guilt (Marteau 1991; Lippman 1992).

Much of the psychological and genetic counselling literature is concerned with what individuals and couples decide and do in the light of given risks. Do 'at risk' couples go on to have further pregnancies? How do probabilistic risk assessments affect their decisions and actions? Are those given 'high' risks (such as 50 per cent) less likely to have more children than those with 'lower' risks (such as 25 per cent)? Do those who embark on further pregnancies use prenatal genetic testing, if it is available, and termination of affected pregnancies to manage the risk of adverse birth outcomes? This literature shows that the relationship between numerical risks, attitudes and intentions, and reproductive decisions and outcomes is complex and varies for different social groups, and even within couples. The decisions people make also diverge for different genetic disorders and reflect changes over time in therapeutic possibilities and the availability of DNA testing (Shihol 1996: 84). Further, while a numerical risk of having another affected child is rarely entirely irrelevant within couples' reproductive decision-making, it is a poor guide to what couples eventually decide or do. Indeed, from the parents' perspectives, such a risk is better understood as a statement about a negative or uncertain future reproductive outcome, since, whatever its value, the numerical risk can also be seen as reducing to a simply binary opposition: either the child will have the condition, or it will not (see also Lippman-Hand and Fraser 1979).

My interest in this chapter is to explore British Pakistani Muslim parents' responses to this inherent uncertainty, clinically expressed as a probability of their chances of having an affected child, and, where relevant, to the offer of risk management in a subsequent pregnancy, for different kinds of genetic condition. Couples' responses to clinical risk information reflect, I suggest, the relative trust they accord scientific versus other sources of knowledge, their attitudes to prenatal diagnosis and termination of pregnancy, and the views of their close kin on these issues. Their responses are also influenced by the nature of their marital relationship, their prior reproductive history, including whether or not they already have any unaffected children, and their attitudes to and experiences of the disorder for which the pregnancy is at risk, including whether it is likely to lead to stillbirth or early infant death, or whether, if the child is likely to survive, it will have physical (*jismānī*, i.e. bodily) rather than intellectual (*damāghī*) problems, or both. In other words, couples' responses to reproductive risk information are, like risk perception generally, structurally and culturally shaped (Douglas and Wildavsky 1982; Douglas 1992). Despite the apparent authority of scientifically derived risk information, social circumstances and moral considerations determine if a given risk is considered 'too high' to take or a risk worth taking.

Broadly, my observations reveal a diversity of attitudes to prenatal diagnosis and termination of pregnancy even within one ethnic and religious group. This finding challenges the clinical stereotype that, for Muslims, termination of pregnancy is always unacceptable (Modell et al. 2000). However, by reporting not on hypothetical scenarios (for instance, on what women say they would decide if they found themselves pregnant with a child affected by a genetic condition of a particular type) but by observing actual clinical consultations and listening to parents' reported experiences of real situations, my observations also identify issues that may be more specific to British Pakistani Muslim experience, because they reveal some of the ways in which assumptions about consanguineous marriages and assumptions about Muslim attitudes to such issues as termination of pregnancy can complicate the presentation and negotiation of reproductive risk.

Gifts from God

Husnain, the U.K.-raised lawyer whose infant daughter's birth abnormalities had no firm diagnosis (Chapter 4) and who was sceptical of 'this cousin marriages and birth defects argument' (Chapter 1), considered her problems a 'test from God', no matter how serious the problems or what the results of clinical investigations might show: 'It is down to religion. It was meant to happen. Even if it was very serious, even if she died, or if she lived but was seriously disabled for the rest of her life, it would not change anything. It is a test from God, a test for us as parents.'

The view that there is a divine purpose behind the births of children with disabilities was shared by several other parents of young children with birth abnormalities, as well as by parents of older children with serious life long disabilities, including behavioural problems. Zahida, who came to England twenty years ago following her marriage, has a sixteen-year-old son, Mukhtar, with no obvious physical disabilities but unsocial, physically aggressive behaviour. He attends a special school, but is sometimes expelled for a week or two at a time for bad behaviour and language; when I met him, he was at home on 'race report' for his racist remarks. To minimise disruption to the rest of the family, at home he has a special room, with a television and play station, but remains difficult to manage, being insensitive to other people's emotions and inclined to hit and punch his close relatives or anyone who comes to visit. Zahida told me: 'When he gets angry, he calls me "Fucking Paki, go back to your country."' Nonetheless, Zahida sees the task of managing him as a God-given test, for which she will be rewarded in the next life. Rather than considering having Mukhtar a hardship (*musībat*), she told me that, 'My God has been very kind to me' and 'shown a lot of mercy', because:

> My God says that people like Mukhtar are higher than angels. Each child that is handicapped is a special gift from God for a special person, a person that God has chosen. God chooses special people for these special gifts. God is very kind. You understand *amānat* (safe keeping). A child or person like Mukhtar is '*Khudā kī amānat*'; God has given him to you for a special time.
>
> AS: Not as a punishment?
>
> No. You know that when you go somewhere, say to another country, you have to answer questions, someone interviews you, checks your papers, your record, your history, to check you are not a terrorist. If someone is allowed through without any checking, what would you think?

AS: That they have some special status.

Yes. It's like that with those who will go into heaven without an interview. Children and people like Mukhtar are those who will go into heaven without an interview. He says, when he gets there he will hit God. But he has no sense. It is the same for all people like that, whatever their religion. They are more respected. Have you heard of the poet Ilama Iqbal?

AS: Yes, why?

There's a *ghazal* (poem):
Tund bād-e-mukhālif se nā ghabrāe uqāb,
Yyh to chaltī hai tujhe ūnchā urāne ke liye
[Eagle, don't be afraid of the violent whirlwind
It is blowing to take you higher]

He is saying, "When it is very windy, the wind will take the birds higher." This means, don't be afraid of difficulties, they will take you higher; all these problems will take you up higher, closer to God.

God made hell and heaven. But, for us, there is a way to heaven. The first important thing is *namāz*. When Mukhtar is very naughty I can't do *namāz*. But Mukhtar needs me. Mukhtar is my responsibility, and this responsibility of him is my test for the next life. And God wants me to pass. I will pass.

Religion, science and authoritative knowledge

Not all Pakistanis would take the view that a disabled child represents a responsibility that is a test from God. Saleem Ullah, father of an eighteen-year-old with learning difficulties, told me that 'Some people say, the parents have been sinful, and that is why their child is suffering.' Like many other parents in my sample, Saleem himself did not take this view. However, parents were generally sensitive to the stigma of having an affected child, particularly when the child was young, sometimes keeping knowledge of the problems concealed even from close relatives (Chapter 7). I also found that some women viewed the births of children with disabilities as punishment for the sin of terminating or preventing a pregnancy (Chapter 6) (see also Miles 1992; Ingstadt and Reynolds-Whyte 1995; Jenkins 1998).

Having thought his son's problems were probably caused by an immunisation, Saleem Ullah had not pursued a possible genetic explanation until now:

It might give my mind a bit of rest to know. It might be easier to live with, rather than wondering about the injection. But a genetic explanation would not change anything. I have not seen any artificial limb that will be better than a limb God has made. Maybe it is the will of All'ah that his brain is

> like that. No one can change it except God. You can try to find out why, but God knows best. Maybe God has done this to make me more responsible.
>
> AS: How do you mean?
>
> He has decided to give you that responsibility. Maybe it is my sins when I was young. I am only here to guide my son along. God can look after him better than I can.
>
> AS: Do you think it could be a punishment?
>
> How could it be a punishment for me? If it is a punishment, it would be a punishment on my son, not on me. He is the one who is suffering. But some people say, parents have been sinful and that is why their child is suffering.

Zahida gave me the example of a successful computer consultant, originally from Lahore, who had a child with problems similar to but more severe than Mukhtar's and was apparently so angry about having such a child that he left his religion:

> He thought that God must be punishing him, and said he could not believe in a God that would do this to him. People said to him, "God has been good to you, made you clever, given you a good job, plenty of money." He disagreed, he said, "God did not give this to me, I built up my brain myself."

Zahida's view of Mukhtar as a 'gift from God' may be one that she has reached over time, as a part of becoming reconciled to being the mother of a child with very demanding, long-term needs. It also reflects the importance of her religious faith in her life now: 'As you get older you think more and more about God, you become more aware that this life is short and will pass, that you could die at any moment, and that you will then be near God.'

Another mother of a teenager with learning difficulties talked of how she had changed in her perception of her son's problems. She described to me the shock and subsequent depression she experienced when she first learnt that her new baby had Down syndrome (the current clinical term for a condition more commonly understood as 'Down's syndrome'), so named after the Victorian doctor John Langdon Haydon Down who described it in 1866. Dr Down compared the characteristic features of this condition with those of 'Orientals' and named the condition 'Mongolism' or 'Mongolian idiocy', reasoning in accordance with Victorian evolutionary thinking that the features of 'idiots' will resemble those of the 'lower' ('less developed') races, the former being people with arrested development (Gould 1980). For Riffat, Down syndrome did not have these connotations; I am told that in Pakistan, unlike in Europe and America, there is no tradition of viewing Down syndrome (or other children with learning disabilities) with the stigma of an 'inferior' racial identity, such as 'Mongoloid' (see Rapp

2000: 292). Learning difficulties do not necessarily have the same associations in Pakistan that they have in the West (Miles 1992). Even so, she felt at first ashamed and afraid to show her baby to others, fearing their negative reactions, and her son's diagnosis plunged her into post-natal depression. In fact, it was the reactions of some of her Punjab-born neighbours that helped transform her perceptions. Riffat's neighbours would come to her home specifically to see her son, to touch or feel him, or borrow an item of his clothing, occasionally giving money or gifts in return or even asking to take him for the afternoon, believing that this would bring them good fortune. They described him as *sāya*, which literally means 'shadow' or 'shade', and refers to spiritual qualities or supernatural powers. At first, Riffat was embarrassed by this interest, but she now says, 'I can't imagine how I would live without him.' She also used to worry that her son did not understand about the importance, for a Muslim, of washing (doing *wuzū*, a ritual ablution, to establish purity) before praying or reading words of the Qur'an. However, her *imām* (religious leader) advised her that if her son feels like reciting the *qalmā* (Islamic confession of faith) while sitting on the toilet, so be it – she should not worry, because 'Your son is *sāya*; he has a special relationship with All'ah' (Shaw 2000b: 102).

A view of clinical or scientific information as not necessarily more authoritative than knowledge derived from religious sources, and that, ultimately, 'only God knows', represents a general issue that runs, in different ways, through many family negotiations of reproductive risk assessments, as the following conflict over the authority of clinical knowledge illustrates. Kaneez, a twenty-one-year-old British-raised marketing trainee, terminated her first pregnancy because prenatal scans, supported by a prenatal genetic test (via amniocentesis), indicated that this pregnancy was 'incompatible with life'. She was also given a standard recessive recurrence risk. Kaneez understood that this represented a 75 per cent chance of having an unaffected child, so she remained hopeful of having a healthy baby, but did not want to become pregnant again 'just yet'. She was glad to return to work after four weeks, to keep her mind busy. In contrast, her Pakistan-raised husband wanted another baby as soon as possible, 'to fill the gap', and had never been convinced that the doctors were right about the diagnosis and thus about the wisdom of terminating the first pregnancy. He had been persuaded by his wife, her sister and her parents that the termination should go ahead because the child would certainly die – 'It is not as if he is a handicapped baby. If God gives you a handicapped baby, you would still love them, and look after them. But this baby was going to die', Kaneez's sister told me – but he remained sceptical. Kaneez's sister had found it difficult to explain to him the diagnosis and its implications: 'He is like our parents' generation in his thinking. He came from Pakistan for marriage. He did not go to school here. He thought the doctors had made a mistake. He thought, God knows, they don't know anything. How can they say?'

There is some general truth in this observation about the views of the older generation and of spouses raised in Pakistan. Clinicians confirmed three-year-old

Sohrab Hussain's problems to be the result of a recessive metabolic condition (see Chapter 4), for which his parents were given a one in four recurrence risk. This risk information was repeated by a genetic counsellor, working with an interpreter, during a home visit at which Sohrab's grandparents were also present. Nevertheless, Sohrab's grandfather remained sceptical that Sohrab's problems were genetic, or 'in the family' for, as he put it, 'we have never seen this thing before' (see Chapter 1). He remembered the initial uncertainty over the diagnosis, that the blood (chromosome) test was 'negative' and the doctors had said there 'isn't a blood test yet' for this particular condition: 'They don't know; it's just a guest [*sic*], innit. Only God knows.' Instead, he speculated that the condition might have been caused by a circumcision operation at which Sohrab lost much blood. That a risk assessment is probabilistic (e.g. a chance of one in four) in itself conveys uncertainty rather than authority; against this, parents often refer to the ultimate authority of God. In part, this reflects the patchiness of many people's knowledge of Mendelian genetics and mechanisms of inheritance, regardless of their ethnic background or level of education.

On the other hand, some of those with experience of a genetic condition in the family have become lay experts in particular conditions, having consulted specialists and read printed information, hospital letters and information available on the Internet. Hamid Ullah, a thirty-three-year-old computer programmer, born and raised in High Wycombe, has grown up with a younger brother with learning difficulties and obesity. For Hamid, genetic science provided a convincing explanation for how a condition not previously seen in the family had originated. Hamid understands that his brother's problems were caused by a chromosomal arrangement in an unbalanced form, which he carries in balanced form and which probably originated with his father:

> Most nurses and social workers think this is to do with consanguinity. It is not. My parents are not related. They are from different castes and from different areas of Pakistan. [Whether Pakistani *birādarī*s (kinship groups) are like castes is a matter of academic and lay dispute: see Shaw 2000a.] Their marriage was arranged by someone who knew my father and someone who knew my mother. My father was getting very Westernised; he'd been over here a long time. Someone who knew my father and who knew my mother's family got the two families in touch with each other. My father's friend, and his family, they thought it was time my father got married, so he did not forget his culture.
>
> There was no illness [this condition] in our family before. My father's father married twice and all this children were OK except my father, who had the translocation, but he was OK, it didn't affect him, and he did not [even] know [he had the translocation] because he had all the genetic information [chromosomes] he needed [and so his own health was

> unaffected]. It was only with my brother that we saw this thing for the first time; he is unique in our family. It is because there is a bit missing from one chromosome, chromosome 15, I think, that is to do with his hunger. And on chromosome 22 there is something that means he can't say 'no'. Like a few years ago, he just went with someone, down the street. Luckily it was OK, the person just brought him back. But he has no moral sense, just instincts.
> I've known about my brother's illnesses for a long time. About ten years ago, I went to a conference in Northampton [in the Midlands, England] on my brother's illness. It is rare: there are about 200 cases in the world, and most of them are in America, not in this country, and most of the people at the conference were Americans. Some doctor had said that the affected children don't live that long, but at that conference I saw that there were people like my brother who looked mature, like they were forty years old. At first, they did not know what ... was wrong with my brother, not for the first nine years. The name was only given at a late stage. The food thing alerted them. And he was mentally slow compared with his physical development. Then they came out with the name of the condition, a letter came one day, but before that there was no name. That was before my father passed away, so he had been told, but I don't know how much he understood. He was illiterate.

On the face of it, at least, there is a striking difference in levels of genetic knowledge between people such as Hamid, on the one hand, and Sohrab's grandfather and Kaneez's husband, on the other. This might suggest a categorisation of responses to clinical risk as 'more' or 'less' religious or scientific, which might correlate, broadly, with place of birth, or, perhaps more accurately, with whether the person attended school in Pakistan or in Britain. On closer examination, though, several additional factors are likely to have facilitated Hamid's acceptance of a genetic explanation for his brother's condition. The condition is not recessive and so does not imply that the family's marriage pattern is to blame, a point to which I return later in this chapter. Hamid has also had much more direct experience of the genetic condition in question, and more opportunities to access genetic explanations, than had either Sohrab's parents or his grandfather. Sohrab was only three years old when his learning difficulties, behavioural problems and obesity were diagnosed as part of a genetic syndrome, whereas Hamid has had over eighteen years' experience of living with his brother. For Kaneez's husband, asked to accept doctors' interpretations of results obtained by ultrasound and amniocentesis, the medical opinion seemed remote – hypothetical rather than real – for he had no previous experience or knowledge of this fatal condition. Many women use ultrasound, considering 'it does not harm the baby', but do not necessarily view its results as definitive; as Hamid's wife put it, in the context of discussion about ending a pregnancy following prenatal diagnosis, 'Sometimes they get it wrong; only God knows everything' (see Chapter 6). Parents who have had experience of an affected child are more attuned to the thinking and procedures of prenatal risk management; otherwise these can seem very alien. Moreover, acceptance of a genetic explanation is compatible with the belief that the birth of a child with a disability has a divine purpose, as Zahida's acceptance of a genetic explanation for Mukhtar's problems illustrates:

> God says this is why I haven't made everyone the same. You know, we are all different, in colour, in age, some thick, some clever. This is so that we can recognise each other and know where we are from. Science says it is from genetics. We went to the genetics clinic. They made a family tree, and they showed how it could have come down in the family because my husband's grandfather (father's father) and my mother's grandfather (father's father) were first cousins. I don't doubt that. I think this is true. But God has a purpose for everything. God has given man sense, and once you know about something you should think and apply your knowledge.

Explanations that invoke infections, accidents or morally reprehensible actions may entail mechanisms that conflict with or conform to genetic theories (see Chapter 7), but, irrespective of this, they may be compatible with the view of many study participants, regardless of whether they were born and schooled in Britain or Pakistan, that ultimately God decides whether someone lives or not, or is healthy or not. Khalida, a British-raised carrier of two recessive mutations – one associated with a fatal condition, the other potentially fatal – asked me rhetorically, 'Does not God decide when to take us away?' Nadia, a British-raised mother of a child affected by a recessive syndrome involving major limb abnormalities, knows she is a carrier of the mutation, and yet she surprised me one day by commenting, 'We still don't know why this happened.' I pointed out that the mechanism of recessive inheritance had been explained, in English and in Urdu, on several occasions in hospital clinics and discussed with me at home: 'Yes, that tells you how, but I still do not understand why this happened.' Genetic explanations, like theories that invoke germs or other environmental causes, provide a mechanism, but probabilistic concepts of chance leave a void that appeals to God's will serve to fill. That genetic mechanisms can be invoked at the same time as people attribute genetic disorders to forces beyond human understanding is, of course, not unique to British Pakistani Muslims. Katie Featherstone and colleagues report that Anglo Britishers affected by genetic disorders often attribute this to fate or destiny, as if in a kind of biological predestination (2006: 69–70, 113).

Sociological theory proposes a fundamental difference between what might be called a pre-modern and a modern view of risk, the former appealing to an external authority, such as God or fate, the latter involving the private negotiations of individuals in relation to expert risk assessments made within institutional structures for risk management (Giddens 1991). This formulation tends to stereotype responses to risk into one of two categories, but in reality people often draw on more than one model simultaneously. Such a typology, moreover, offers little insight into the factors that influence whether or not people will accept the invitation to 'manage' reproductive risk. Kaneez's brother-in-law's view that the doctors had 'made a mistake' did not determine the outcome of his wife's pregnancy; it was one of many considerations in the final decision to terminate (despite the stereotype associated with a patriarchal pattern of family authority that the husband's point of view prevails). Equally, as we shall see, Hamid Ullah's articulation of a genetic explanation for his brother's problems does not necessarily entail acceptance of genetic prenatal diagnosis; as he told me, 'knowing the science does not always help you decide what to do'. Zahida believes that 'God has a purpose for everything', but she also believes that 'God has given man sense, and once you know about something you should think and apply your knowledge.'

In my informants' views, scientific knowledge is distinguished from moral choices and action. There is, thus, an inbuilt resistance to the message to 'reduce' or 'manage' the risk of adverse birth outcome contained within the structures for managing birth and infant health in contemporary modern society, despite the emphasis on informed choice and individual responsibility. Moral choices and actions, moreover, are made in relation to a number of factors – social, medical and emotional as well as ethical or religious considerations, as I detail in the following sections. While clinicians may tend to gloss Pakistani Muslim clients' decisions as 'stemming from religion', particularly if the decisions entail resistance to risk management, there are many non-religious reasons why a couple might 'take the risk'. Likewise, the view that a child is a gift from God and a test of one's faith does not necessarily preclude consent to 'risk management' during another pregnancy.

Preventing birth anomalies: social, medical and emotional considerations

A desire to avoid the birth, or another birth, of an affected child is sometimes uppermost in couples' responses to risk information. Parents may make a firm decision to prevent another pregnancy or to use prenatal diagnosis in the next pregnancy. Certain features of their risk and reproductive history make this decision more likely: if the diagnosis and risk assessment are for a serious condition involving medical problems and learning difficulties, if they already have a living child with serious problems and special needs and if they have other, unaffected children too and think they would be unable to cope with another affected child. In such circumstances, the scenario of having another affected child is imagined 'with a degree of certainty as unmanageable' (Lippman-Hand and Fraser 1979: 331). Zahida, who viewed the task of Mukhtar's safe keeping as a blessing from God, was pregnant with her fifth child when Mukhtar's condition was diagnosed and she learnt of the one in four recurrence risk. Terrified by the idea of having to manage a second affected child, in addition to three other children, especially as her husband was often in Pakistan on lengthy visits, she agreed to a prenatal genetic test. This showed an unaffected baby, but because of the reproductive risk she requested a sterilisation (a procedure to make her infertile by tying the Fallopian tubes) after the birth. Likewise, Riffat, who viewed her son with Down syndrome as a blessing from God, accepted amniocentesis and would have ended her next pregnancy if the test had shown another affected child. In the process of deciding what to do, she consulted a woman *pīr* (religious specialist) and explained her family situation: she already had three children, she had been depressed after her affected son's birth, her husband was often absent and she did not think she could cope with another affected child. Her *pīr* told her that All'ah would not punish her if she went ahead with the test, because she had a duty to care for her existing children. In both of these cases, the presence of other unaffected children was an important factor in decisions to prevent another pregnancy or to prevent the birth of another affected child.

Another common response to a reproductive risk is to say, 'We have made a decision to postpone a new pregnancy for a few years.' Kaneez's sister's desire to wait a few years may have been, in part, a response to the distress of making a decision to terminate a pregnancy deemed 'incompatible with life'. A decision to postpone another pregnancy is also often a response to risk for a condition affecting a living infant, where the prognosis is uncertain and where parents are unsure about their ability to cope. Neha is a young British-raised woman whose first child's limb abnormalities were noted at birth as part of a serious recessive syndrome. When asked, soon after his birth, about their reproductive intentions, she and her husband said they wanted to concentrate on caring for their son, for whom a series of operations were being discussed. Nadia, whose daughter's limb abnormalities were detected prenatally, intended to postpone another pregnancy for a few years because of the stress of managing their daughter's problems, which have involved half a dozen corrective operations. Nighat Sadiq recalled that, when Bilaal's condition was diagnosed, she was told she had 'high chances' of having a child similarly affected with learning difficulties and metabolic problems requiring a lifetime's special diet:

> I had no intention of having another baby, because I have high chances. That is one reason for our slow time to have another baby: nine years was a long time. We just did not want to think about it. And it is not fair to the child either, is it? He is suffering at the moment. If you can avoid it, then it is better. I mean, that's how we look at it.

Significantly, she recalled a recurrence risk that underlined her desire not to repeat the experience of coping with an affected child: her husband remembered being given a one in four risk, but Nighat contradicted him. 'Three out of four,' she interrupted. 'No, one out of four,' he corrected. 'The point is', her husband explained, 'we did not have another child for a long time after that. We were too frightened the same thing would happen again, and they would not be able to do anything.' There was and still is no 'cure' (Chapter 4) and no early prenatal genetic test (Chapter 6) for Bilaal's condition.

Here, the recalled inflated recurrence risk may be less an indication of wrong information or misunderstanding than a clue to parents' emotions when they are or have been caring for a child or infant with serious medical problems. Farook Anwar is a twenty-seven-year-old, college-educated computer programmer married to a first cousin who speaks very little English and came to Britain from Azad Kashmir four years ago. They have a three-year-old son, but lost two daughters in early infancy to a fatal recessive condition. Just after the second infant death, Farook Anwar recalled that when the first baby died:

> We were told that we had a three in four chance that the next baby would have similar problems. A three in four chance is high, but people don't like to think about that, they turn a deaf ear, and I did not take it seriously ... After this, we do not want to have more children, not for five or six years at any rate. We have been today for birth control.

During this conversation his wife lay on the sofa and scarcely spoke: 'She is very upset. She feels she cannot produce healthy children; she cannot perform the function for which she is here. I do not blame her. It is a cultural thing that she feels like this.'

Taking the risk: fertility and the importance of having children

Sometimes, though, the early death of an infant may be associated with a new attempt to have a healthy baby, as in Sofia's case (Chapter 4). Lippman-Hand and Fraser (1979: 335) suggest that, in such cases, it is not so much that an infant death removes the 'expected burden' of emotional and physical energy spent on caring for an affected infant, but that the death limits uncertainty, particularly parents' uncertainties about their ability to manage another child, healthy or not. Thus, an infant's death may facilitate the decision to try again.

It would be difficult to overestimate the importance of having children within most British Pakistani marriages and family life. In general, a wife's pregnancy and childbirth indicate the success of a marriage. Conventionally, childbirth secures the position of a new wife in her husband's household, while childlessness renders it insecure. Sofia's four unsuccessful pregnancies (the miscarriages having not escaped her mother-in-law's notice) led her parents-in-law to suggest that their son took another wife. Occasionally, genetic risk may provide grounds for dissolving a marriage that is shaky for other reasons. A woman clinically identified as a carrier of two genetic conditions but already clinically depressed and unhappy with her marriage interpreted this risk as meaning, 'I can't have children.' In many cases, though, the desire to have children overrides the fear of having another affected child, particularly if the couple have no children or have only one or two, and want a large family. Indeed, in these circumstances parents may consider it better to have a child with a disability than to have no child at all.

Wanting to have a large family, or at least to give an existing child a sibling, can be an important element in parents' responses to recurrence risk. When Farook Anwar learnt of the recurrence risk when their first daughter died:

> I thought, what are they talking about? How do they know it? They said it is because we are first cousins, but there had not been anything like this in our family before. Plenty of people marry cousins without having handicapped children, and some people have handicapped children without marrying cousins. So we decided to go for it. Perhaps it was selfish, but we wanted our son to have a brother or sister to play with.

Lippman-Hand and Fraser suggest that, for American couples who have received genetic counselling, the presence of an unaffected child in the family diffuses parental responsibility to make a reproductive decision: 'Parents frequently commented how a living child needs a brother or sister – another child was necessary. To some extent, this permits them to downplay their own role in making a choice – it is the thing that has to be done' (1979: 335). In Farook's case, too, it provided another rationale for 'taking the risk', in addition to his scepticism of the consanguinity thesis.

Just as the observation that 'plenty of people marry cousins without having handicapped children' is evidence that the birth of an affected child is not inevitable in a cousin marriage, so too, the presence of an unaffected child in the family demonstrates that the birth of an affected child is not inevitable. A reproductive risk assessment represents a risk, not inevitability. In this situation, 'the idea that an abnormality need not occur is emphasized' (Lippman-Hand and Fraser 1979: 335).

Khalida and her husband already had two unaffected children when their third baby died within a few hours of her birth from – as they learnt later- a recessive condition involving structural problems. Their next pregnancy produced a healthy baby, but he died suddenly at nine months from a second recessive condition, involving a metabolic problem undetectable by prenatal scans. The couple had been planning to have four or five children – they had already bought a large car to transport them in – and attended the genetics clinic because they were still considering having more children: 'We want to know if we are carrying anything that might affect a future pregnancy.' The clinical geneticist gave them a combined risk for two genetic disorders, but first explained some basis genetics:

> Chromosomes contain genetic information (genes) in two copies. Each partner passes on one copy of this information to a child. Sometimes changes or mutations occur in this information and usually these do not matter because the copy inherited from the other partner compensates for them. But, if there is a mistake in the gene, there is a 50 per cent chance you will pass on the mistake. [This is a statement about the chance of passing on any mutation, and not a statement of the parents' risk of having an affected child.]

She then explained the inheritance of each of the conditions, saying that, for each, both parents' chromosomes contain an identical mutation, giving a 25 per cent chance of a child being affected in another pregnancy. The parental consanguinity meant, 'You have probably inherited the gene from a common ancestor and they've come full circle and met up again.' Combining these risks:

> This gives a one in four chance of each disorder: this means the risk goes up, to one in two or 50 per cent.[1] There is a risk that the child will have both conditions, and a chance that a child is a carrier of one or the other. And when they grow up, they may want to find out, especially if they marry outside the family. The chance would go up if they marry a close relative ... But one in four is a significant risk, even though there is a chance that the baby is OK ... especially where there are two conditions.

Recalling this information a couple of months later, Khalida was sceptical of the recurrence risk because it seemed to imply she had no chance of having a healthy child, and yet, 'I am still married to the same person':

> KA: We were told we had a fifty-fifty chance of having one or the other. We were told it is normally one in four. The doctor, she says it goes up to fifty-fifty. But the things are not related. You're put under so much stress. What do you do? There's no chance of a healthy baby – a fifty-fifty one way or the other. Doesn't that sound scary?
>
> AS: that can't be right, because you have two healthy children. It can't be that you have no chance of a healthy child.
>
> KA: That's what I say. We have had the other two children checked for [the metabolic problem] – scans, X-rays, there's no sign of it, and one of them has had a blood test ... I am still married to the same person – how can they say now that I have a fifty-fifty chance of one or the other, and I have two healthy children? I don't believe in them. I don't believe in this stuff that it is genetic. It is bad luck. I accept that, when something happens, but not that it is genetic. They try to say that it is your fault because you are married

to a cousin. If they did not know we were cousins, or if we weren't cousins, they would not say it is genetic. In our culture, there are more people married in the family than out, but you don't see this going on with every family. They say this, and they scare you. They scare you that this will happen again in the future. We have two children and we want a big family. It scares you. It does scare you.

Just as the emotionally draining experience of serious abnormality can lead to parents making inflated recollections of probabilistic risk, so too their desire to have children or to have more children, and the doctor's recognition of this desire, can mean that patients and doctors may emphasise the chances of having an unaffected child in their presentation or recollection of recurrence risks. The doctor talking to Khalida, above, considered 'one in four is a significant risk, even though there is a chance that the baby is OK', perhaps because Khalida's risk is in fact for two different conditions. In other cases, clinicians may say that another way of considering a recessive risk is as a 'higher' chance (75 per cent) of an unaffected child, as Kaneez's sister had understood her risk – thus offering hope. Liaqat Ali, a twenty-five-year-old medical technician, and his wife, a first cousin who came from Pakistan five years ago, have one healthy daughter, but then lost a baby to a rare recessive condition. They were advised of the recessive recurrence risk, but were keen to have another child: 'So we tried for another baby. It was a worrying pregnancy, as there were no tests available. A week before the birth, I asked the gynaecologist, "What is the chance of this happening again?" He said, "It is like me telling you I am going to the moon and back."' The gynaecologist had tried to be reassuring, but, sadly, this child was similarly affected and died in infancy. Common sense seemed to suggest to Liaqat Ali that they would be unlikely to be unlucky a third time. Reassured by his paediatrician that 'the risk is no greater than before', he felt hopeful, believing 'the chances should be less and less' with each subsequent pregnancy:

The paediatrician said we had been very unlucky, that there is the risk element that it will happen again, but it is OK to try for a baby, the risk is no greater than before. He said, 'It is unlikely the dice will land again on a six and a six.' But, if we had known, we would have stopped, for three or four years at least. All that time, we were trying to fill that vacuum up, to replace the lost baby. But instead, the vacuum got bigger and bigger. In the probability sense, the chances should be less and less, we thought it would be less and less, when the next baby was born. But it was not. The girl who did the EEG (electroencephalogram) for this baby was the same one who did it for the other two. I could see from her face; I did not need to wait for her to tell us the result.

As the English proverb 'Lightning never strikes twice' suggests, it is difficult for us to accept that chance has no memory (Wexler 1979). Here, Liaqat Ali's reasoning also seemed to be that increasing the number of attempts at a successful pregnancy will increase the chances of being lucky, rather akin to buying lottery tickets. He later used the same reasoning when he enquired about fertility treatment for his wife to stimulate multiple ovulations and conceptions.

These interpretations of recessive risk underline the limits of probabilistic thinking when applied to real-life reproductive decisions, for, while Mendelian probabilities remain the same with each conception, risk information is always given and received in a social and cultural context. Having experienced three infant deaths from the same disorder, Liaqat Ali now wondered, in the light of such bad luck, if the odds might in fact be more heavily stacked against him than with the 'standard' recessive recurrence risk, for reasons perhaps beyond medical explanation. He felt the risk information they received gave a false sense of hope; at first, they understood this was a 'one-off' genetic disorder, perhaps thinking that a 'one in four' risk meant they had already had their one affected child, and so tried for another baby. The fact that the risk was described each time as 'no greater than before' may have led him to conclude that the chances of another affected child would diminish, as if their bad luck was being used up, 'We thought that our bad luck would be over and the next child would be OK … In the probability sense, the chances should be less and less, we thought it would be less and less, when the next baby was born.' The couple's response now was to postpone another pregnancy, at least for a few years, and to return to Pakistan to escape from the constant reminders of their losses.

'We have completed our family'

Occasionally, couples respond to the uncertainty of a recurrence risk with a statement to the effect that they do not want more children, rendering the reproductive risk irrelevant. Again, certain features of their reproductive history make this response more likely: if the diagnosis and risk assessment concern an already teenage or older child, or if the child is the youngest of several siblings. Saleem Ullah's son was eighteen when his father requested a genetics appointment to establish a cause for his son's problems, and, as the eldest of five children, the risk assessment seemed irrelevant, because 'we have completed our family'. Likewise, for Nusrat, whose teenage daughter has mild learning problems, the reproductive risk, which was in any case imprecise because of uncertainty over the diagnosis ('possibly a "one-off", with low recurrence risk, and possibly a one in four'), was of no concern, for Nusrat has four children and has completed her family. Three other sets of parents of boys diagnosed with neurofibromatosis type I (NFI), a dominant condition with a 50 per cent recurrence risk if it has not arisen *de novo*, were also unconcerned about the risk to a subsequent pregnancy because, in each case, the affected child was the youngest of four or more children of middle-aged parents who had completed their families. In two cases, the parents seemed relatively untroubled about the condition, for it did not appear to be 'in the family' and its presenting features seemed relatively mild. In a third case, the diagnosis explained only some of the child's many medical problems.

Although parents who have completed their families may consider reproductive risks irrelevant, clinicians counselling such parents will usually also raise the issue of future reproductive risks to the children of the affected child or children, should they marry. They may also mention the risk of recessive conditions in the as-yet unborn children of an affected child's unaffected siblings, as possible carriers of the same recessive mutation, particularly if these siblings were to marry relatives such as first cousins, who might also be carriers. For many parents of young children, these seem remote concerns, but the issue may come to be perceived as important with older children or where marriages are being considered (Chapters 7 and 8).

Not deciding, 'unless I have to'

Rather than making a decision to avoid a risk or deciding to proceed with another pregnancy despite a risk, another common response to a clinical recurrence risk is indecision about a future pregnancy. Such a response may involve the use of methods of contraception that the couple recognises as unreliable. Lippman-Hand and Fraser describe this as playing 'reproductive roulette': 'the couple engages in a form of contraceptive risk taking', which, they argue, is not an irrational choice or necessarily an indication that the genetic counselling is unsuccessful (1979: 336). Rather, such non-decision, especially in the absence of prenatal diagnosis, is a response to the seemingly unsolvable problem of whether or not the couple could cope with an, or another, affected child, because it 'removes personal responsibility for conception' (Lippman-Hand and Fraser 1979: 336). If a pregnancy ensues, it was unplanned, accidental; if decisions are to be made, they can be made later, in the pregnancy or after the child's birth. The youngest of Rukhsana's three children is nine years old, has learning difficulties and is very difficult to manage. Rukhsana would like another child, but does not want another affected child. She knows a prenatal genetic test is available and thinks she might use it in another pregnancy, but is unsure whether or not she would be able to terminate another pregnancy (see Chapter 6). She is unhappy about using the contraceptive pill or an IUD (intrauterine device), preferring her husband to use condoms, but he dislikes this method of contraception. In addition, he remains sceptical about the recurrence risk, saying if they have a child, and what the child is like, is 'up to God'. If she does become pregnant, she says, she will decide what to do.

A statement that we will 'wait a few years' can also hide greater underlying uncertainty, often combined with a desire for more children. As discussed in the previous chapter, doctors in genetics like to know what couples' intentions are, and may even ask patients to inform them if they decide to try for another child, so that they can find out if a prenatal test is or would be available, but for patients this can seem like 'asking their permission', as Khalida put it. While waiting and not deciding, both clinical and family circumstances may change and being unable to make a clear decision at one point in time does not mean that a decision will not be made later. Nadia and her husband had told the clinical geneticists that they would wait a few years before having another baby, given their one in four risk of having another child with major limb abnormalities. Already, their affected child had undergone four lengthy surgical operations. But Nadia became pregnant sooner than she expected – their contraceptive use had not been foolproof. The prenatal staff then arranged early scans and further genetic counselling to discuss the risks, and offered a genetic test (via amniocentesis), which, for Nadia, was out of the question because of the (1 per cent) risk to the baby and because she felt she could not terminate an affected pregnancy. In fact, as it emerged, the couple had not discussed these options between themselves, finding the subject too painful, and it was only with the assistance of an interpreter and counsellor that they were able to consider each other's views. Nadia's husband, in England for about six years, felt the decision was ultimately his wife's, but thought that if there was evidence from either scans or genetic tests that clearly showed an affected baby, then it would be better to stop the pregnancy, to reduce future suffering for all concerned – himself, his wife, the unborn child and their existing children and the wider family. Asked if the timing of a termination, and hence of genetic tests, would be an issue (see Chapter 6), he replied, 'No, it would be a medical decision, not one made on religious grounds.' Afterwards, he told me that this had not been his view in the first pregnancy when early scans had detected limb abnormalities: 'Our view was that a child is a gift from God; that was all there is to it. But now I know what suffering there is.' He thus now brought a more nuanced understanding to the negotiation of risk in this subsequent pregnancy. Further discussion with the doctor revealed that amniocentesis could, in fact, be postponed until after the next prenatal scan, which would give fuller information about the foetus, and as it turned out the scan showed no limb abnormalities and the couple decided against amniocentesis. As Nadia's husband put it, 'The risk is now something less than one in four, so we do not want to tip the balance even a little in the other direction.'

Resisting religious stereotyping: 'I don't believe in abortion. It's not because of religion, it is personal.'

While doctors seek to be sensitive to patients' views about managing risk in a subsequent pregnancy, patients' views are not necessarily fixed but may change over time with experience. Moreover, patients' decisions to use or not to use a prenatal test or therapeutic abortion are not necessarily derived from religion, as Nadia's husband's comment above indicates. In fact, patients are sometimes very sensitive to health workers' assumptions that resistance to genetic testing in pregnancy must be related to their faith.

Before I met Hamid Ullah, a health visitor warned me he is 'very religious … for him, everything is in the hands of God; he turned down the offer of amniocentesis when his wife was pregnant'. Some months after their twins were born, Hamid and his wife Humairah requested a genetics appointment to clarify their sons' genetic status (blood samples for chromosome analysis had been taken at the birth). Hamid also wanted to go over the inheritance of the condition, so that he could explain the genetic risk to other family members. In the exchange that followed, the doctor wanted to mention the boys' future reproductive risks as unaffected carriers of a chromosome rearrangement and to ensure that the parents were informed about the options for managing risk in another pregnancy:

> *Consultant:* Your children are OK, because they both have the correct amount of genetic material. But you will have to be concerned for when they come to have children.
> *Humairah:* Is there a difference between them?
> *Consultant:* Not in their chromosomes 15 and 22. Both of them have the same balance; there is no difference between the two of them. [To Hamid] Your boys are like you, and they will be faced with the same possibilities when they have children that you are faced with now … You might want to have more children and then you can test for whether there is this condition when you are pregnant.
> *Hamid:* Yes, I know. [But what] I want to know [is] how did this come [about]? … I understand it came from my father, but how?
> *Consultant:* It probably originated with your father, that the 15 and 22 chromosomes got mixed up, some of one of his two copies of chromosome 15 went on to one of his chromosome 22s when he was formed as a baby. The chromosomes have to divide and recombine, and mistakes can happen, just by chance. He was OK, he still had enough information, the 15 was balanced. But your brother, he had too little of chromosome 15 and was missing the eating-control genes …
> *Hamid:* Can any of our sons' children by chance get normal chromosomes, and then the mental disorder would disappear?
> *Consultant:* Yes, it could be that, by chance, they pass on only the normal 15. They have the same possibilities as you. The other thing I should say is that now they are offering preimplantation testing for some translocations like these. If it is against your religious belief …
> *Hamid:* [Interrupting her] Personal belief.
> *Consultant:* If it is against your personal belief to have a test during pregnancy …
> *Hamid:* [interrupting her again] By then, the baby is there, isn't it? The test could kill it; they said so…

> *Consultant:* [ignoring the interruption] … you can consider pre-implantation testing.
> *Hamid:* how do they do that?
> *Consultant:* When the egg meets the sperm, there are eight days before it is implanted in the womb. This can be done outside the body: the egg and the sperm meet and are then planted in the body. You have to do it before you get pregnant, and it is therefore more artificial. They take your eggs and sperm outside and put them together.
> *Hamid:* How do they get the woman's eggs?
> *Consultant:* They use a catheter through the belly button to the ovaries, or sometimes they take it in through the vagina, to harvest the eggs. They are offering it for some translocations.
> *Hamid:* Dr. X [his paediatrician] will tell us more, if we want to know.
> *Consultant:* Any more questions?
> *Humairah:* What is our blood group and the boys' blood group?
> *Consultant:* Well it's probably B positive, most Asians are B positive, I am. But the blood group has nothing to do with this syndrome. It is not connected with this.[2]

Having stated the possibility that, in another pregnancy, a baby might have an unbalanced translocation, the doctor invites the couple to consider two means of managing this risk: prenatal testing, which implies a termination of pregnancy if the child is affected, and primplantation genetic diagnosis, 'if it is against your religious belief to have a test during pregnancy'. Aware from clinic notes that the couple turned down amniocentesis in their first pregnancy, the doctor feels it is important to detail the options for risk management. Preimplantation genetic diagnosis (PGD) is available for a limited number of conditions for at-risk couples who want to avoid having an affected child but who do not want to terminate a pregnancy. It involves prenatal genetic diagnosis performed before the implantation of the embryo in the womb, thus avoiding the need for termination. It is considered likely to be useful for couples who, for religious reasons, consider termination of pregnancy unacceptable. However, many of those who consider it do not go ahead, because of the low pregnancy rate or potential misdiagnosis (for which prenatal diagnosis is usually also offered and often declined, after PGD) or because the idea of destroying embryos is unacceptable (Franklin and Roberts 2006).

Hamid immediately resisted the suggestion that his discomfort with termination stems from religion, stressing this is a 'personal belief', but seemed to feel a justification was necessary – unlike the clinician, since she proceeded to explain PGD. Hamid returned to this topic when I talked to him several months later, justifying his rejection of amniocentesis in his wife's first pregnancy:

> I don't believe in abortion, not because of religion. It is personal. I feel that the baby inside is a living thing, however small it is. When they ask, I have never said this [to them], but I think, how can [they] people do it? The doctors say, 'Do you want to know?' I have said, 'No, there is not anything to discuss.' Imagine, you are a carrier, what would you do if you knew, in the first month or in the first three months, that one of your children will have this illness? They call it termination: to terminate, to abort, to stop. How can you justify this in the first month? How can you justify it in the first three months? The legal limit, how do they justify that? It is just money and politics.

Hamid went straight on to talk about contraception, perceiving certain forms of preventing pregnancy to be as problematic as prenatal diagnosis to prevent the birth of a child with a genetic disorder, if they similarly involved potential harm to fertility, the mother or the unborn child:

> I was talking to a Christian at work, and he was against women taking the contraceptive pill. He says it is wrong because you are killing the eggs. I've got nothing against the pill, because you're not killing a life, and I said to him, some eggs disappear naturally anyway. But he was adamant. Saying to me, you're a Muslim, you shouldn't even be contemplating it. He thought that condoms are OK because the sperm are not the same as the eggs. I can't remember why. I'm also against [contraceptive] injections ... I remember, now, what my Christian friend was saying: the pill is a drug, so it is not like condoms. It is doing physical harm. Sometimes women cannot get pregnant after they have been on the pill for a while and it can cause illnesses. So I wouldn't want to put my wife through it. A condom is just a piece of plastic. There are none of the physical damages. I have read that the eggs get weak if you've been on the pill. If the eggs are weak, and you put them with the sperm, the child is weak.

He then acknowledged that his views initially stemmed from religion, but added that he has since thought through the reasons for his discomfort with prenatal testing:

> When I was asked about whether we should check the babies before they are born, I said no. At that time, I thought it was in God's hands. Apart from that, I did not think much about it, but now I've thought more, and I think, how would I have felt if I was being rejected, if my parents decided to terminate me? If I had known, and if my child had this thing I would still have had him, as long as she [my wife] agreed. Our consultant paediatrician, he said, this can happen. It can happen to you, that you have

> a child like your brother, and you can find out beforehand. I said, No, thank you. If you know it is affected, they think it is too much work to have a handicapped child. How do they know it is going to be so much work? You might decide to do so much work anyway, to earn more money, however your child is, and your child might be healthy and still suffer. If you have a child like that, you might get blessings from that child. But society has taught us to expect perfection.

Thus, he would describe his earlier rejection of amniocentesis as a personal decision, made because of the risk of spontaneous abortion: he did not want to put a potentially healthy first pregnancy at additional risk. Humairah agreed with this view, but put a religious gloss on it by saying she would not want any test that might result in losing the baby, for this, according to her religion, would be sinful. Nevertheless, for both of them, the risk of having a child with the same condition as Hamid's brothers was a genuine concern stemming from direct personal experience. Humairah told me, later, that her husband 'worries a lot, because there is a big difference between having a child that is handicapped (*mazoor*) and having a child that is not. But he also says, and in our Islam it is like this, that the kind of child you have is in the hands of God.' Humairah's comment points to the importance of context in statements about religious versus personal belief. In talking to his wife and to senior members of his family and local community, Hamid might use a religious idiom; when discussing the issue with me or the clinic doctors, he used a more individualistic form of reasoning:

> Some people say leave everything in God's hands, but I think you've just got to use your common sense. Science done in the proper way is good, because without science you wouldn't have medicine. You would not have aeroplanes. Human beings have been given the knowledge. You have to use it. It is the same with the knowledge of these defects. You have to use your common sense.

Hamid's sensitivity to religious stereotyping seems to me to represent a rejection of a view of Islam as rigid and unchanging. It does not necessarily follow from the belief that the kind of child you have is 'up to God' that human intervention in reproductive processes is, by definition, illegitimate in Islam (see Chapter 6). Rather, in relation to the use of these technologies, clinicians and patients are negotiating relatively uncharted moral territory (Rapp 2000). In these negotiations, people's positions vary with context and experience. At the same time, Hamid's sensitivity also appears to reflect the wider stigma of a Muslim identity in the contemporary political context of the rise of Islamic fundamentalism. Yet it is not that clinicians always stereotype Muslims' responses in ways that preclude considerations of clinical options; as we saw above, the consultant speaking with Hamid was keen to raise the option of PGD. After this consultation, Hamid told me that, while his 'common sense' told him that prenatal diagnosis with a view to terminating a pregnancy was wrong, he was not automatically against preimplantation diagnosis; he thought it 'a bit cold' but, other than that, admitted, 'I don't know what I think about that.'

Assumptions about consanguinity

Rather similar issues arise regarding the impact of the public discourse of genetic risk in consanguineous marriage upon patients' negotiations of reproductive risk and the clinical presentation of risk information. The elevated risk of recessive disorders with parental consanguinity is not just a 'theoretical' or epidemiological risk but has specific clinical implications within families where marriages tend to be with consanguineous kin when a recessive diagnosis has been made. The wider public health debate over consanguinity as a 'cause' of birth defects in Pakistani children has had the effect of stigmatising cousin marriages and giving the impression that 'genetic' or 'inherited' means 'in the family'. This, in turn, can generate personal scepticism of 'the consanguinity thesis' in ways that complicate the communication of clinical diagnostic and risk information. The fact that his brother's condition is not recessive seemed to make it easier for Hamid to accept a genetic explanation, but significantly Hamid began his account of the inheritance of this condition by emphasising that 'most nurses and social workers think this is to do with consanguinity. It is not. My parents are not related'. Sohrab's grandfather was sceptical that Sohrab's problems were genetic, saying, 'We have never seen this thing before' (Chapter 1), at least partly because of the implication, drawn from the wider public health discourse, that the parental consanguinity, in a family in which it was usual to arrange such marriages, was 'responsible' for his grandson's condition. The clinicians had simply noted but had not remarked on Sohrab's parents' consanguinity during the consultations I observed.

The stigma associated with being a consanguineous couple or having a history of consanguinity in the family seems to reflect deep-seated concerns within mainstream British society about consanguineous marriages that are not specific to clinical genetics and may not be expressed by clinical geneticists themselves during clinical consultations (Chapter 1). Although reproductive risk assessments are the professional responsibility of clinical geneticists, three consanguineously married couples in this study told me that they had been told by other medical specialists from other departments, before their genetics referral, that they had a one in four risk of having another affected child. The child's condition, in these cases, was presumed to be recessive, and the parents said their consanguinity had often featured in clinical discussions of their child's problems. As it turned out, the subsequent genetics clinic assessment confirmed a recessive diagnosis in two of these cases, but the third was established to have arisen from a *de novo* dominant mutation with no recurrence risk for any subsequent pregnancy.

When she was born, paediatricians noted that Nisha had some unusual features in her scalp, an asymmetrical head, *café au lait* spots and a marked curve (scoliosis) of the spine, but because she went to Pakistan for three years from the age of six months, she was 'lost to follow-up', as a genetic nurse-counsellor put it. Now nearly four years old and 'back in the system', she was being treated for her curved spine so that her internal organs could grow better. She had been slow to walk and talk and had some rather unusual facial features, so was referred to clinical genetics. Her mother's brother and her maternal grandmother brought her to the appointment, because her mother was at work and her father was still in Pakistan, awaiting an entry visa. The consultant took a family history, recorded without commenting on the consanguinity and examined Nisha by removing her shirt to pay particular attention to the spine but leaving in place the *tāvīs* (amulet) she wore round her neck (which Nisha's mother and grandmother had obtained, to counter Nisha's fears 'of green things in trees', from a *pīr* in Pakistan who had advised that Nisha never remove it). The consultant thought Nisha's problems might be genetic or congenital (originating 'from birth'), arranged for blood tests, urine tests and X-rays, and said she would see the family again if she could confirm the cause.

Afterwards, Nisha's grandmother insisted there were no problems at birth:

> GM: The doctors checked her and they did not notice anything, they said she was fine. At birth, her spine was straight (*kamar sīdhī thī*).
> AS: What about the marks on her scalp?
> GM: They took the *pānī* (water) out of her head with a syringe, they said the hair might not grow there, but it was nothing to worry about.

Resisting the idea of birth abnormality, Nisha's mother thought the spinal problem began in Pakistan, with many episodes of fever, perhaps typhoid, that had 'remained inside [Nisha's] body', followed a period of paralysis (*fālij*). Her grandmother speculated that injections given in the U.K. before Nisha was six months old (such as routine childhood immunisations, which were incomplete when Nisha went to Pakistan) had initiated a problem that was exacerbated by taking Nisha to different doctors in Pakistan:

> We got *ilāj* from one doctor. The next day we went to a different doctor. That is our mistake … And in Pakistan, they give you two injections before they ask you anything. Here they ask first … There is a hospital for treatment for bones where we live, but we did not know we had to get this treatment. We did not know till this year that there is something wrong with her back. We thought the paralysis was the result of a fall. That is what one doctor told us.

Their resistance to the idea of a genetic or congenital problem might be linked to the fact that the clinicians in the U.K. had not, at the time, discussed the features they had noted at Nisha's birth with her mother, who speaks little English, perhaps assuming there would be time for this and for genetic investigations during 'follow-up'. In addition, the family had been told by a medical professional that Nisha's problems were caused by 'too many close marriages in the family', as Nisha's college-educated auntie (her mother's brother's wife, a distant relative, recently arrived from Pakistan) explained:

> Nisha has problems because of too many close marriages in the family. The blood is the same each time. It is not just that her mother's mother and her father's father are sister and brother, but they themselves are the progeny (*aulād*) of first cousins (i.e. Nisha's great-grandparents' fathers' were brothers). Apart from this, the same blood comes again from Nisha's mother's mother and Nisha's mother's father, because her mother's father is a brother of Nisha's great grandfather. The blood is too close if the children of two brothers marry. Nisha's problem is because the blood is the same, all the way back; our family blood does not change (*hamārī nasal kā khūn nahīn badaltā hai*). The doctor said that the blood should change – one or two generations is OK, but not three generations.
> AS: Which doctor?
> NA: The one we saw last week, she asked about the blood relations between the parents and grandparents when we got Nisha's plaster put on.

As in many other local families, so too in Nisha's family, consanguineous connections can be traced for some generations, but the 'closeness' of blood connections was not the explanation for Nisha's problems offered at the genetics clinic, where the consultant geneticist was in fact working towards confirming a diagnosis of a dominant condition, likely to be a new mutation. Nevertheless, prejudging Nisha's problems as caused by consanguinity seemed to impede Nisha's grandparents in accepting the idea of any kind of genetic problem. Several months later, anticipating Nisha's father's arrival in the U.K., the consultant geneticist asked if the parents would consent to a blood test to establish any risk of the same problems recurring in another pregnancy, but Nisha's grandfather was adamant:

> GF: She was not born with this problem, it happened later. These things happen at any time in life, people get sick at any time in life. Do the doctors not die? Is that not true?
> AS: It is true. People can get ill for many different reasons, sometimes for inherited reasons, at any time.
> GF: It is not because it is in the family. This is the first case.

As discussed in Chapter 1, many people consider that a genetic or inheritable condition must be already visible or known 'in the family' for it to be genetic, rather than something that can appear for the first time, unknowingly passed across the generations by unaffected carriers of recessive conditions or arising as a new mutation. In the above extract, my comment to Nisha's grandfather failed to convey the idea that a genetic condition is not necessarily inherited, even though it may be inheritable. In fact, his response, 'It is not because it is in the family. This is the first case,' is an accurate clinical summary in this instance. The genetic investigations confirmed no recurrence risk with this *de novo* mutation, although Nisha herself could have affected children.

Conclusion

This chapter has discussed some limitations of taking at face value the view, often expressed by Pakistani Muslims, that the kind of child you have is 'up to God'. In the first place, to follow a sociological typology that might classify such views – alongside the recently documented Anglo-British beliefs in fate or destiny (Featherstone et al. 2006) – as 'pre-modern' in contrast with apparently 'modern' articulations of genetic theory as an explanation for medical or intellectual problems fails to convey the complexity of responses to genetic risk information. It also gives little indication of how, in individual cases, social circumstances and personal views shape responses to risk information, and how these responses in turn can be changed by circumstance and experience.

The view that a disabled child is a 'gift from God' or that the kind of child you have represents 'God's will' might seem to preclude the prevention of adverse birth outcome. However, just as such views do not preclude the therapeutic management of genetic conditions (Chapter 4), so too the religious positions on the permissibility of prenatal testing and termination are more complex than is often assumed (see Chapter 6). Moreover, the point beyond which human intervention in processes deemed to be the result of 'God's will' is unacceptable varies between individuals and from case to case and is influenced by social circumstances; a decision to undergo prenatal genetic testing or to terminate a pregnancy may be made on explicit social or medical grounds, rather than with reference to religious ethics. The place of religious views in the negotiation of reproductive risk is therefore very variable, despite the emphasis that clients may place on 'God's will'.

Documenting this diversity of engagement is important because clinicians may assume that the view that 'everything is up to God' precludes engagement with medical science and such an assumption may lead to prenatal services being withheld from Muslim clients (Modell et al. 2000). During my fieldwork, several women asked me if I had noticed whether white women are offered scans, prenatal tests and termination of pregnancy more often than Pakistani women and whether this might explain why there are more children with congenital and genetic abnormalities and learning difficulties among Pakistanis. My fieldwork was not designed to answer this comparative question. Nonetheless, my presence as an interpreter or observer during some clinical appointments may well have facilitated discussion of sensitive issues that might not otherwise have been discussed, or that might have been mentioned but not discussed in any detail, the topic, instead, perhaps, being drawn to a close by a patient remarking that a birth outcome is 'up to God'. While clinicians must respect such views, it is also important for equitable service delivery that all options are discussed with clients, even if such discussion does not lead to a different choice.

I have also described some of the ways in which the stigma associated with cousin marriages can complicate the presentation and discussion of risk information. Like dominant mutations, recessive mutations also occur by chance, but, because recessive conditions are caused by inheriting a mutation in the same gene from both parents, clinicians usually emphasise that having an ancestor or ancestors in common makes it more likely that both parents carry a mutation on the same gene. This emphasis on the marriage pattern, with the implication that it has 'caused' the problem in question, feeds into the public discourse of consanguinity and genetic risk, which is thus often experienced by patients as stigmatising, even where clinicians have no intention of judging or blaming patients for their marriage pattern, or where, as one consanguineously married father put it, 'we keep an open mind'.

Notes

1. In fact, the clinical risk was revised and established to be rather more complicated than a one in two risk reached by adding two risks of one in four. The revised risk was a nine in sixteen chance that a child would be unaffected, which is close to a one in two risk but reached in a different way. At the clinicians' request, I explained this at the end of the interview, drawing a diagram to show how the following risks are calculated: the risk of a child being affected by one condition or the other is 6/16, of being affected by both conditions is 1/16 and of being affected by neither condition is 9/16. In this case, the chance of an unaffected child being a carrier of neither condition is 1/9, a carrier of both conditions is 4/9 and a carrier of one or the other condition is 4/9.
2. Humairah possibly associates 'blood group' with the blood test done on her sons at birth, which was in fact a chromosome test. This is another confusion that may arise over 'blood tests' in chromosome or molecular genetic analysis, as discussed in Chapter 4.

CHAPTER 6
FORETELLING AND MANAGING INFANT DEATH

During my fieldwork, infant death emerged as a central concern for some parents. Certain rare recessive disorders have lethal effects, resulting in pregnancy loss, early infant death or shortened life expectancy. Ten of the couples recruited to this study lost eighteen babies between them as stillbirths, neonatally (soon after birth) or during the first year of life; this excludes miscarriages, which some women had experienced repeatedly. In all but one or two cases, the identified cause was a lethal recessive condition, reflecting national findings that attribute part of the excess infant mortality among British Pakistanis to lethal recessives. Five couples had experienced an infant death two or three times from the same recessive condition and in one family two babies died within the first three months of life from one recessive disorder and a third death at nine months was caused by a different condition.

This chapter highlights some of the emotional, social and practical ethical issues these experiences raised for the parents. The 'foretelling' of infant death refers to the fact that the parents were forewarned that their baby had a fatal genetic or probably genetic condition during the pregnancy (in 12/18 cases) or at or soon after the birth (in 5/18 cases). Just one infant death occurred 'out of the blue': this was the nine-month-old baby, and a genetic diagnosis was made afterwards. As a foretelling of early death, or at least of serious life-threatening problems, the prenatal or immediate post-natal diagnosis of a fatal abnormality has psychological and social consequences for the parents. Prenatally, it raises the issue of termination of pregnancy; post-natally, it may necessitate decisions about the withdrawal of life support from an infant in intensive care.

A dominant biomedical perception of Muslim women users of British prenatal services is that they will not consider termination of pregnancy on religious grounds. A national confidential inquiry into the uptake of thalassaemia screening found that many medical professionals believe that there is no point in offering prenatal diagnosis to Muslim women because termination is unacceptable in Islam (Modell et al. 2000). In other words, religion is perceived as a significant constraint on British Muslim women's use of reproductive technologies. This perception is also reflected in anthropological scholarship that suggests Islamic religiosity is increasing in parts of the Muslim world in ways that threaten women's rights

(Shafik 2001; Abu-Lughod 2002). A second perceived constraint on British Pakistani women's autonomy is that of the family, and the hierarchy of gender and status within it, in mediating women's access to contraception and prenatal facilities. On occasion, husbands or other senior family members such as fathers-in-law have prohibited women from terminating a pregnancy, sometimes on threat of divorce or death, and mothers-in-law have intercepted their daughters-in-laws' access to or use of contraception or prenatal diagnosis. Against this background, the question of how the individuals and couples in my study negotiate the practical ethical issues raised by the pre- or early post-natal diagnosis of fatal abnormality is particularly relevant.

Within the Muslim world and for many British Muslims, Islamic teachings on the control of reproduction constitute a very important element in how people negotiate the use of modern reproductive technologies, including those of prenatal genetic diagnosis and termination of pregnancy; this reflects the more general influence of Islam in governing the proper conduct of daily life. Such teachings have a particular force in that they are seen as having authority beyond the couple or the family and universal validity within the *ummah*, or global Muslim community. However, what is less immediately evident is that there is also some uncertainty and disagreement over what constitutes the Islamic position on such issues as termination of pregnancy; indeed, many people may be unaware of a religious opinion that allows termination of pregnancy under certain circumstances (Ahmed et al. 2006b). Moreover, what people actually do, in these situations, does not necessarily reflect their understandings of religious teachings (see also Gameltoft 2001). What is the relationship between Islamic teachings and what individuals or couples do in practice, in the negotiation of the real-life situations in which they need to make a practical ethical decision? What is the role of an opinion from a religious leader such as an *imām* (Muslim priest) or a *pīr* (saint) or another religious source in the negotiation of the practical ethical dilemmas following a pre- or post-natal diagnosis of a fatal abnormality? In these negotiations, how do the teachings of religion or religious experts relate to other sources of opinion and advice, such as the expert knowledge of medical practitioners (obstetricians, paediatricians, genetic counsellors, etc.) or the authoritative knowledge of senior kin or other close relatives? And how does the immediate context of family and local Muslim community influence the way these dilemmas are handled?

This chapter makes three related points. It begins by demonstrating some ambiguities and differences of opinion over the Islamic position on issues such as termination of pregnancy and the withdrawal of life support from infants in special care. Many of my study participants would assert that Islam forbids termination of pregnancy under any circumstances, but an alternative, albeit locally muted, Islamic discourse permits termination in early pregnancy in the case of serious abnormality. Secondly, while decisions about whether or not to terminate a pregnancy are made against a background of competing discourses about its acceptability (and a dominant discourse of disapproval), in practice, a particular course of action may be contemplated or justified on biomedical, practical or emotional grounds (and sometimes all of these) as well as, and sometimes without, reference to Islamic teaching (reflecting, for instance, a desire not to repeat a previous painful experience of infant death or childhood disability). Thirdly, the material presented here underlines the importance of the context of family and community within which these decisions are made. On the one hand, my observations support a relational understanding of autonomy, as shaped by the interests and opinions of other members of the family and justified with reference to the authority of Islam. On the other hand, they support a view that recognises that individual needs and desires are not necessarily those of the wider family and underline the importance of respecting the confidentiality and privacy of the individual or couple in their encounters with clinical services.

In what follows, I include views of parents of children with physical and intellectual disabilities and of people with close kin with affected children, but I draw mainly on case material relating to the ten couples whose infants died during the first year of life. None of these couples actually terminated a pregnancy, a point that might seem to support the dominant medical view that ending a pregnancy is unacceptable in Islam. However, my material indicates that the perceived Islamic restrictions are a contested arena in the case of serious abnormality. In particular, I detail one woman's failed quest for an Islamic justification for ending a pregnancy, which was followed by an especially traumatic delivery of a baby with multiple abnormalities, who died shortly afterwards. Shakeera's experience highlights the need for incorporating within public discourse awareness of Islamic views that permit ending a pregnancy in cases of serious, fatal abnormalities.

Whether women and their partners would experience less psychological harm if they terminated a fatally abnormal pregnancy rather than carrying it to term and delivery, however, remains an open-ended question, particularly where doubts remain as to the accuracy of the medical diagnosis or the ethics of ending a pregnancy in these circumstances. Indeed, as I show, there may be psychological benefits in delivering a baby that lives for even a short while, particularly where this is likely to facilitate the social recognition of pregnancy loss. The final part of this chapter considers the implications of cultural and religious beliefs associated with personhood in the context of pregnancy loss and funerary rituals for the medical management of childbirth where the baby is not expected to live.

Rendering abnormalities visible before birth

The practice of prenatal ultrasound examination is common and regarded as routine in most developed countries. Although many serious abnormalities remain undetectable by ultrasound scanning, particularly without any known family history to inform and direct the sonographer's gaze, the ultrasound examination nevertheless permits an ever-increasing amount of information to be obtained about the health of a foetus. Sometimes described as a dating scan, a mid-trimester ultrasound examination can estimate foetal age and indicate the presence of twins and the position of the placenta. It can also provide information about possible physical problems in the foetus by looking for development abnormalities or for 'markers' of known abnormalities (Boyle et al. 2003). An observed or suspected abnormality can then be investigated further with subsequent scans or prenatal genetic tests using amniocentesis or CVS.

These recent innovations in prenatal care are part of the ongoing transformation of prenatal and maternity services in the developed world since the mid-twentieth century; twenty years ago, ultrasound was offered only to women at higher risk of abnormalities because of their age. Routine use of ultrasound has had the effect of making a pregnancy tentative, or only provisionally normal, until given the all-clear by medical professionals (Rothman 1986; Press et al. 1998). As feminist critics have noted, developed systems of antenatal and obstetric care contain a contradiction: they exist to support women in having healthy babies, but are based upon a medical view of pregnancy and childbirth as potentially pathological, requiring screening and supervision (Taylor 1998). Whether this empowers or harms women remains an open question. Women's attitudes to the increasing use of medical technology indicate a general ambivalence to medicalisation and a pragmatic engagement with prenatal care involving 'selective compliance' (Abel and Browner 1998; Lock and Kaufert 1998: 16).

Most women in my study considered the scan a normal part of routine prenatal care, performed 'to check the baby is OK' and unlikely to harm the foetus. Women who had previously had a baby with a birth anomaly were anxious about their ultrasound examinations, fearful that these might 'give bad news', and, like Sofia in Chapter 4, sometimes delayed their first antenatal appointment, frustrating prenatal and genetics staff, who advise 'at-risk' women to make early contact in a subsequent pregnancy. While the idea of checking that a pregnancy is normal implies that it might not be, women without any previous experience of a birth abnormality were generally unprepared for the possibility that ultrasound might render visible abnormalities that would otherwise have remained concealed until the birth or until the pregnancy miscarries, in that they had not thought through what they would do in this event. This observation is also true of the wider population: Teresa Marteau and colleagues found that couples are often unaware that a scheduled ultrasound examination can provide information about the health of their foetus (Marteau et al. 1993). In my study, information about abnormalities provided by routine ultrasound came as a shock to women with no prior experience of a problematic pregnancy or no known family history of a genetic condition. In these women's recollections of their experiences of the scan, it was usually the expression on the face of the sonographer that gave the first indication that something might be wrong. The emotional distress of this realisation is heightened in women's reports of being alone during the scan. Shakeera, twenty-six years old, born and raised in the U.K. and married to a first cousin, was pregnant for the first time when she learnt at an early scan that there was a problem:

> My husband was in Pakistan, because his Mum was ill. There was this Indian guy doing the scan, and he went very quiet. I was praying. He says, 'there seems to be a piece of fluid in the lungs.' There was no one with me, because my sister was still trying to park the car and I started to cry. The Indian guy brought a consultant, and the consultant said, 'It is best to send her to Oxford because they have better machines there for scans.'

Miriam, twenty-seven years old, born and raised in the U.K. and married to a first cousin, already had two healthy daughters when she went for a second routine scan in her third pregnancy. Her earlier scan had indicated that 'everything was OK', so her shock was coupled with an initial disbelief that anything could be wrong:

> They first thought there was a problem at the twenty-week scan. Before that, I thought everything was OK. I was happy. I was well and full of energy. My husband and the girls were waiting outside because my eldest daughter hates hospitals and would not come in. I still remember that day and how I knew they knew. You just know from the way they look at the scan. The man doing the scan paused, took a while, then he went out of the room, saying he wanted to speak to someone senior. He said he can't be 100 per cent sure but he thought he had picked up something. I burst out crying. I thought I had done something wrong. I didn't believe them at first. I thought, 'They don't know what they are telling me, the baby is OK.'

Suspected abnormalities require a second opinion and even then it is likely that women will be referred to the regional hospital where there are facilities for more detailed scans than are available in the local hospital. Miriam was seen in the regional hospital the following day:

> The next day, they sent me to Oxford ... I don't know nothing about scans, but even I could see, then, there was something wrong. The Oxford doctor was very shocked at what he saw; it is 'very striking', he said. Basically, everything was outside the body – all the organs were in the wrong place, all the body parts. They listed everything they could see. They did not see the eyes: they wrote – eyes 'not seen' on the report. Then they went through the options.

In other cases, the significance of what has been observed on the scan, such as 'fluid in the lungs', is less immediately conclusive. Shakeera's follow-up scan took place two days later in Oxford, where she recalls being told, 'There is definitely water in the lungs, but it can disappear, though sometimes it doesn't. Come back in two to three months.' Either way, the prenatal visibility of a possible or a conclusive abnormality draws women into a treadmill of more intensive management of their pregnancy. Shakeera's narrative details the increasingly complex medical issues raised by subsequent scanning of her pregnancy – showing the continuing presence of water in the lungs; suggesting and then confirming a heart abnormality, for which the option of post-natal surgical correction was mentioned; and finally revealing fluid on the baby's brain, raising serious questions about the viability and delivery of this baby:

> When I went back they found there was again water in the lungs and it had increased. It was still too early to look at the heart, because the baby was too small. They gave me another appointment, and when I went back they looked at her heart and said there might be abnormalities in the heart. They said it would be best to do an amniocentesis, and I agreed. They said the results of that were fine – the chromosomes were okay, and there was no Down syndrome or anything. Then I had another appointment in Oxford, and this time they said they could see an abnormality in the heart – normally there are two arteries that pump the blood, but with her heart there was only one artery and it pumped from one side. They said if the baby was born they would operate. They also said the heart was pushed to one side because there was so much fluid … The next two scans showed that there was a little fluid on the baby's brain. Then, at the following scan, they said there is a lot of fluid in the brain. The baby's brain is not going to be properly formed. At that point it was too late to abort.[1] They said the birth might be difficult to do naturally, because the brain will be too big – the head is the size of an adult's, because of all the liquid. But a Caesarean would mean risks to later pregnancies.[2] They said, 'If the baby doesn't survive, you will have put other pregnancies at risk' ['without good reason' or 'needlessly' is implied here]. They also said that they would not be able to do a usual Caesarean, because to take the head out they would need to cut in two ways, across and up the belly, and they said my belly might rupture in another pregnancy. Then they said there is another procedure. They would put in a shaft and drain the fluid off the brain, and that way I could have a natural delivery. The choice was that or a Caesarean. They did the shaft. I asked the doctor, 'How many times have you done this before?' He said, 'Once or twice.' That did not make me feel confident. Anyway, they drained 2.5 litres of pinkish fluid off the brain. I was in so much pain, but after draining the water … I could feel a huge difference. That evening they decided for me to be induced, and I had her the following morning.

Having first focused on the medical issues raised by the regular ultrasound scanning of her pregnancy, Shakeera then commented on the emotional impact of being confronted in advance of her child's birth with the possibility of its death or having serious handicaps. Her pregnancy became an experience of grief for the loss of normal pregnancy and the child not yet born, mixed with hope that the doctors were wrong. Her account reveals her increasing sadness and isolation as a new problem seemed to be revealed with each scan, setting Shakeera apart from even her close kin, such as a sister-in-law experiencing a trouble-free pregnancy and her parents, who continued to say, 'Everything will be all right':

> I didn't want to eat, or to dress up, I'd wear dark clothes all the time. I didn't tell anyone at work. Some of my work colleagues knew I was pregnant, and I said I was sick and tired – but they did not know about any of the problems. Then my older brother said, 'Take your pregnacare tablets.' My sister-in-law was pregnant at the time, and her child was fine, and I used to envy her. She ate fruit, and took her pregnacare tablets. I never told her what I was feeling. She used to talk about babies a lot, even though she knew I was going for extra scans. I think she didn't really understand. She would say, 'What are you going to do? Breastfeed?' ... Every scan was another shock, another disappointment. I used to lie down and cry. But my Mum would say, 'Just pray, and everything will be all right.' My Dad said, he would say, 'The doctors aren't always right. It will be OK. Don't worry.' I have faith in God that everything will be fine, but I had to prepare myself. There were so many abnormalities.

In a discussion of ethical approaches to the practice of prenatal ultrasound examinations, Robert Boyle and colleagues have argued that couples who want information about whether their foetus has a major or minor abnormality have a right to such information but that couples also have a right to remain ignorant of this information 'especially where it may cause some harm' (Boyle et al. 2003). The harm they detail concerns what they define as 'unnecessary distress' associated with ultrasound findings of indefinite, uncertain medical significance. Informing parents about probably insignificant markers of possible abnormality, they argue, can adversely affect parents' long-term perceptions of their child or affect the child itself by rendering it 'abnormal'. Similarly, defining a prenatally detected 'unusual' structural feature as abnormal, providing grounds for terminating a pregnancy, may also have adverse psychological effects on living relatives who share the same feature as a family trait. To respect couples' right to remain ignorant, especially of information 'that may cause some harm', they suggest routinely asking couples to choose one of three options: a non-detailed scan to check the dates and for the presence of twins and the position of the placenta; a more detailed scan that also looks for physical problems; or a scan that, in addition, looks for markers of abnormalities. These options, however, would carry a major caveat: if a scan detects an abnormality with 'definite implications' for the health of the foetus, then the parents will be told, even if they requested a non-detailed scan. Not to inform the parents or not to investigate further a finding with serious implications would be medically negligent – whatever the psychological distress caused to the woman or couple.

This suggestion for giving couples information about their foetus is aimed at reducing the harm associated with giving medically 'unnecessary' information. Even if they had not wanted such detailed information, Shakeera and Miriam would have had to have been informed about the problems noted on the scan, since these had 'definite implications' for the health of the foetus. In other cases, the significance of observed abnormalities may not be clear-cut. An indication of abnormality often requires a second opinion and the body language of the person doing the ultrasound can indicate to the parents that an abnormality is suspected – as Miriam put it, 'You just know from the way they look at the scan' – so it may be difficult to shield parents from receiving 'unnecessary information'. Rather, the process of asking a couple how much information they want from an ultrasound might highlight the inherent contradiction in prenatal scanning; in an era of low infant mortality, small family size and high expectations of infant health, it will focus attention on the possibility of abnormality. Further, while some women might choose not to have a detailed scan, my fieldwork indicated that, although women are often unprepared for the possibility of an abnormality, they nonetheless expect ultrasound to detect everything that might be wrong with a baby. Twenty-three-year-old Neha was extremely angry when she first learnt after her son's birth that he had limb abnormalities that had been missed by prenatal ultrasound, implying that she would have terminated the pregnancy had she known; indeed, she suspected medical negligence. At other times during my fieldwork, women voiced suspicions that Pakistani Muslims were being offered fewer scans and prenatal tests than white women (see also Chapter I and 'Conclusion' to Chapter 5). This perception may be based on inequalities in access that reflect, among other things, health professionals' prejudice that there is 'no point' offering prenatal tests to people who believe that a birth outcome is 'up to God'. Clearly, ensuring equitable access to and providing appropriate information about the available prenatal technologies are important issues for service providers in a multi-ethnic context. In addition, I found that British Pakistani women who had received information about a problem with their pregnancy were most concerned about the practical ethical problem of whether or not to continue with the pregnancy in the knowledge of a serious abnormality.

Considering terminations: differences of opinion

When Miriam learnt at her twenty-week scan performed in the regional hospital that her baby had many serious abnormalities, that 'basically everything was outside the body', she was told unambiguously that the baby would not survive. This gave her two options: to end the pregnancy or to carry on with the pregnancy and give birth to a baby that would be stillborn or die very soon afterwards: 'They said that whatever I decided there was no chance that the baby would survive, but also, whatever I decided, they would support me. But I was twenty weeks gone, so I could not terminate. It is an individual thing. Maybe if I had known earlier, my decision would have been different, but that was my decision.' Miriam described her response, that at 'twenty weeks gone' it was too late to terminate, as 'an individual view' rather than one representing an Islamic or religious standpoint; if she had known earlier, she said, she might have decided differently. I found that several other women likewise thought an early termination would be acceptable, but that they could not envisage having a later termination, after they could feel the baby moving. Nighat, a thirty-six-year-old college-educated mother of two boys, one of whom has learning difficulties, said that, when she became unexpectedly pregnant for a third time, she would have terminated this pregnancy if an early genetic test had been able to demonstrate conclusively that the foetus was affected:

> I had been through it all with my son. I was so scared the same thing would happen again. They had told me to tell them if we planned another baby, so I went to the consultant and she offered me an early test, where they take something from the womb. I can't remember what the test is called. But then they changed their mind, because, they said, they would not be able to tell me for sure if the baby is affected or not. They said they could not tell me until the very last, not until after four or five months, if the baby would have any problem. I was very upset by that. I mean, they told me I could have some tests when I was four months pregnant, and if I want, you know, to lose the baby after that [she is speaking hesitantly now, and uses the Urdu idiom for termination: *zāiā karnā,* literally to 'lose' or 'waste' the baby] but it was a very late stage. I just did not want ... There is no point ... [in a test] after four months ... I wouldn't mind going for the very early stages.

Neither Miriam nor Nighat described their views on ending a pregnancy as religious. Miriam's emphasis that this 'is an individual thing' could be interpreted as an attempt to avoid religious stereotyping, rather like Hamid Ullah's comment, in Chapter 5, that his objection to terminating a pregnancy was 'personal'. The feeling that an early termination is more acceptable than one performed after the mother can feel the baby move is shared by many women, regardless of ethnic or religious background. It is, moreover, consistent with an Islamic position on ending a pregnancy, discussed in more detail below, which accepts early termination within the first three or four months or 120 days of pregnancy, before 'life' (*ruh*, soul, spirit) is breathed into the child (what, in English usage, used to be called the 'quickening'), but which considers termination after this time to be sinful.

On the other hand, a widely held local view prevails within local discourse that termination of pregnancy is unconditionally *gunāh* (sinful) at any time – before or after the 120-day period – or else that it is only permissible if the mother's life is in danger. In Shakeera's case, doctors raised the option of terminating the pregnancy after scans had shown the continuing presence of water on the lungs and confirmed a heart abnormality. Frightened by the idea of having a child with serious disabilities, Shakeera thought she might end the pregnancy at this point, but was equally frightened by her mother's insistence that termination of pregnancy, even where the foetus was expected to have serious abnormalities, would be *gunāh* (sinful) and tantamount to murder:

> The doctors really scared me, they would say, have an abortion. At one point, I thought I might, even before the scans showed the fluid on the brain and by then it was medically too late to abort. My husband said he would support me, whatever I decided. But my Mum said that, in our religion, termination is a sin, it is murder and God will punish you after death – unless it is certain that the mother will die. If the mother's life is at risk it is justified because, if the child lives and the mother dies, who will look after that child? The child will be a problem. But otherwise they say it is not allowed. My Mum said she would look after the baby if it was handicapped – I was terrified of ruining my life by having a handicapped child. My Dad told me to pray. He said, 'The doctors aren't always right. These things are in the hands of God.'

Shakeera's Pakistan-raised husband would have supported her had she chosen to end the pregnancy. Yet Shakeera also felt strongly that her mother might be right – that to end the pregnancy would indeed be sinful unless Shakeera's own life was clearly in danger. Among the several books written in English about Islam and kept in her parents' front room, there was one to which Shakeera had referred for guidance. In it, a section confirmed that termination of pregnancy is only allowed if the mother's life is threatened, for then there would be no one to care for the child; ending the pregnancy would then represent the lesser of two evils. This view prevailed among other older, pioneer-generation migrants from rural Punjab and Azad Kashmir and among some younger adults. Sofia, who has lived in England for four years, considered that 'to stop the pregnancy, even early on, is *nājāiz* (illegitimate) – that is the word you use for a bastard – it is not allowed in our religion'. Hamid's wife Humairah, who has lived in England for three years, told me, in the context of a discussion of her own risks of having a child with major learning difficulties: 'You cannot waste the baby (*bachche ko zāiā karnā,* i.e. terminate the pregnancy) because when the chromosomes from the mother and from the father mix together the baby starts and there is a soul: you cannot kill the soul, that is sin (*gunāh*) and God will punish you.

What does Islam say?

These snapshots of local perceptions indicate variation rather than consensus in understandings of the Islamic position on abortion, but they also show that the topic of abortion is surrounded with a strong sense of disquiet. This disquiet stems, in part, from an understanding of Islamic teachings regarding the use of reproductive technologies constructed in opposition to what is perceived as Western morality regarding use of these technologies. It also derives from an understanding that, according to Qur'anic teachings, certain kinds of activity are intrinsically wrong.

In her contribution to a volume presenting the case for family planning in world religions, Sa'diyya Shaikh argues that instances of contemporary Muslim resistance to contraception and abortion, such as illustrated by the vociferous antipathy expressed by leaders in some Muslim countries towards the 1994 United Nations family planning and population control initiative, should be understood in the context of post-colonial power relations:

> Over the past several centuries the shift in the balance of power between Islam and western powers has contributed to a polarised 'Islam vs. the West' schema. In the current era, this is exacerbated by the fact that Euro-American cultural forms, through the processes of globalisation, are perceived as encroaching and increasingly threatening to Muslim societies. Within this context family planning, contraceptive usage, and access to abortion are regularly framed as either a conspiracy by western powers to limit the growth and power of the Muslim world or as a reflection of the permissive sexual mores of western society. Thus, the issues relating to birth control are submerged within a larger minefield of political and cultural polemics. (Shaikh 2003: 106)

This offers a framework within which to read the work of such scholars as Pakistan's Maulana Maududi, whose argument that family planning and contraception contradict some of the basic premises of Islam is also underpinned by a patriarchal gender ideology in which women are morally inferior to men and confined to roles in the domestic sphere (Maududi 1974; Shaikh 2003). In contrast, Shaikh argues, the historical treatment of contraception and family planning within several traditional Islamic sources reveals a legacy of thinking on these issues that takes a more complex, less defensive stance.

Islam is often defined as providing guidance for the conduct of all aspects of everyday life, particularly as expressed in Islamic *shar'īa* law. The *shar'īa* law consists of social and ethical guidance originally worked out by scholars in the second century and constructed from several sources. Its two chief sources are the Qur'an, regarded as the Word of God as revealed to the Prophet Mohammad (in the final and most perfect revelation in a series of revelations to earlier prophets), which offers general and specific guidance on the handling of legal, social and political questions, and the Prophetic Traditions, comprising the *sunnā* and the Hadith, which provide details of how the obligations and prohibitions in the Qur'an should be interpreted. The *sunnā* (literally 'customs') comprise a collection of social and legal principles derived from Hadith, which are sayings of and stories about the Prophet told by his Companions, originally handed down by oral tradition. Following a system called *isnād* ('backing'), individual Hadith have been authenticated by Islamic scholars and classified as reliable, good or weak. To establish meaning where the Qur'an and Traditions are ambiguous, Islamic jurists also use two other processes: *qiyās* (analogy), which involves applying to a new problem the principles underpinning an already agreed point, and *ijmā* (consensus), the unanimous opinion of Islamic scholars, the *ulamā*. The development of *shar'īa* law has resulted in seven schools, six of them associated with Sunni orthodoxy, which accounts for the majority (between 80 and 90 per cent) of the Muslim world, and one constituting the Shi'a branch; each recognises the Qur'an, the *sunnā* and analogical reasoning (in some form) as key sources, and across all there is substantial agreement on key issues.[3]

The Qur'an and Traditions are unambiguous and explicit on many doctrinal and practical issues, such as the five 'pillars' of Islam (the confession of faith, prayer, alms-giving, fasting and pilgrimage) as outward expressions of belief in All'ah, but are ambiguous or implicit on such issues as contraception and termination of pregnancy. Islamic scholars may make a judgement and arrive at a legal solution on issues on which the primary sources are ambiguous (*ijtihādī* issues) by means of the process of *ijtihād*, which involves interpretation, analogy or reasoning informed by the spirit of the Qur'an. Their religious opinions, known as *fatwas*, determine whether a particular action is obligatory (*wajab*), recommended (*sunnā*), permitted (*mubah*), disapproved (*makruh*) or prohibited unconditionally (*harām*). Any religious scholar may offer a *fatwa*, but in Egypt, for instance, the government recognises only three official sources. One of them, the Al-Azhar university, is 'considered by most Muslims to be the center for Islamic education in the Muslim world' and so *fatwas* issued from there 'have great weight throughout the Arab countries as well as [the] non-Arab Muslim world' (Inhorn 2003: 96)

The process of reasoning, moreover, is not confined to scholars who issue *fatwas* but also rests with the individual, who is invested with moral agency, in accordance with the foundational principles of Qur'anic teachings about God and humanity. The central principle is that of *tauhīd* or the unity of God: that God is one, and he has no partner. From this stems the Qur'anic concept that each person belongs to God and must use their capacity for knowledge and reasoning (*fitrah*) to know God, most importantly through the exercise of their moral agency (*khilāfah*) (see Rahman 1980: 18; Shaikh 2003: 107). The emphasis here is on an individual's knowledge and understanding, their personal and social responsibilities and their powers of choice: the human being is God's trustee, his *khalīfah* or moral agent, working to fulfil God's purpose.

Such a view permits a more nuanced Islamic approach to family planning, contraception and abortion, as *ijtihādī* issues on which the Qur'an and Traditions do not offer unambiguous teachings. Opponents often base their views on a 'literal' reading of the Qur'anic injunction not to kill one's children: 'Kill not your children, on a plea of want, we provide sustenance for you and for them' (Qur'an 6: 151, quoted in Shaikh 2003: 113). An alternative reading puts this text into historical context by considering it a response to the pre-Islamic practices of burying alive female infants: it can thus be read as a condemnation of misogyny and infanticide and not of family planning (Rahman 1982: 286–87).

Those opposed to family planning also frequently argue that to intervene in reproduction represents the thwarting of God's will, an assertion of one's own will against God's, and this counters the spirit of Islam, which demands trust in God (Omran 1992). As Shakeera's father had said, 'These things are in the hands of God.' The following verses support this argument:

> There is no creature on earth, but its sustenance depends on God. He knows its habitation and its preservation. (Qur'an 11: 6)
> And whoever is conscious of God, He will find a way out [of difficulty] for him, and He will provide for him in a manner beyond all expectation, and for every one that places their trust in God, He alone is sufficient. (Qur'an 65: 2–3).

An alternative reading is that, while the belief that ultimately everything rests with God is central to Islamic belief, it does not necessarily follow that this absolves human beings from taking active responsibility for themselves and for others. Indeed, such a conclusion contradicts 'the very fundamental Islamic notion of human *khilafah* ... [which] includes using the faculties of reason, judgment, and God-consciousness ... to plan one's life, to seek out sustenance, and to strive actively for the well-being of self and society in relation to the challenges of our age', including those posed by population growth (Shaikh 2003: 114). There are Qur'anic verses and Hadith that address the combination of human agency with trust in God; indeed, 'family planning, including contraceptive usage, may be seen as [an] extension of the human capacity to plan, to respond to, and to actively make choices in terms of contextual needs and emerging realities' (Shaikh 2003: 114).

Historically, Shaikh notes, the majority of the Islamic legal schools have permitted coitus interruptus (*azl*) as a contraceptive method, with the wife's consent, while in the ninth century, medical and legal discussion concerned whether or not the husband's consent was necessary for the use of female contraceptive techniques (see also Musallam 1983; Omran 1992). In the medieval period, the overarching permissibility of contraceptive practice is evident also in the voluminous, detailed research conducted into the medical and legal aspects of contraceptive use (Musallam 1983). The scholar Al Ghazzali (d. 1111), for instance, supported decisions to use contraception for reasons that included avoiding financial and psychological hardship (Farah 1984). Rather than representing a Western conspiracy aimed at limiting the Muslim population of the world, Shaikh considers this Islamic argument in favour of family planning to be of direct relevance to solving the current socio-economic problems faced by the world's growing population. Summarising a survey of contemporary conferences and publications by Islamic scholars on the permissibility of contraception, she notes that the key arguments involve 'an application of Qur'anic ethical principles to the perceived needs of the age', including promoting ease and quality of life, not hardship. Contraceptive practices 'that temporarily avert pregnancy' are analogous to *azl* and therefore permissible, while those resulting in permanent infertility are not, except under exceptional circumstances (Shaikh 2003: 114–17). In addition, while the views of religious experts may be helpful, she stresses that 'in Islam, the individual believer retains the right to make her own decisions on the basis of being a moral agent (*khalifah*). These decisions need to be informed by the primary sources and the Islamic principles of justice, human well-being, mercy, and compassion, where freedom is always accompanied by moral and spiritual responsibilities' (2003: 119).

Regarding termination of pregnancy rather than contraception, there is less consensus in Islamic teachings, which historically range from unqualified permission to end a pregnancy before 120 days to unconditional prohibition (Musallam 1983: 57–59). The issues here concern the moral status of the foetus, the process of foetal development and the stage at which the foetus can be considered human. Muslim scholars refer to two particular Qur'anic verses in this regard, one suggesting stages of development, the other embellishing on this idea:

> He creates you in the wombs of your mothers
> In stages, one after another
> In three veils of darkness
> Such is All'ah, your Lord and Cherisher. (Qur'an 39: 6)
>
> We created the human being from a quintessence of clay
> Then we placed him as semen in a firm receptacle
> Then we formed the semen into a blood-like clot
> Then we formed the clot into a lump of flesh
> Then we made out of that lump, bones
> And clothed the bones with flesh
> Then we developed out of it another creation
> So Blessed is Allah the Best Creator.
> (Qur'an 23: 12–13, quoted in Shaikh 2003: 120)

An authenticated Hadith offers a more specific time frame for foetal development, culminating in the transformation of the foetus into a human being:

> Each of you is constituted in your mother's womb for 40 days as *nutfa* (semen), then it becomes an *alaqa* (clot) for an equal period, then a *mudgha* (lump of flesh) for another equal period, then the angel is sent and he breathes the *ruh* (spirit) into it. (Muslim, Book of Qadr, Hadith no. 4781, quoted in Shaikh 2003: 120)

These sources provide the basis of teaching that 'ensoulment' (or animation) happens at 120 days, when the foetus is significantly transformed into a human being by the angel breathing the spirit into it; as the Qur'anic verse suggests, 'Then we developed out of it another creation'.

Most interpretations of the Islamic position prohibit termination after 120 days unless the foetus threatens the life of the mother or where the pregnancy is harming an already suckling child or where the foetus is expected to be seriously deformed (Omran 1992: 192). However, views differ on whether termination is permissible before animation (Ahmed et al. 2000: 382). Shaikh states that there are four different positions in classic Islamic law relating to termination before 120 days: (1) unconditional permission; (2) conditional permission for an acceptable medical or social reason; (3) strong disapproval (*makruh*); and (4) unconditional prohibition.[4]

This range of positions reflects both respect for the potential of human life and a concern to view the well-being of the foetus in relation to that of the mother, the family and the wider society. Even within a single locality, religious leaders may take varying positions, some saying there must also be medical grounds for termination before 120 days, others being less dogmatic. In High Wycombe, one Pakistan-trained *imām* told me termination of pregnancy was justified on social grounds in the case of unmarried girls, for otherwise the child would be illegitimate; this provides a 'reasonable cause', which also justified abortion in nineteenth-century Hanifi scholarship (Shaikh 2003: 123). Balancing social and ethical considerations, in 1998 a *fatwa* from Al-Azhar University in Egypt permitted abortion of pregnancies following rape (ibid.: 122). Foetal abnormality is included among other 'reasonable causes' for terminating a pregnancy within the first 120 days in *fatwa*s from Islamic states such as Kuwait and Saudi Arabia (Abel Haleem 1993; Alkuraya and Kilani 2001). In Iran in 2000, a *fatwa* was issued permitting abortion of foetuses at less than ten weeks when testing positively for thalassaemia, and another permits it in the first trimester of pregnancy for reasons that include the mother's health and foetal abnormality (Shaikh 2003: 122)

In Pakistan there has been no state-authorised *fatwa* equivalent to the Kuwaiti or Saudi opinions, and evidence suggests that people are often unaware that there are Islamic views that permit termination of pregnancy, either conditionally or unconditionally, before 120 days. Nonetheless, authoritative statements by

Muslim scholars can influence parents' decision-making in the light of a diagnosed abnormality. When a city-based prenatal diagnosis service for thalassaemia was introduced, couples who were initially hesitant to use it were reassured when two well-known religious scholars confirmed that termination of an affected foetus before 120 days of gestation was permissible (Ahmed et al. 2000: 382).

In the light of this range of views, I want to return now to Shakeera's story. Caught between the fear of having a child with serious disabilities and the knowledge that her parents would not support her in having a termination (although her husband would) Shakeera talked to her sister. Her sister suggested that Shakeeera consulted a sister-in-law whose experiences had been rather similar to Shakeera's, and whose husband is an *imām* who did his religious training in Egypt. Shakeera learnt from her sister that this couple's first child had died a few hours after birth from a genetic condition, their next two children were unaffected, but, when, in the fourth pregnancy, a scan showed another affected child, the couple chose to terminate the pregnancy. Shakeera thought: 'if she did it, I could. But she just did not want to talk about it with me, I think because my parents didn't know about it, and my sister-in-law and her husband wanted to keep it quiet. I wanted her backing, but she didn't want to talk about it.' As this indicates, the fear of local disapproval can powerfully inhibit open discussion on this sensitive issue. In fact, it was only after her baby was born, had died and was buried that Shakeera heard about an alternative religious view on termination of pregnancy where the baby has a fatal abnormality from a woman who, as is customary, came to the house to offer condolences:

> That's when I realised that's why my sister-in-law had an abortion, but she didn't want to explain this to her parents, or to my parents. Just now, when I was in the kitchen and you were in the bathroom, I said to my Mum you had come to talk because you are interested in knowing if a Muslim woman can terminate a pregnancy. She said, '*istighfār-ull'ah!*' That's like what you say when someone does something wrong (it means something like 'God, have mercy'). That is what she said when I told her my sister-in-law had it done. It is a shame that people don't discuss these things. Why don't they discuss it on digital, or on TV? Or even have some leaflets about Islam and abortion. So many people don't know what to do. They say Islam has a solution for everything. So why are there no guidelines for this?

Personal circumstances, community context and exercising moral agency

Knowing the formal Islamic scholarship on the issue of abortion is not, however, the only consideration in couples' negotiations of prenatal foetal abnormality. Shakeera's story points to the importance of having 'backing' from an authoritative source such as a trusted relative or someone with religious authority, especially for a decision that counters prevailing opinion. Even then it can be difficult for individuals to make a decision that they know will be disapproved of by parents, other close kin or neighbours.

There may be doubts about the accuracy of the diagnosis, especially if it concerns a first pregnancy where there is no prior experience or family history of the suspected condition. As we saw, Shakeera continued to hope the doctors were wrong even after scans showed fatal abnormalities; she considers she would terminate were she to face this situation again, because, despite 'preparing' herself, the experience of giving birth to a tragically malformed baby was so traumatic:

> They'd said [in the last two scans] that the baby's belly had something connected to it, part of a rib ... When I saw the rib coming from the belly button, I was so scared. I didn't know if I should pick her up. Her head was huge compared to her face, all the skin went in because they'd drained the fluid. Her head was cone-shaped, like a pyramid, not round, she looked very abnormal. Even the nurse felt so scared when she was delivering her that she had to ask for assistance [breaks down into tears].
>
> My husband and the nurse saw her first.[5] I thought my husband was going to faint. I had not seen her head. I looked at him and thought maybe he is just scared because he has seen what has happened. Then I saw her head. I looked at my husband and asked, 'Have you seen her head?' He said nothing at all. Then the paediatrician came and said there is nothing we can do. I didn't even kiss her ... [tears]...
>
> The doctor asked, have you got a name for her? My husband told them her name. They took me upstairs to the en suite and I sat there with her. I was desperate for my family to come. I thought they would tell me what to do. Then my family came. My Mum picked her up and said she was beautiful. I remember her coughing once, but she did not make movements. She was in my brother's arms when she died. He was whispering, 'She has gone really cold' and at that point I knew she had passed away ...
>
> I expected it, but I was never really ready for it. I thought she would be OK.

In another case of a first pregnancy, a marketing trainee in her twenties, married to a first cousin, decided on a late termination of a pregnancy after it was shown to have multiple structural abnormalities 'incompatible with life'. In this case, she was supported by her sister and parents, whose reasoning hinged upon a distinction between a baby that would die at birth and a baby that would have a life as a handicapped child, but her husband remained sceptical about the diagnosis. Her sister explained:

> She carried the baby for six months but the doctors said the baby would die within an hour or two of being born because they found many things wrong with him. They said he might live only half an hour. It was not a

> fifty-fifty situation. He would certainly die. His heart was wrong, his liver was wrong. His kidneys were very large. His stomach was full with kidney. He would not live for more than a couple of hours. My sister thought it over, and her parents, and the family. We did not want her to carry for nine months a baby that would die. It is not as if he is a handicapped baby. If God gives you a handicapped baby, you would still love them, and look after them. But this baby was going to die. My sister said she would think it over. The next morning, she rang me to say her husband won't let her go through with it. He wants to keep the pregnancy. He is like our parents' generation in his thinking ... He did not go to school here. He thinks the doctors had made a mistake. He thought, God knows, they don't know anything. How can they say? Then I spoke to him and explained and he agreed.

Several months later, the parents were still grieving for the baby they might have had, and the sister felt responsible, wondering if she and her parents had advised wrongly: 'I made her make the termination. I don't know if I made the right decision. Someone told me the other day that they had been told they had a high risk of an abnormal baby, but they kept it, and the baby turned out to be fine.'

From a medical perspective, a 'high-risk' pregnancy in the probabilistic sense – where there is, for instance, a recessive or dominant recurrence risk (of one in four or one in two) of a serious problem – belongs to a wider realm of uncertainty than a pregnancy in which markers of serious or fatal abnormalities have been seen on prenatal ultrasound and perhaps also confirmed by a prenatal genetic or chromosomal test. This distinction is often lost in local discourse, in which stories circulate about pregnancies deemed 'high-risk' that result in perfectly healthy babies. Nonetheless, as discussed in Chapter 5, circumstance and experience, particularly a previous experience of having a child with serious behavioural problems or multiple disabilities associated with a limited life expectancy, can prompt women to consider terminating such 'risky' pregnancies, even in the absence of a 'positive' prenatal diagnosis. These cases can be viewed as instances in which women exercise their moral agency, but may also become cautionary tales against the termination of pregnancy. Shamim, who has two healthy children, has also lost two infants to an unnamed condition, presumed recessive, and was very worried by the prospect of having another affected child when she became unexpectedly pregnant again, learning this during a routine check of her IUD. The doctors, she said, 'told me that I had a high risk' (they gave a one in four risk) and made an appointment for ending the pregnancy. As the date approached, 'I asked my mother-in-law, and she said, "No, don't do it" and told me she had a termination once, in Pakistan, and this is why her daughter developed a mental illness. God had punished her. So I told the doctor to cancel the appointment; it was not easy to do but I found the courage.' She did not feel she had been coerced by the clinicians to terminate; on the contrary: 'They had a duty to tell me that the risk was high and to offer me a termination. I did my duty too. I thought about what I was afraid of and I found courage. When our son was born, our GP brought us flowers. I could see she had tears in her eyes.'

The locally dominant discourse of disapproval means that a decision to end a pregnancy can be socially and psychologically problematic, making the couple vulnerable to disapproval from some members of their family or community. Riffat, who viewed her son with Down syndrome as a blessing from God (Chapter 5), terminated a later pregnancy because she felt she could not manage another affected child, especially given her family circumstances, and this time consulted only her husband. Lying on a trolley recovering from the anaesthetic, she recognised one of the porters as a Pakistani neighbour and noticed that he glanced at her identification tag. The following day, this man's wife came to her home; Riffat protected herself by denying she had been in hospital, suggesting the man was mistaken.

In response to the potential for gossip, women may arrange with their doctors for terminations to be performed somewhere other than in the local hospital. In such circumstances, sometimes women who end a pregnancy tell their relatives that the baby 'fell' (*bachchā gir gayā*), employing the euphemism for a miscarriage, to avoid the suggestion of their own agency in the process. Alternatively, they may tell their doctors that 'abortion is forbidden in my religion' or 'my mother-in-law won't allow it', thus closing negotiations rather than proceeding further into this morally risky territory. Another strategy is to tell relatives that a decision was 'medical', as if the matter was decided for them by the doctors (despite the professional philosophy of non-directiveness). One young Pakistan-raised mother whose first child died after four days in intensive care and whose second child was stillborn told me they would 'do what the doctors say' if genetic tests, which became available for the condition in this family during my fieldwork, found evidence of the same fatal condition, her phrasing playing down her own agency. A decision to end a pregnancy on medical grounds may thus be made without any explicit reference to religious teachings. As we saw in Chapter 5 (in a comment from Nadia's husband), mothers' and fathers' views on the acceptability of genetic testing and ending an affected pregnancy may change in the light of experience of caring for children with disabilities, such that they may become more open to the idea of termination in a subsequent pregnancy than they would have been had they never had a disabled child themselves. I have suggested here that in practical terms these decisions require not just professional respect for the privacy of the couple but discretion in the couple's negotiation of communication in the family and locality, given the moral disquiet associated with the subject of ending a pregnancy.

The withdrawal of life support

A similar disquiet surrounds the negotiation of death when it becomes clear to medical staff that infants born with fatal abnormalities supported in the special care baby unit will not survive. As with the issue of termination, the reality is more complex than the stereotype that Muslim parents would, under no circumstances, do anything that might be interpreted as assisting death, as the following case illustrates. Talib is the young father of a premature baby supported for three months in intensive care, whose wife speaks very little English. He was eventually asked by the doctors to decide if medication should continue and if the baby should be kept alive with a ventilator. He turned for advice to a *pīr* (spiritual guide, saint) known to his family for generations, who happened to be visiting Britain:

> Often, people say things to a *pīr* just to get an opinion that suits them. I wanted him to understand. He stayed there about half an hour. I think he was disturbed by what he saw. He said he thought it would be wrong to make her die, but it would be wrong to increase her suffering. So I said to the doctors, just keep the tubes and medicines, but don't do anything more, no ventilator now. It is up to her, we will see if she has the will to live or not. And I could see, with her mouth open, no control, that it was too much for her.

Relating this experience to me soon afterwards, Talib stressed this was a personal decision and one that he felt he would be able to live with. His reasoning was that the doctors had done what they could and his *pīr* had reassured him that he had not done anything sinful that could be considered murder. However, he had not told close family members; the rest of the family simply understood that the baby died. Two years later, I talked with him about whether tissue samples had been taken for research from this baby, since the clinicians thought they might now be able to perform a genetic test on stored tissue (which might also result in a prenatal test). Our conversation led to a discussion about death, post-mortems and the ritual treatment of the body, during which Talib asserted that it would be wrong, under any circumstances, to withdraw life support. Remembering what he had told me during our previous conversation, I asked if he therefore distinguished medication and tubes from ventilation, but rather than answering this question, he asked for my reassurance that he would not be identifiable from my research reports; I reassured him and let the subject drop. During my fieldwork, three other couples consented to the withdrawal of life support from their severely handicapped infants, after the medical problems had been explained; they, too, had simply told their relatives that their babies died. This, I suggest, is a strategy to avoid further pain in what is already a painful experience, in view of the moral ambiguities posed by the intervention of human agency into processes that are usually talked about as being 'up to God'. An individual or couple's moral agency, itself the outcome of ethical struggle, can be at odds with a dominant 'public' or family view, which may offer less scope for negotiation and in relation to which the individual or couple risks public censure.

Grief and the social recognition of pregnancy loss

The emotional impact of a medical diagnosis 'foretelling' infant death, prenatally or after birth, is complex and not necessarily lessened if couples choose to end such a pregnancy or withdraw life support, particularly if doubts remain about the accuracy of the medical diagnosis or the religious acceptability of intervening in processes considered 'up to God', even where couples have made a responsible, morally informed decision. The emotional impact of infant death is profoundly shaped by the social and moral contexts in which it occurs and for British Pakistanis this includes disquiet over 'ending a life'. It also concerns the social value of having children and the particular social implications of unsuccessful childbearing for women. The emotional impact of pregnancy loss may also be related to aspects of the social recognition of the loss, particularly as these are expressed through conventions of mourning and funerary practice in which ideas about whether the foetus or newborn baby is fully a person play an important part.

Pregnancy loss may be especially acutely felt where marriage and motherhood provide the dominant positive image for women. A common local understanding was that the emotional impact of pregnancy loss – miscarriage, abortion, stillbirth or early infant death – is less for women who already have living children. Miriam, who already had two daughters when her son was stillborn, said that, if this had been her first pregnancy, 'I think I would have gone crazy. I would have thought, "I'm a failure. My husband is going to divorce me." But I have two healthy children. My heart goes out to those people who have this happen for the first time.' While recent psychological studies challenge this assumption (Jackman et al. 1991; Slade 1994), it is also clear that social and cultural context can profoundly shape these experiences. As we saw in Sofia's case (Chapter 4) and in many societies, reproductive failure has serious implications for women's lives. In rural north India and Pakistan, pregnancy loss is shameful and polluting (as is menstruation), while infertility or the lack of any surviving children constitutes grounds for divorce or taking another wife (Jeffery and Jeffery 1996b: 17, 24; Shaw 2000a: 215–20). Yet the psychological literature (which is large in comparison with anthropological studies of miscarriage, stillbirth and neonatal death) is equivocal on this point, perhaps because it draws largely on Euro-American research and does not explore the implications of diversity in social and cultural context (Cordle and Prettyman 1994; Robinson et al. 1994; Statham and Green 1994).

In both popular and academic contemporary Western psychology, there is also an understanding that the emotional burden of bereavement is easier to bear, if not lessened, when a death is socially recognised by family and community, including through funerary rites. Nancy Kohner and Alix Henley, describing the experience of late miscarriage and stillbirth, write that 'the loss of a baby is the loss of a person', noting that parents' grief is thus at least in part about adjusting to their lost identity as parents of that child (1991: 9). However, a cross-cultural perspective reveals that the relationship between infant death and grief is complicated by culturally variable ideas about what defines personhood. If a baby is not defined as a person and its loss is thus not marked as the loss of a person, it may not be mourned in the same way.

In societies where maternal and infant mortality rates are high, miscarriage and stillbirth seem to be given little social recognition. This observation, coupled with women's reluctance or inability to discuss an experience of failure where childbearing is a woman's primary role, may account for the relative ethnographic silence on this topic (Cecil 1996a: 2). A lack of social recognition for pregnancy loss also seems connected with the idea that a foetus acquires human status only late or ambiguously in pregnancy and with the recognition of an individual as a person only at or some time after birth. In a striking study of life in Brazilian slums, Nancy Scherper-Hughes notes that 'mothers may be slow to personalise the infant, to give it a name, or ... to baptise the child' (1991:1145, 1992). Writing about rural north India, Patricia and Roger Jeffery (1996b) note that infant death is mourned only briefly, pregnancy loss is ritually insignificant and early miscarriage does not constitute the loss of a child because a child becomes 'rooted' in the womb only at three months; before this time, vaginal bleeding is a delayed period, not a lost pregnancy. In south-east Tanzania, the loss of premature or malformed infants is not elaborately mourned because such infants are not considered human; indeed, the human status of an unborn child is ambiguous and can only be known at birth when a midwife checks the baby for defects (Wembah-Rashid 1996: 89–90).

It is an anthropological truism that emotional expression is socially and culturally shaped. As Richard Huntington and Peter Metcalf write: 'Cultural difference works on the universal human emotional material ... the range of acceptable emotions and the constellation of sentiments appropriate to the situations of death are tied up with the unique institutions and concepts of each society' (1979: 43; see also Abu-Lughod 1986: 206). Thus, it might follow that, if stillbirth and miscarriage are not regarded as the loss of a child, the loss itself might be less painful. Nancy Scherper-Hughes suggests that the gradual processes of maternal attachment to children that she observed in the Brazilian slums constitute 'individual and collective defences' against infant death, enabling 'death without weeping' (1991: 1145, 1992). In rural north India, Patricia and Roger Jeffery (1996b) observe that women speak of what Western doctors would define as miscarriage and stillbirth with a notable lack of emotion in comparison with the distress with which they recalled the deaths of toddlers and children.

Against this view, a lack of formal or informally expressed emotion does not necessarily indicate a lack of emotional distress. As Jeffery and Jeffery note for rural north India, mothers 'had little opportunity to mourn their loss openly or at length' (1996b: 29). Rosanne Cecil's edited volume on the anthropology of pregnancy loss suggests that, even where a miscarried or stillborn foetus is not considered a baby or a person and its loss is not ritually mourned, the experience remains distressing for women. Elderly Northern Irishwomen's recollections of miscarriage in the early twentieth century, at a time of high but declining rates of fertility and perinatal and maternal mortality, reveal personal, emotional pain and distress despite the lack of social significance attributed to their experiences at the time (Cecil 1996b). Wembah-Rashid notes of contemporary south-east Tanzania that the loss of only briefly mourned premature or malformed babies nonetheless causes women considerable distress and anxiety because of the importance of reproduction. The bereaved couple are consoled by relatives and friends and 'are encouraged to forget the loss and look ahead with courage and enthusiasm because they possess the potential for having babies' (Wembah-Rashid 1996: 92). In my study, as I detail below, several U.K.-raised British Pakistani women spoke of the distress caused by late miscarriage or stillbirth, as well as by late termination for fetal abnormality, as noted above, all of which are given only brief ritual and social recognition.

Historical context also plays a role in shaping and changing ideas about the value of a pregnancy.[6] The Northern Irishwomen in Rosanne Cecil's study who recalled their experiences of miscarriage in the early twentieth century were particularly aware that the meaning and management of miscarriage and premature birth had changed dramatically in the course of their lifetime. Had their miscarried pregnancies happened later in the century, when, with the availability of new technologies of life support, what was lost was more highly valued, then some of their premature babies might have survived. Despite a lack of legal, lay, clerical or medical consensus over when a foetus becomes human, recent developments in reproductive medicine enabling very premature babies to survive do seem to be associated with radical changes in perceptions of the status of the foetus and the newborn (Cecil 1996b). In my study, for several young U.K.-raised British Pakistani women who experienced stillbirth, the lack of social recognition accorded by their family and community for their loss was itself a source of distress and contestation. For these women, as for the women in Rosanne Cecil's study, the lack of ritual recognition of their loss contrasted starkly with the rituals associated with an adult death.

Rituals of death, *janāza* (funeral) and burial

Shakeera's daughter, Sofia's son (Chapter 3) and Talib's daughters are among the infants buried in the in the Muslim section of the local cemetery, set into a hillside fairly close to the town centre. As you walk through the cemetery with its well-maintained paths, the upper part of it that is allocated for Muslim burials gradually becomes visible because, in contrast with the other graves, the tombstones all face east, towards Mecca. The face of a deceased person must face the Ka'ba in Mecca and the legs must face the opposite way (and likewise in sleep; thus beds and sofas are placed so that a person can lie with their head towards Mecca). The number of Muslim graves is comparatively small, because the bodies of most deceased adults, especially men who were born in Pakistan, are usually returned to Pakistan as the 'homeland' (*apnā mulk*) for burial in cemeteries located at the edges of migrants' villages of origin, alongside other members of their *birādarī*. Bodies are preferably buried in Pakistan so that, as people say, relatives there can see the deceased person's body and pay their respects for one last time before burial and *sawāb* (blessing) will accrue to the deceased person's account with God (which will be weighed up on the Day of Judgement) through the prayers of the many kin who will visit the grave; fewer people, I was told, visit the local cemetery in Britain, because fewer people are buried there (see Shaw 2000a: 100, 278; see also Gardner 2002, on the burial overseas of British Bengalis).

Although this attitude to place of burial is common among pioneer-generation migrants, some younger U.K.-born adults say they expect to be buried locally. Increasingly, British Muslims are being buried in specially designated Muslim burial sites, usually established after negotiations with local authorities (Eade 1996). Locally, these burials include some women and men whose expressed wish was to be buried where their children are settled and some whose children decided, sometimes contrary to parental wishes, to bury their parents locally so that they could visit their graves (Shaw 2004). Some of the highly decorated tombstones have inscriptions that offer insights into these aspects of the migration and settlement history of this community.

Perhaps the most striking feature of the Muslim cemetery, however, is the fact that, alongside the lines of adult graves, there is a roughly equal number of lines of smaller graves – I counted a total of 176 small graves – in which infants and children are buried. Some of these are unmarked grassy mounds of earth but many have elaborately decorated tombstones carrying inscriptions that bear witness to the brevity of the child's life – noting a death that occurred a few moments, hours, days or months after birth, or marking the short life of an older infant – thus registering the profound sense of loss experienced by the parents.

According to Muslim belief, the bodies of deceased Muslims should be buried as soon after death as possible because the soul remains in the body and continues to suffer, at least until burial. Talib explained it this way:

> Once a Muslim person has died, their body will feel pain and torture until the body is put in the ground and given back to God. Even then, their suffering may continue, especially in the first forty days, and that is why we pray for that individual, to relieve their pain and suffering. That pain to the soul is greater than any you would experience in life.

Consequently, although embalming is common practice when corpses are returned to Pakistan for burial, some people are highly critical of the practice, maintaining that in Islam, a person should be buried where they die, in accordance with the requirement for burial as soon after the moment of death as possible. Talib would have preferred his father to be buried locally; it was ironic, he said, that such a pious man, who had never touched alcohol in his life, had to suffer in this way after death. Likewise, autopsy should be avoided: as Talib put it, 'A post-mortem amounts to cutting up the body. With any Muslim family, if an elder dies, they say no to the post-mortem.' British law requires post-mortems in cases of unexpected deaths, including of infants, and in these cases bodies may not be returned for weeks or months, causing considerable distress to relatives, although some coroners who work with Muslims try to return bodies quickly (Gardner 2002: 200). Khalida was very upset that she had to wait for a post-mortem following the sudden and totally unexpected death of her nine-month-old son:

> They wouldn't release his body for ten days, so we could not have the funeral until then. I spoke to the coroner ten times, to find out why it was taking so long. It was probably because they couldn't understand what had happened. They were looking for something, like abuse. But there was no abuse. You won't find a single case of abuse among the Pakistanis. No one would do that to their children, they value them too much.

In this case, Khalida understood that the tissue samples that were retained for use in mutation research would be released later, so that the family could hold a memorial, but she continued to worry that these might be disposed of without parental consent.

Where a neonatal death occurs under medical surveillance, a post-mortem is not usually required, so this was not a concern for the parents in the remaining (7/8) cases of infant death in my sample: these parents and doctors had known of the fatal or potentially fatal problems during the pregnancy or at or soon after birth. Nonetheless, some parents were asked to consent to a post-mortem or at least to the storage of tissue samples or umbilical cord blood for diagnostic purposes or mutation research (a cord blood sample may be sufficient for research, rendering a biopsy or post-mortem unnecessary). Talib thus agreed to a biopsy of tissue, which eventually enabled a genetic diagnosis, while withholding consent to a post-mortem, believing that further suffering would accompany this more invasive procedure and wanting the bodies returned intact in preparation for the Muslim funeral (*janāza*).

A body released from hospital premises is usually taken directly to the mosque so that it can be prepared for the funeral (*janāza*); there are no 'laying out' facilities for Muslims in British hospitals.[7] Less often, the body is returned briefly to the home, where female relatives have already gathered to chant, pray and thus mark the bereavement, before being taken to the mosque. Islamic funerary rituals require the body to be properly prepared with a ritual bath (*ghusal*) and then wrapped in unstitched white cloth. It is not usual practice to place the prepared body in a coffin except if the body is being sent to Pakistan, or unless the relatives specially request one. The *ghusal* is done by close female relatives of a deceased woman and by close male relatives of a deceased man, using the purpose-built facilities of the local mosque. In some parts of the U.K., knowledge of how to prepare the body for a funeral has 'passed from the domain of the family, to that of private mosque-sponsored functionaries' (Gardner 2002: 200); in east London, the *ghusal* is performed by Muslim undertakers. However, in High Wycombe and Oxford, although bereaved kin of the deceased sometimes say they lack full knowledge of how to prepare the body, in the cases I know of, relatives performed these rituals themselves, drawing on the knowledge and experience of older members of their community. Shakeera's mother, mother's sister-in-law and husband's mother's sister performed Shakeera's daughter's *ghusal* at the mosque. They placed her body in a coffin because her body seemed too small and vulnerable without one, and then brought her to the house, so that the female relatives gathered there could see her, and so that Shakeera could see her again (newly delivered women are required to stay indoors for forty days) before the coffin was taken to the mosque for the *janāza*.

Janāza refers to the prayers read before burial. These prayers are performed exclusively by men, are led by the *imām*, and usually take place in the mosque. In High Wycombe, *janāza*s are performed in the largest and most central of the three mosques (each is located in a key area of Muslim settlement and all three are administered through a single organising committee) because it can accommodate the largest number of mourners. Even so, if a very large number of people are expected to attend, the *janāza* prayers may be performed in the cemetery at the side of the grave, as is the usual practice in Pakistan. Women do not attend *janāza* prayers, which can only be read by men, but may read other prayers in a separate section of the mosque. If the *janāza* is held outside, women sometimes wait at the edge of the cemetery but may not enter it.

If the body is to be dispatched to Pakistan (usually with the assistance of Pakistani funeral services), two *janāza* prayers may be performed: the first in England and the second at the village cemetery (*qabristān*). If the body is buried locally, as is the case with infant or child funerals, the grave is usually first marked with a board bearing the person's name and after a year, the relatives will order a more permanent gravestone. Often these are ordered in Pakistan, where religious verses can be carved into the tombstones, and then brought to England; I am told that it is easier to get smaller-sized tombstones through customs than large ones (see also Imran and Smith 1997). Talib's two daughters have beautifully carved tombstones made in Mirpur city; Shakeera's husband's parents in Pakistan have ordered a tombstone from Pakistan and her husband will bring it when he next visits his parents. Some parents visit their child's grave regularly: Shakeera was doing so weekly during my fieldwork; Khalida returned early from a trip to Pakistan so that she could be by her son's grave on the anniversary of his birth. Other small graves are less well tended, and women may be fearful of attending the cemetery alone, for fear of *jinn* (named in the Qur'an as part of All'ah's creation), who can cause harm and are believed to lurk in lonely places.

Other personal mementoes include photographs of the dead baby. While the English generally consider it macabre to photograph or even view the body of a deceased beloved relative (photographs of the dead being more usually associated with the 'extraordinary' events of war, terrorism or environmental disasters) in Pakistan and among British Pakistanis it is common practice to take photographs of the dead – of adults and children – to remember them by. Nearly all of the parents whose children had died showed me their child's death photographs. These included images of tiny premature babies in special care, with life-supporting tubes attached, and images of these same babies wrapped in white, in readiness for the *janāza*. Parents of older infants and children usually had many more photographs, taken at different stages of their child's life: Khalida's daughter was making a 'memory book' at school for her dead baby brother.

However, while personal mementoes are important, the *janāza* constitutes the crucial, socially recognised ritual marker of the infant's life, however brief, because it fully acknowledges the social and religious identity of the child. As Rosanne Cecil writes, a funeral 'may be considered to be the formal expression of the community's loss of one of its members. It affirms the worth of the deceased in the eyes of all those who participate' (1996b: 187). As a commemorative ceremony, the funeral's significance extends beyond the occasion of the ceremony itself and also extends to the living participants, for it acknowledges their loss and affirms their continuing worth within their community (Connerton 1989: 44). It is thus both socially and emotionally important for the closest kin of the bereaved.

Unmarked deaths: *azān*, naming and personhood

However, the *janāza* is not performed for babies that have not drawn breath and so does not accompany a late miscarriage or stillbirth. If a baby has not drawn breath, it cannot receive the *azān*, which marks a new baby as a Muslim; *janāza* cannot be performed for a dead baby that has not received the *azān*. *Azān* refers to the words of the Muslim call to prayer, which may be heard five times a day in High Wycombe in homes that have a radio connection to the mosque. To mark a newborn as a Muslim, soon after the birth a senior male relative of the child customarily speaks the words of the *azān* into the child's ear. The *azān* can only be performed if the child is breathing and can be done if the baby draws 'even one breath', but cannot be performed for a newborn baby who has stopped breathing. A baby is thus not formally recognised as a Muslim person without the *azān* and *janāza*, despite the Qur'anic concept of ensoulment at 120 days.

The *janāza* is a crucial social event in marking the child's identity as a Muslim. Without it, the death of an infant is accorded considerably less social recognition. As Miriam put it:

> If he had drawn even one breath, then we would have had a funeral, and all the family would have been there, and he would have been buried in the Muslim section of the cemetery. But no, sometimes, it's like he never existed. One Pakistani couple, I heard, their baby was born dead, and they just left it in the hospital and went home.

This lack of social recognition, dramatically illustrated by the story of the couple who left their stillborn baby in the hospital, reflects the shame and embarrassment surrounding miscarriage and stillbirth in the parts of rural Punjab and Azad Kashmir that many Wycombe Pakistanis are from. Against this background, a U.K. doctor's clinically motivated enquiries, during a prenatal or genetics clinic appointment, about a previous experience or family history of miscarriage may seem inappropriate: when one young U.K.-raised husband replied that he thought his mother had experienced miscarriages, his Pakistan-raised wife stopped him, saying quietly in Panjabi, 'You should not talk about such things.' Shrouded in silence, these lost pregnancies also leave no visible trace: I was told on several occasions that, in Pakistan, a miscarried foetus or dead baby is buried not in the cemetery but outside the boundaries of the village.

There are striking parallels here with the invisibility of pregnancy loss in Rosanne Cecil's historical account from Northern Ireland:

> The ritual of baptism not only gives a child a name but marks its entry into society as a full member. If a child died before baptism it was believed to have gone to limbo, a place where the light of God never shone. Until the 1960s, unbaptized and illegitimate children in Ireland were not usually buried in the consecrated ground of churchyards because the Catholic Church did not regard them as part of its community. (Cecil 1996b: 181).

With no public burial, there would be no pre-burial wake involving family, friends and neighbours and the house would be empty of visitors.

Miriam and her husband have various informal and private markers of their child's personal and religious identity. They gave him a beautiful Muslim name, and believe that a stillborn child born to Muslim parents is Muslim, even without receiving the *azān*. They also took his photographs before he was sent for post-mortem and although they were advised not to see him again before his burial (taking this advice is something Miriam regrets). He is buried in the snowdrop garden, a relatively recent memorial garden for miscarried and stillborn babies, which is located not in the Muslim section but at the lower edge of the public cemetery. Miriam and her husband have visited his grave there several times. The fifteen or so graves of babies born to Muslim parents are set apart from the others in the snowdrop garden and are distinguishable by being unnamed and unmarked, though some still carry the numbers that enable parents to identify them; in contrast, some of the other small graves have name plaques, tombstones and flowers.

The lack of local community recognition of the baby and thus of its loss can be a source of considerable distress for the mothers, as several U.K.-born women articulated. Basharat, a U.K.-raised woman married to a cousin from Pakistan, whose first baby was stillborn, was upset and angered by the way even her close kin failed to acknowledge his personhood: 'My husband and parents would not recognise him as a person to be named, because he had not drawn breath. So I named him myself. He is buried in the snowdrop garden.'

There may be a difference between U.K.-raised and Pakistan-raised adults in their attitudes to miscarriage and stillbirth that reflects changing ideas about the status of the foetus or newborn baby. All women recalled with detail and emotion babies who had been named and buried, but the few older and younger Pakistan-raised women with whom I raised the subject of miscarriage and pregnancy loss tended to be reticent or matter-of-fact on this topic. Sofia did not mention her miscarriages to her mother in Pakistan, for fear of making her anxious about Sofia's security in her in-laws' house. In contrast, younger U.K.-raised women generally raised the topic with me themselves, one woman saying it was only when she told her mother about her miscarriage that she learnt her mother had experienced one too. Similarly, the older Northern Irish women in Rosanne Cecil's (1996b) study had not talked to their daughters or to other younger women about their miscarriages or stillbirths. Two other women said they felt they could not talk openly about miscarriage or stillbirth with the close female kin they had nearby. Miriam felt she could only talk to her husband: 'There is a lot of shame about these things. Our people should own up and admit that these things happen. Then when something goes wrong they don't talk about it and that is really sad. I ended up blaming myself for it.' Miriam had heard of two other cases – one of stillbirth, the other of a late miscarriage – in the few months since her own experience but had not talked directly to the women concerned:

> My cousin, I met her and it was clear she did not want to say anything about it and I did not like to ask, it did not seem appropriate. But I wonder how she is feeling. The baby was not full term. It was born dead at six months. They did not say if it was a boy or girl and I did not ask. I presume it's in the snowdrop garden but I don't know for sure. I don't think she has talked to anyone in the family though I think she will have talked to the hospital staff. She is just twenty-one.
>
> The other, she is a friend, or rather a friend of a friend. I thought she'd had her baby as it was due a month before me and they noticed something at the scan too. She has taken it really badly. It was her first pregnancy and she had been married a long time. She lost the baby at six months, but I don't know exactly what was wrong or what happened, only that the baby died at six months … people don't open up. Her baby is in the snowdrop garden.

The silence shrouding these experiences can also make it difficult even for women like Miriam who are fluent in English to seek professional support:

> All the hospital care was above average, and they do give you phone numbers for if you want to talk to someone. When they gave the numbers I wanted to ring, but I was scared to. Now it is all right, face to face, I can talk, but, when your letter came, my husband said, 'Phone her,' but I was scared to. I think you need someone to check on you after something like this has happened ... It's the women who don't speak English that I feel most sorry for. Who can they talk to? Where can they visit? There should be somewhere at community centres, there should be some counselling. But counselling, the very idea, they think it means you are pathetic and they say they don't want it ...[8] they completely conceal it but it is an emotional and psychological burden. Luckily for me, my husband did not feel he had to hide anything – even he, at one point, cried – and he is not the sort of person to show anything, and we talk about it. We cannot talk to anyone else but we can talk to each other. But people to whom this has happened first time, I can't see them getting any support. They just get on with it and hope the next one is fine. In Pakistan it is even harder because there are no scans, no facilities there and it must all be hidden as if it does not happen at all ... It happens there too, of course, but no one opens up.

Parents of babies born prematurely or expected to die soon after birth may worry about whether the baby will breathe or not, and, if it is likely to die, whether *azān* can be done in time. Fahmida's son lived for two hours, received the *azān* and had a *janāza*; when a similarly affected sister was born two years later, the family were prepared for the possibility that she would die soon, and ensured she received the *azān*. In addition to losing a son at nine months from one recessive condition, Khalida lost a daughter within two hours of her birth and a son one hour after his birth to a second recessive condition. Since the second condition could be detected (by a skilled sonographer) by prenatal scan, the parents were prepared in advance of the birth for the possibility of death and ensured these infants received the *azān*, were named and had a 'proper' funeral (*janāza*). Knowing in advance that her daughter was likely to die soon after birth, Shakeera was very anxious that her father, who was expected to do the *azān*, would reach the hospital on time: 'My Dad did still do the *azān*, but he had been a bit later getting there,' she told me.

A prematurely delivered baby cannot receive the *azān* if he or she does not draw breath. Samina's first baby was born at thirty-six weeks by Caesarean section, and lived for a few more days in intensive care, received the *azān*, was named and is buried *upar* (above) in the Muslim section of the cemetery. But Samina's second child was stillborn and is buried *nīche* (below) (in the snowdrop garden). Samina believed that if the doctors had delivered this baby at thirty-six weeks by Caesarean section she would have lived, at least long enough to be named and have a Muslim burial. She raised this concern with a doctor in her next pregnancy, and was told that in fact her second baby had already died *in utero*, so an early Caesarean would not have affected the outcome. (Doctors are also unwilling to perform a Caesarean section to deliver a dead baby, or one that is sure to die, because of the risk to the mother; see note 2). In the next pregnancy, there were no indications of abnormality but Samina nonetheless wanted 'full medical management' with an early Caesarean, 'so that they can get the baby out early, while it is still breathing'. As her doctor explained, medical staff would not perform an early Caesarean in the absence of any indications of abnormality, because a premature delivery carries risks to the baby.

Conclusion

Two areas of constraint have been identified by medical practitioners and academics in relation to British Pakistani women's access to and use of prenatal services and the termination of pregnancy. The first concerns religion, particularly the idea that to end a pregnancy or assist in ending a life is inherently sinful and that intervention in processes that are 'up to God' counters the spirit of Islam, which demands trust in God. The second concerns family, particularly its gendered power dynamics and the authority of senior kin. In this chapter, I have described the complexity and challenges associated with both of these arenas of constraint in parents' negotiations of the difficult decisions that follow the diagnosis of a fatal abnormality in pregnancy or a premature birth. Regarding religion, while the dominant local religious discourse defines termination of pregnancy as a sin, an alternative, religiously justifiable view recognises its acceptability within 120 days or on medical or social grounds. Despite the lack of open public discussion of Islamic positions that accept termination of pregnancy, different views prevail even within one family. There is a need for more information on Islam's stance on termination of pregnancy for severe or fatal conditions (see also Ahmed et al. 2006b: 255). Parents' deliberations and negotiation of these issues, as documented here, indicate a desire for religious guidance that does not simply replicate the views of the older generation but recognises the novelty of the dilemmas that have been produced by means of prenatal surveillance and technologies of life support. These negotiations may be described, I suggest, as the exercise of moral agency with reference to the Islamic concept of *khilāfah*, which involves interpreting Islamic principles in the light of both an understanding of traditional religious sources and new environmental conditions (Shaikh 2003).

However, the idea of reinterpreting traditional sources remains anathema to many Muslims; thus alternative Islamic discourses on such issues as the ensoulment of the foetus and the permissibility of ending a pregnancy and assisting death remain locally muted. Further, there may be significant differences between what a woman understands as permissible in theory and what it would mean in practice to end a problematic pregnancy. Moreover, while carrying to term a baby that is likely to die at or soon after birth carries an emotional cost, so does terminating a pregnancy, especially where doubts remain as to the religious permissibility of abortion and the accuracy of the diagnosis. Carrying to term a fatally abnormal pregnancy also raises a further set of issues concerning the ambiguous personhood of a miscarried or stillborn baby.

My material also demonstrates the influence of the wider family in the negotiation of these issues. For many men and women, it is important to have 'backing' from an authoritative source. For women, this often includes their parents or sisters or a mother-in-law, and without such backing a particular choice may not be made. At the same time, these processes frequently challenge the conventional understanding that female authority is subordinate to male. As we have seen, a husband's approval or disapproval may be secondary to the views of other kin, or husbands may offer their support for whatever their wives decide, or a woman might take a particular course of action (such as naming a stillborn baby) despite disapproval from a husband and other kin. These processes may also illustrate transformations of gender dynamics associated with marriage migration, particularly where Pakistan-raised men marry British-raised women (Charsley 2005; see also Mahler and Pessar 2001, Pessar and Mahler 2003).

Some of the incidents narrated here are also examples of how men and women may exercise their moral agency without the knowledge or approval of their wider family, such as their parents or in-laws, for instance by saying that they 'lost' a pregnancy (*bachchā gir gayā*, 'the baby fell') when they chose to end it, or saying that a baby died while in special care where the death involved a decision to withdraw life support. These illustrations of an individual or couple's autonomy challenge the conventional anthropological construction of South Asian kinship that contrasts Western individualism, according to which a person is understood as separable from their interactions with others, with the 'relationality' of South Asian kinship (see, for example, Marriott and Inden 1977). As Janet Carsten (2001) observes, this contrast seems to have been too starkly drawn. In the analysis of moral decision-making, Western feminist theorists have made the case for introducing the concept of relational autonomy (Mackenzie and Stoljar 2000). My analysis of British Pakistani parents' practical ethical decision-making supports the argument that autonomy is always exercised in a social and moral context, as the outcome of interactions with significant others with whom on going relationships must be sustained, but it simultaneously places individuals and the dilemmas and choices they face at the forefront of the analysis. Aspects of the detailed personal narratives presented here also augment recent challenges to the conventional picture of South Asian arranged marriages – as involving relationships between families or households rather than between individuals, and in which the marital relationship is subordinate to the interests of the *birādarī* – that point to the agency of individuals regarding choice of marriage partner (as discussed in Chapter 3; see also Shaw and Charsley 2006). In noting the anguish of couples in relation to the diagnosis of serious abnormality in a pregnancy and the birth and death of babies with fatal problems, this chapter also indicates some of the ways in which these experiences are private to the couple, rather than shared with the wider family. This issue is explored more fully in the next chapter.

Notes

1. The gestational limit for termination on medical grounds is twenty-four weeks. There is no time limit on termination for fatal abnormalities, but late termination is more difficult, involving feticide by injection and an induced labour.
2. A Caesarean section (C-section) involves removing the baby after surgical incision into the abdomen and uterus. It is not recommended in the absence of medical indicators, because of the risk of complications for the mother and the baby, and it is not recommended for women planning several children because it increases the risks of placental problems in subsequent pregnancies.
3. Of the four international Sunni schools, the Hanafi (the oldest) today predominates in Pakistan and the Indian subcontinent; the Shafi predominates in South-East Asia, the Maliki in North and West Africa and the Hanbali in Saudi Arabia. There is also the Zaidi school in Yemen and the Abadi school in Oman (Al Aqeel 2007). The Shi'a school of thought predominates in Iran, as well as parts of Iraq and Lebanon. Shi'a orthodoxy follows the Sunna of the Prophet, but repudiates the traditions associated with the first three Caliphs, three of the Prophet's Companions, and accepts only those associated with Ali, the fourth Caliph and the Prophet's son-in-law and nephew. In the late 1990s, significant divergences emerged between Shi'ite and Sunni opinion on third-party gamete donation (Inhorn 2006)
4. Within Sunni Islam, the Zaidi school and some Hanafi and Shafi scholars give unconditional permission, with the Hanbali school permitting the use of oral abortion-inducing agents within forty days of conception; most Hanafi and Shafi scholars give conditional permission; some Maliki jurists strongly disapprove, and some other schools, with more limited following, unconditionally prohibit termination of pregnancy within 120 days (Shaikh 2003: 121–22).
5. Traditionally, in rural Pakistan, husbands would not be present at their wives' deliveries, but there is evidence that this practice is changing for at least some couples. As one husband said to me, 'If you stay outside, the midwives think you don't care.'
6. In eighteenth-century England, a construction of their pregnancies as 'little more than blood' was an important part of the legal defence for single women charged with murdering their newborn babies, who would otherwise have produced bastard children (Johnson 1996: 210).
7. In contrast, such facilities are provided in a major hospital in Oslo, Norway, providing an interesting example of integration and ritual variation (Doving 2003).
8. The local authority provides a trained counsellor who is fluent in Panjabi, but, as the extract shows, there are cultural and practical barriers to some women accessing this service. Miriam had associated the letter I sent about my research, which I followed up with a phone call, with the opportunities for counselling provided by the hospital.

CHAPTER 7
GENETIC SCREENING AND THE EXTENDED FAMILY

Introduction

A unique feature of a genetic diagnosis is the precise ways in which it implicates the affected person's close biological relatives. Genetic material – by which, here, I mean nuclear DNA, located in every cell of the body – is transferred in equal amounts via the gametes (the mother's egg and the father's sperm) to a child. From this, the extent of shared DNA in relationships between biological relatives can be calculated. Parents each contribute half their genetic material to a child, so an individual shares 50 per cent of their DNA with each biological parent and sibling (their 'first-degree' relatives), 25 per cent with their grandparents, nieces and nephews and aunts and uncles (their 'second-degree' relatives) and 12.5 per cent with their first cousins. Thus, the probability that an affected person's relatives will share the same mutation is 50 per cent for first-degree relatives, 25 per cent for second-degree relatives, 12.5 per cent for third-degree relatives, and so on.[1]

The genetic model of inheritance is informed by and reaffirms ideas widespread in Western models of kinship – those of Europe and America – about how relatedness is constructed through biology, particularly in the acknowledgement of the bilaterality of kinship, which refers to having relatives on the mother's and the father's 'side' of the family (Goody 1983; Strathern 1992; Davison 1996). The assumption that biological and social kinship broadly correspond has long characterised Euro-American kinship (Strathern 1992); as anthropologist David Schneider has put it, for Euro-Americans, 'kinship is defined as biogenetic' (1968 [1980]: 23). The idea that biology 'underpins' kinship in the Euro-American tradition pre-dates the rise of modern genetics; indeed, Mendelian genetics probably took the form it did because of the prior bilaterality of European kinship (Richards 1996b; Featherstone et al. 2006: 7). Euro-Americans are often amateur geneticists and folklorists in their interests in tracking how particular personality types, exceptional abilities, or distinctive physical appearances 'run' in their families across the generations (Bouquet 1996; Richards 1996b; Edwards 2000).

Yet it does not follow from this that Euro-American understandings of biological relatedness necessarily correspond with relatedness as defined in genetic theory. Within Euro-American kinship, what constitutes the crucial biological link, or the one deemed natural, does not in every case map on to a model of genetic substance passed from a genetic mother and father (genitor and genitrix) to a child. Patrilineal links may be prioritised over matrilineal ones in the recording of ancestry, as in the Anglo-American surname tradition (whereby a child is given the father's second name and a woman takes her husband's surname on marriage). Similarly, patrilineality is prioritised in the breeding of racehorses, where speed and ability are believed to be inherited from the stallion (Cassidy 2002). Alternatively, biological ties may be understood to include or be constituted through links other than those of shared DNA (or 'blood'), such as by breastfeeding and gestation. What makes someone a relative is a matter of social practice, of parenting, care giving and giving gifts as well as, and sometimes more than, biology (Hirsch 1993; Edwards 2000). As cases of genetic non-paternity, gamete donation and transnational adoption illustrate, biological ties are not always aligned with the social. In such cases, cultural processes are frequently deployed to realign the social with culturally defined natural connections between kin. In a Californian infertility clinic, for instance, prospective mothers using techniques of IVF with donated eggs and gestational surrogacy 'naturalise' their claims to motherhood in biological idioms, even though gestational surrogacy and egg donation are fragmenting the meaning of biological motherhood (Thompson 2001). The idea of kinship as rooted in the natural facts of biology is thus not 'given' but socially and culturally constructed (see also Franklin 2001; Franklin and McKinnon 2001; Howell 2001).

Beyond the conventions of Euro-American kinship, while genetic ties are often understood as relatedness by blood (as implied by the term consanguineous, which means literally 'of the same blood'), the idea of 'sharing the same blood' does not always follow a genetic model. Within a patrilineal kinship system, blood may be understood to link men more strongly than women across generations. This idea occurs in the belief of a group of Gujarati musicians in the U.K. that their musicality is passed on down the generations by means of the blood of their male ancestors (Baily 1993). It also underpins the South Asian concept of caste, according to which particular qualities are associated with particular kinds of families and are retained across the generations by marrying within the caste (Ostor et al. 1982: 59). Elsewhere, biological ties may be understood in non-genetic terms, or social and spiritual connections may be prioritised over the biological. In Melanesia, for instance, although mother and father contribute to the nurturing of a child, conception is perceived as resulting from the entry of an ancestral spirit into a woman's body, the ancestor providing 'generative agency' and the foetus forming from ancestral spirit combined with maternal blood (Weiner 1976; Franklin 1997: 60). Here, the parents' respective reproductive contributions to a child are understood in ways that reflect the wider social environment in which a child is produced, rather than reduced to the 'cellular model' of conception that informs genetics (Franklin 1997: 61).

The variation and complexity of social and cultural understandings of relatedness have a number of important implications for the expansion of genetic diagnostic technologies in contemporary medical practice. They highlight the cultural specificity of the genetic model of shared DNA, which is often erroneously assumed to be widely shared by people across the globe. This cultural specificity means that the risk implications of a genetic diagnosis for a person's biological kin will not necessarily be understood by everyone in the same way: the kinship implications cannot simply be 'read off' from a genetic model of shared risk, because they will be mediated by people's prior understandings of what defines a family and of what constitutes the natural or biological ties between kin. For clinicians providing diagnostic and risk information for clients using genetics services, this raises a key question about how far clients' ideas about who is family and how kin are connected correspond to the genetic model.

The question is fundamental to the construction of clinical models of shared risk and to communicating this risk within the family. When a genetic diagnosis is made, clinical geneticists can identify at-risk relatives of the proband (the person about whom the diagnosis is made), using the family tree (pedigree) drawn up in the genetics clinic. This pedigree, initially constructed as a diagnostic tool in conversation between the clinician and her patient, is based on patients' descriptions of the kinship links between relatives (see Richards 1996b: 253–58). As such, it is often a partial map of the full range of the patient's genetic connections with kin. Patients may mention only those relatives who are important to them or whom they see regularly, omitting others who may be genetically close but socially distant; they may forget exactly how some kin are related and approximate their kinship relationship; they may conceal certain consanguineous connections to avoid revealing a disjuncture between social and genetic paternity; and they may simplify complex consanguinity (such as where people are related to one another in more than one way) so as to ease the clinician's task of mapping them on to a standardised A4 sheet, or for fear of medical disapproval of complex consanguinity. Thus, both at the diagnostic or research stage (which usually requires DNA samples to be collected from those believed to be biologically related, such as parents and siblings) and in connection with identifying potential carriers in the family, the definition of family is socially and culturally circumscribed.

From a clinical perspective, the implications of a diagnosis for other biological relatives (as represented in the clinically constructed family tree) also depend on the type of diagnosis made (see also Introduction). Thus, the diagnosis of an unbalanced chromosome translocation condition in a child of unaffected parents raises the possibility that one parent is a healthy carrier of a balanced translocation and that this parent's siblings might also carry balanced translocations and be at risk of having affected children. The diagnosis of a variably presenting or late-onset dominant condition in a child or adult implies that (unless the mutation is *de novo*) one parent and perhaps that parent's siblings and one of their parents are carriers at risk of developing the condition.

A recessive diagnosis in a child of unaffected parents establishes both biological parents as carriers of the mutation, giving them a 25 per cent risk of having another affected child. A recessive diagnosis also implies a probability (of 50 per cent) that any sibling (brother or sister) of each parent is an unaffected carrier of the mutation. This risk is particularly relevant where marriages occur within the family, such as between the children of siblings, because, if both partners carry the same mutation, they too would have a 25 per cent risk of having an affected child.

A recessive diagnosis also implies a probability (of two in three) that any sibling of an affected person is an unaffected carrier of the mutation for the condition. As shown in Figure I.1 (page 17), each time they conceive, each parent passes on either their unchanged gene (A) or the mutation (a) via the gametes (egg and sperm) to the child. Each child inherits one of four possible combinations: in one, the child inherits both copies of the mutation and is affected (aa); in the three other combinations (aA, Aa, AA), the child is unaffected, but in two of these three combinations (aA, Aa), the child has one mutation and one unchanged copy and is therefore a carrier. As Figure I.1 shows, any unaffected sibling of a person with a recessive condition therefore has a two in three chance of being an unaffected carrier of the mutation and, therefore, of being at risk of having affected children should they marry another carrier of the same mutation.

The diagnosis of a recessive X-linked condition has gender-specific implications: it generally only affects boys, who have no second X chromosome to compensate for the effects of a mutation or rearrangement on the X chromosome (see Figure I.3, page 20). A diagnosis implies that the mother is an unaffected (or, with some X-linked conditions, mildly affected) carrier, at risk of having further affected sons, and of having unaffected carrier daughters who would be at risk of having affected sons; sisters, too, could be unaffected carriers at similar risk. The term 'carrier' therefore implies a risk for a genetic condition that can be direct, entailing mutations or chromosome rearrangements that cause a condition in the carrier, or indirect, involving mutations or chromosome rearrangements that do not cause a genetic condition in the carrier but could cause it in their close kin (children, parents or siblings, etc.). Ambiguity over the meaning of 'carrier' can spill out into family members' perceptions of familial risks.

In clinical genetics practice in the U.K., doctors expect the proband (or their parents or guardian) to initiate the process of telling other relatives that they might be at risk of carrying or having a genetic condition, a process clinicians call 'disclosure' of risk information or genetic test results. Following the principle of non-directive counselling, clinicians do not insist that disclosure occurs, nor do they themselves undertake to inform their patients' family members about their genetic risk. The term 'cascade screening', first used in the 1960s in connection with tracking carriers of cystic fibrosis, is sometimes used to describe the process by which clinicians identify potential carriers from the family tree and offer them genetic risk estimates or carrier tests, but this usually requires the proband to secure their relatives' consent to be contacted by a genetic counsellor, as well as to consent to their genetic information being shared with relatives. If genetics doctors or counsellors are contacted by the relative of a patient known to have a genetic condition, they will not reveal information about their patient without the patient's consent. Occasionally, patients explicitly do not want genetic information shared with their relatives and this form of non-disclosure can create dilemmas for doctors: should they sometimes break confidentiality to inform relatives of their risk (Leung et al. 2000; Clarke et al. 2005)? Does the familial nature of genetic information mean that genetic information is exceptional to the extent that the argument for the right to individual privacy does not apply? If so, who should take on the responsibility of identifying relatives and informing them of their potential carrier status and of the opportunities for clinical risk assessments or carrier tests – the proband, or their parents, or their doctors?

A key problem with the idea of disclosure and the arguments generated by clinical concerns over non-disclosure is the assumption that disclosure has actually occurred and that it is unproblematic. What exactly does communicating genetic risk information or test results within the family mean? Who constitutes the family to be disclosed to, given that a family may be constituted in many socially and culturally variable ways? Who takes on the responsibility of telling? Who is actually told, and how, when and what are they told? In South Wales families identified through genetics clinic referrals as having or potentially sharing risk for a genetic condition, relatives hold complex and sometimes contradictory ideas about the inheritance of a genetic condition and interpret risk information in the light of these ideas (Featherstone et al. 2006). They do not necessarily retain the details of an inheritance pattern after they leave the genetics clinic. Their 'passing on' of risk information may simply involve mentioning that 'it', without naming the condition, is 'in the family'. Perceptions of who is at risk may be based less on medical models than on the scrutiny of relatives across the generations for indications of risk, sometimes based on shared traits such as personality type. With this kind of family surveillance, risk communication is rarely a discrete, one-off event. Occasionally risk information is 'blurted out' but more often people take a 'drip-drip' approach, giving partial information that builds slowly over time, sometimes over many years (Gregory 2006). The process is also contextually shaped by being rooted in the events and practices of everyday kinship, dependent on finding the 'right' time and occasion, sometimes prompted by the introduction of a new member into the family (Featherstone et al. 2006; Gregory 2006). It is also often strongly gendered. Women rather than men may shoulder the responsibility of informing kin, as has been shown in work on the communication of risk for genetic breast cancer (Hallowell 1999), and as is also true of conditions such as Huntington's disease which are not seen as 'female' conditions (Richards 1996c).

The South Wales study identifies two main sources of influence over processes of genetic risk communication within the family. One, reinforcing the findings of several other British studies, concerns patients' everyday ideas about inheritance and risk for genetic disease, which are informed by and inform mutual surveillance within the wider family. These ideas are often based on prior family experiences of health and illness and can suggest patterns of risk where, according to the genetic model, none exists, or can overlook risk where it does (Featherstone et al. 2006; see also Davison 1996, Richards 1996b). The second concerns the practical morality and popular psychology that inform the sharing of risk information. Regardless of their understanding of inheritance and risk, people assess how different family members will cope with the burden of genetic risk information when they think about whether and with whom risk information should or should not be shared, and their conclusions often result in the withholding of risk information (Featherstone et al. 2006).

How far are such observations also relevant to British Pakistani understandings of inheritance and patterns of risk communication within the family? This question is of academic and practical importance, given the ethnic diversity of contemporary Britain, the discourse of recessive genetic risk relating to British Pakistanis and the significance of preferential cousin marriage in many populations worldwide. Nevertheless, little empirical work on everyday understandings of inheritance and genetic risk communication has explicitly addressed cultural or ethnic diversity. The existing literature contains two hypotheses about the significance of cultural difference for genetic counselling. One highlights the potential for alternative models of kinship, specifically those departing from the bilaterality of Euro-American kinship thinking, to provide cultural blueprints for thinking about inheritance that are at odds with genetic theory, and calls for more research on this question (Richards 1996b; Meiser et al. 2001). The other, focused on British Pakistanis, proposes that cascade screening will be particularly effective with British Pakistani families in which a recessive condition has been diagnosed, if genetic counselling focuses on the parents of the affected child and is then 'with appropriate sensitivity', extended to the parents' siblings and other kin (Darr 1997: 94). This view draws on a model of the British Pakistani *birādarī* (extended kindred) as a closely interdependent unit, linked by ties of consanguinity, affinity and descent, which will facilitate communication about genetic risk, in contrast to the more individualistic structure of the white Anglo-British family (Darr 1997).

I begin this chapter by discussing British Pakistani ideas about inheritance, the nature of the biological links between parents and children and patterns of inherited characteristics in the family, and go on to argue that, while cultural models may be important in shaping and sometimes inhibiting clients' understandings of clinical risk information, direct observation and personal experience can challenge or change these understandings. Communication about risk within the family is only partly a matter of knowledge about inheritance; it is also powerfully influenced by context, timing and the nature of relationships between kin. Indeed, considerations of context and timing often work against the communication of genetic risk information within the family, combined with the fear of gossip, especially in this particular cultural context in which fertility is highly valued. In other words, genetic counselling is not necessarily any easier within extended Pakistani *birādarīs* in the U.K. than within other patient groups

Everyday ideas about biological inheritance

The idea of patrilineal descent that prevails across North Africa, the Middle East, around the Mediterranean and in South and East Asia, including Pakistan, exerts a strong influence over British Pakistani concepts of social identity (as discussed in the Introduction). It also informs ideas that would seem to prioritise male generative agency in the production of a child. The metaphor of the male seed (*bīj*) and female earth (*zamīn*) recurs within numerous ethnographic reports from 'almost all over northern and central India, and in some parts of eastern India' (Böck and Rao 2000: 6). There is also an apparent justification in a Qur'anic verse, 'Your wives are as a tilth unto you, so approach your tilth when or how ye will' (Qur'an 2: 223). Yet defining British Pakistani everyday understandings of biological inheritance in the context of clinical genetics referrals proved rather more elusive.

During clinical genetics consultations, I was sometimes aware that, when a doctor described recessive inheritance, the genetic theory of an equal contribution of male and female reproductive substance sat uneasily alongside a family's theories of the causes of a child's problem. After a consultation in which the doctor had explained the inheritance of a child's recessive condition, the Pakistan-born mother asked me to repeat what the consultant had said and then interrupted my exposition with the question, 'Are you saying the material from the mother and father is equal? Does the father not give more?' (*Bāp kī taraf se ziāda nahīn miltā?*) On another occasion, a woman fluent in English and Urdu with whom I was discussing the translation of a leaflet on recessive inheritance asked me, 'So the baby gets material from both sides? So it has to come from the father and the mother? I thought it just came from the father. I had never known that.' In the context of a discussion of marriage arrangements, a woman who had lost three children in infancy to a recessive disorder and understood she had a one in four recurrence risk told me she thought it would be safer to marry her daughter to a maternal rather than to a paternal relative, saying, 'If the fathers [of the boy and girl] are brothers, there is the most danger.'

When I asked what constitutes the material (*mavād*) of biological inheritance, 'that which a baby gets from its mother and from its father', the most common response was that this was blood; blood was thus the vehicle and constituent of genetic substance, or DNA. Jamila, an Azad Kashmir-raised mother of a teenager with learning difficulties, told me, 'A baby is made from the blood of the father and this mixes with blood from the mother.' Several other women described foetal abnormalities or pregnancy loss as the result of blood 'not mixing'. Occasionally, those who had previously attended genetics clinics used genetic terminology to describe biological inheritance. Hamida, whose brother-in-law has a chromosomal condition, described conception by saying, 'The chromosomes from the mother and father mix together and the baby starts.' Others with experience of a single-gene disorder in the family used the term gene rather than blood to describe conception, and explained unsuccessful pregnancy as a consequence of when 'the genes did not match'. The technical English, Urdu or colloquial Panjabi terms for what, in genetic theory, is the male and female genetic contribution to a child, via the gametes, namely the sperm (Urdu: *mada-e-taulīd,* literally 'material of procreation', or Panjabi: *manī* or *mazī*, for sperm, or, more euphemistically, *pānī*, 'water', or *mard kā pānī*, 'water from the man') and the ovum, or egg (Urdu: *baizā*), were much less often used. In fact, semen is often understood to be very concentrated blood, in some accounts, one drop being equivalent to a hundred drops of blood and its strength determining a child's sex (Shaw 2000a). Older Pakistan-raised women tended to be hazy about what the mother's generative contribution might be; they told me that to speak about such things is shameful, especially before marriage. Amira, forty-five years old with a child with a dominant condition, told me, 'Even after marriage you don't find out what the words are. It is the same for a girl and for a boy, but here in England, for our children, it is different; now they learn from school and they know all the words.'

Yet both women and men stressed the importance of the biological link between mother and child, especially the influence of gestation on the health of a baby. One young Pakistan-raised woman forcefully countered my suggestion that a man's generative contribution to a child might be greater by telling me in Urdu (using the English word 'gametes') that a teacher in Pakistan had told her class that:

> The gametes from which a child is made come equally from the mother and father [and] the mother's contribution is greater; she said it is not that the father's contribution is greater. In fact, the mother's contribution is greater ... because for nine months the child grows in the mother's body; it does not grow in the man's body. For nine months the mother does not have periods and [that] blood goes into the baby. The mother's health and the food she eats in pregnancy are also very important for how the baby develops. For these reasons, the baby gets more from the mother than from the father. When our teacher told us this, we felt shame that she was talking about such things. We looked down and hid our faces. She told us we should not feel shame. She said she was telling us this because one day it would be useful for us to know.

Patterns of inherited characteristics

While one cultural blueprint thus prioritises patrilineal inheritance, this is not the only idea on which people may draw in understanding the biological links between parents and children. People's observations of shared family characteristics did not reflect a theory of patrilineal inheritance so much as recognise a range of possible inheritance patterns. Sometimes people remarked on same-sex inter-generational resemblances – a daughter being like her mother, a son like his father (see also Fischer and Lyon 2000: 306); more often parents described characteristics as being transferred from either parent to a child, regardless of sex. Rukhsana, thirty-two years old and in England for thirteen years, described her son as 'dark like my husband, [but] he talks like me and eats like me' and her daughter as 'fair like me, but ... has her Dad's eyes ... And her hair is not like mine, it is thin and silky, like her father's sister's hair.' In several families, characteristics that included having blue-grey eyes, having pale skin or only giving birth to boys were described as 'skipping' a generation, showing up in grandchildren, on the basis of observed family resemblances. This range of observations is remarkably similar to those noted among white Anglo-British families (Richards 1996b; Richards and Ponder 1996) and implicitly recognises a male and a female genetic contribution. Despite the complex consanguinity of many Pakistani kindreds, people also sometimes talked about characteristics as being on their 'mother's side' or their 'father's side' of the family, as we shall see in Najma's case below.

Such observations of patterns in the inheritance of characteristics over the generations can suggest a template for thinking about genetic risk that singles out particular kin as susceptible in ways that may conflict with genetic theory. In research in South Wales in connection with predictive testing for late-onset genetic conditions, Charlie Davison (1996) notes that people with a family history of a genetic condition may consider only those descendants of the affected person who share a similar body type or personality to be likely to develop the condition. Katy Featherstone and colleagues show in their South Wales fieldwork that everyday ideas about a condition's inheritance rarely map on to the medical model and imply that some relatives rather than others are at risk in ways that are at odds with genetic theory. For example, a woman whose husband and father-in-law died of a fatal cardiac condition worried constantly that her two-year-old son would inherit the condition, as the next male descendant, and thought she would worry less if she had a daughter, even though according to genetic theory the condition can affect either males or females (Featherstone et al. 2006: 88). Thus, contrary to the initial expectation that cascade screening would have the advantage that family members will already know something about the inheritance of a disorder 'in the family' (particularly if it is serious or life-threatening), a family history of a genetic condition does not necessarily facilitate the communication of genetic risk because the family may already adhere to a different model of inheritance and risk.

Patients' everyday understandings of inheritance and risk rarely emerge within the genetics consultation itself (Featherstone et al. 2006). As we saw above, patients sometimes asked me after they had left the genetics clinic to repeat and explain inheritance patterns that doctors had described but on other occasions they gave no indication that the clinical information did not match their own understandings. Patients may appear to have understood a pattern of inheritance and risk during their genetics consultation but may not retain this information, its significance sometimes only becoming clear much later (ibid.). In the following case, Najma and Nadeem's experience of seeking genetic testing at first seems to represent successful risk communication within the family, since their request for a genetic carrier test was made on the basis of knowledge of a family history of a genetic condition. In fact, as I learnt eighteen months later, their understanding of who was at risk followed a patrilineal model that was only later challenged by experience.

Najma and Nadeem

Najma and her husband Nadeem requested a genetics appointment because two of their second-degree relatives – the son and daughter of one of Najma's sisters and one of Nadeem's brothers – have a recessive metabolic condition associated with problems in hormone production. None of their other married brothers and sisters had any affected children, and the only other reported family history, probably unrelated to the recessive condition, was of an unusually-shaped nose, in the daughter of one of Nadeem's brothers and in a son and daughter of another of his brothers. The clinician told Najma and Nadeem that they have a one in sixteen chance of having an affected child. This probability is reached by multiplying three probabilities: that each partner is a carrier, and, as carriers, that they will have an affected child (i.e. $1/2 \times 1/2 \times 1/4 = 1/16$). The clinician also arranged for carrier tests to refine this risk assessment, because, if only one partner is a carrier, the couple would not be at risk of having an affected child (although a child might be an unaffected carrier). The testing took some time. Besides requiring blood for testing from both partners, it required the affected niece and nephew and their parents to consent to giving blood samples, which they willingly gave. A few months later, the results showed that Nadeem is carrier and Najma is not.

This apparently successful screening and testing on the basis of a family history conceals the fact that Najma's understandings of inheritance and risk were, and for some time continued to be, at odds with the medical model of recessive inheritance. Eighteen months after her genetics consultation, Najma told me she had not understood that both parents must be carriers for a child to be affected with this type of condition:

> We thought my husband's family were carriers … through the men. My sister is married to my husband's older brother. Two of her children have

> [the condition]. My husband's two younger brothers each have children with a congenital nose defect. So it was in my husband's family because this is where the problems were. This is why I thought any children I have with my husband might also be at risk.

Her theory was entirely consistent with the observed evidence of genetic and congenital problems in the family until something happened that transformed her understanding. One of Najma's sisters, who had an unaffected son, gave birth to a baby girl who had the recessive condition. For Najma, 'This was a total shock. It was not even in our dreams that she or her husband could be carriers.' Since this new baby's father is Najma's maternal first cousin – her mother's sister's son – Najma and her sisters had thought there was no risk, because they had understood the condition could only arise in a descendant, through men, of their mother's brother, not in the descendants of any of their mother's sisters:

> My sister [the one with the affected baby] always said it was in our husband's family, not on our side of the family. We thought it was only our uncle [Najma's Mum's brother, who is also her father-in-law] who had passed it on to his sons and one of them had passed it on to my niece and nephew. We thought it went through the men, in the male line. Now I know that this is wrong. We did not realise there has to be a wife who is a carrier for the kids to have got it ... It was such a shock. The stress has been incredible – realising it is in our side of the family too, not just in my husband's side. People always say, 'not in our family'. Originally, we thought only my husband is a carrier and that he got it from his father, my Mum's brother. We did not think that my Mum could be a carrier too, or her sisters, but now we know she is, she must be, and she has passed it on to us and we are carriers – at least, two of my sisters are – they must be, because they both have affected children. My sister, the one with the affected baby, is gutted. She has not even told my Mum that there is something wrong.

Understandings of inheritance and illness causality

This story suggests that it may be useful for genetic counsellors to elicit patients' everyday understandings of the inheritance of a condition where there is a known family history, and to work with these ideas to explain risks to other biological kin. For instance, in Nadia's case, showing how a pattern of inheritance that recognises 'there has to be a wife who is a carrier' is consistent with the initial manifestation of the condition in the family, but in fact highlights a wider spectrum of potential carriers than would be predicted from a unilinear model, might have given Najma's sister prior warning of her risk and enabled her to consider the options of prenatal diagnosis and, in this case, prenatal therapy, because prenatal hormonal treatment is available to reduce this particular condition's effects. However, as noted above, this raises difficult questions about who should be responsible for communicating genetic risk information in the family. Moreover, in many other cases, there is no family history to elicit and work from, because the affected person is, in the majority of cases, 'the first and only sufferer in the family' and there is therefore no prior knowledge of the inheritance of the disorder (Pembrey 1996: 77). In relation to recessively inherited conditions, such as cystic fibrosis within Anglo-British families 'where sibships are relatively small,' the number of cases may be too few 'to make up a pattern that family members may recognise' as something that 'runs in the family'. 'This is even more likely to be the case if the condition is variable in its symptoms and has been poorly diagnosed in the past. Thus many couples are quite unaware that they or their families carry cystic fibrosis mutations until a child is born with the condition' (Richards 1996b: 261).

Similarly for many of the British Pakistani families in this study, despite their generally larger family size, the condition diagnosed was reported to be the first case. People often told me, 'We have never seen this thing before,' and since many of the observed conditions are rare they would not have been diagnosed in rural Pakistan (Chapter 4). Furthermore, receptiveness to genetic information and thus to its significance for the wider family is much more than simply a question of providing information about the condition's mode of inheritance, but is influenced by the wider social and cultural context of risk communication, which includes the prevailing understandings of the causes of the problem. Najma, born and educated in Britain, had been urged by her affected niece to seek a carrier test and accepted that the condition affecting her niece and nephew was genetic. Nonetheless, Najma's understanding of 'genetic' was also shaped by the wider discourse of genetic risk in consanguineous marriages: she had believed the condition in her family was caused by marrying in the family and had delayed seeking a carrier test until after her first child was born for fear that 'these people are going to think badly of me because I am married to my cousin'.

Most other referrals to clinical genetics occurred not because of a relative's insistence but as part of the routine management of birth anomaly without any previous known family history. In such cases, the observed condition was often understood by the family to have resulted from one or more of a range of spiritual and environmental causes, such as those associated with accidents or infections. Even where a condition is recognised as genetic or associated with 'the blood' (as in the idea of 'bad blood', for instance), it may be considered mutable or temporary, like an infection, as sometimes illustrated by the interchangeable use, in Panjabi, of the English word 'gene' and the Urdu/Panjabi word *jerasīm,* which means 'germ'. Such ideas can, however, change with new information and over time, as understandings of illness causality and awareness of genetic risk and therapeutic possibilities change, as the following story of a family's awareness of thalassaemia illustrates. Thalassaemia is a serious, recessively inherited disorder of the blood, for which carrier testing and prenatal diagnosis are available.

Ikra

The youngest of four children, Ikra was born in Britain twenty-one years ago. Her thalassaemia was diagnosed when she was six months old. Ikra's brothers and sister are all now married and have had thalassaemia carrier tests. Yet, at the time of Ikra's birth, Ikra's parents, who are from rural Azad Kashmir, had not heard of thalassaemia and did not appreciate its seriousness. As Ikra told me:

> They did not know [anything about this condition] or else they did not want to know. No one else they knew was having treatment, blood transfusions or anything like that. In Pakistan they don't really diagnose these sorts of illnesses. If I had been born there, I would have died. At least my parents took the medical advice seriously – I know one or two other Pakistani children with thalassaemia, and they are left to cope on their own. And my parents understood that they could have another child with my illness, and did not have any more children, even though they thought that this illness was 'God's will', that 'if it's going to happen, it's going to happen'. Anyway, they already had four children. Other parents sometimes don't believe it, or don't want to. But my parents did not understand the genetics – the risks for others in the family. When my eldest brother's marriage was being arranged to his father's brother's daughter, they said nothing about the risks; it was the same later, when my younger brother got married to his mother's sister's daughter, and my sister got married to her Mum's sister's son. I realise now that this is because they did not understand. They are not educated, they are not literate and they did not have any interpreters then. It took a very long time.

Ikra's parents' difficulties with assimilating the risk information were compounded by their lack of modern medical knowledge of thalassaemia and by the problems of communicating technical genetic information across language barriers. However, that they had understood their own reproductive risk but not the risk that other relatives might be carriers is not unique to people of their ethnic and social background, or to those without higher education or fluent English. White Anglo-British parents of children diagnosed with recessive conditions are likely to remember the one in four risk of having an affected child from the genetic counselling they receive, but rarely recall the risk of two in three that they will have an unaffected child who is, like themselves, a carrier of the mutation (Snowdon and Green 1994). Assimilating such information is largely a matter of context and timing. Within my study, parental concerns always focused on their child's current medical problems and the implications of the diagnosis for the child's future health. Sometimes parents also worried about future reproductive risks, but the wider family implications of the diagnosis seemed a more remote concern.

In the genetics consultation, too, discussion of a diagnosis in a child rarely focused in detail on the family implications. Clinic doctors may mention the implications for other kin such as unaffected siblings, as potential carriers of the condition, and parents may respond by saying, 'We don't need to think about that yet.' Doctors may also not emphasise risks to other family members if a diagnosis is uncertain or if the causative mutation has not been identified and carrier or prenatal tests are unavailable. It may also seem inappropriate or insensitive to raise the issue if a couple appears not to have accepted the diagnosis as genetic, or because they are grieving for a dead child or are preoccupied with caring for an infant with many medical problems. Clinicians may also be wary of raising the issue of risks for other family members, including children, if the condition is variable in its presentation and there is currently no treatment for it, for to do so may simply raise anxieties. Parents might want children to have a genetic test, to establish their carrier status for a recessive condition, or to check whether their genetic constitution means they will, or are likely to, develop the signs of a genetic condition, but doctors may be reluctant to arrange such tests in the absence of clear clinical signs of a problem, for fear of prematurely or unnecessarily labelling the child as having a genetic condition, at least if the child is too young to give independent informed consent. Given such considerations, it is more usual for clinicians to note the implications for other relatives in a letter to the parents and to the general practitioner, who will file it for future reference. 'At-risk' relatives of an affected child or adult may then seek genetic advice and genetic tests, if appropriate, when they are older, have more awareness of the genetic nature of the condition and are considering marrying and having children themselves. Thus, the communication of risk information is very much a matter of context and timing, as well as of knowledge – even within the more formal context of the genetics consultation itself.

This process does not preclude an affected individual, their parents, a sibling or other relatives scrutinising the wider family for signs of the condition, across the generations. When one nine-year-old son boy was diagnosed with the dominantly inherited condition neurofibromatosis type I (NF1), on account his having more than a few patches of darker skin pigment on his torso, freckling under his arms and learning difficulties, the clinicians thought the condition had probably arisen in the family for the first time because there were no signs of it in the parents. Nonetheless, the boy's mother's cousin told me that she had become worried about her four-year-old son after hearing about the diagnosis in her relative's boy. She asked me to inspect the two patches of darker pigment she had noted on her son's neck; I told her there is probably nothing to worry about but that she should see her GP if she is worried.

In the case of a late-onset recessive neurological condition affecting Akhtar's brothers, Akhtar told me that he has no worries now that he might develop the condition himself, but had worried in the past, when his brothers began to show the signs of the condition:

> My beliefs are so strong because of All'ah ... that I don't think like that. In Islam, death comes to everyone. You don't think of your illness or death as out of this world. It is natural. So I don't tend to think I am going to get ill like them. Though when they became ill, I had lots of symptoms too – pains, a bad back, a bad neck. To begin with, I felt lethargic. Then they did a blood test and could not work out what to call it. I looked over at the doctor's notes and he had written 'abnormal'. I used to have TB [tuberculosis] and my Dad had TB and I asked them if the TB could explain the blood result, but they did not say so and did not explain it.

He also has worries about his children, especially his eleven-year-old son, whose unusual way of walking suggests the same neurological problem and causes him to be bullied at school. 'It looks to me like he could have the same problem, but at a younger age,' Akhtar told me. Since the causative mutation for this condition has been found and a predictive genetic test is in principle available, Akhtar asked his GP for a genetics referral for his children, thinking that, although a confirmatory test would not cure the condition, it might be helpful to know:

> If you have it that is your destiny, it is one of the tests that you are given by All'ah. The family as a whole is a test on my parents, whether you are a strong believer, or a half-hearted believer. It may be that we can't alter this, if you have it, you have it. But, if my son has it, we can tell the teachers, and they can deal with the children who are calling him names and giving him a black eye.

The clinicians, though, thought the boy too young and his symptoms insufficiently clear to justify a predictive test which, if positive, would bring the stigma of having a genetic condition and they suggested that a genetic diagnosis should not be necessary to persuade the boy's teachers to control the bullying at school. Yet, at home, it seemed that this boy was already identified and identifying with his affected uncles, with whom he likes to spend his spare time.

Privacy and non-disclosure of test results

Within a family, relatives may be unaware how much other relatives worry about their potential carrier status, sometimes attributing them with disbelief or lack of concern about their risk. During my first conversation with Ikra, she described her eldest brother's views about thalassaemia carrier testing as quite closely matching their father's, that 'if it's going to happen, it's going to happen'. Her brother had married a first cousin from Pakistan about twelve years ago, and at that time he apparently knew about his sister's illness but did not believe he could be at risk. He now has three unaffected children. Ikra did not know if he had been for a carrier test: 'I have no idea, possibly he had, and just did not say.'

Two years later, Ikra told me that there had meanwhile been further discussion of thalassaemia carrier testing in her family. Ikra had discovered that her eldest brother had, in fact, after discussion with his general practitioner, been referred for carrier testing just after he had got married, and had learnt that he was not a carrier. She thought this explained why he was not worried for his children, and why he continued to be sceptical about the risks. Yet, she said, privately he must have been sufficiently concerned to ask his GP for a referral for carrier testing, although he had said nothing about this to his parents or siblings at the time.

A person sufficiently motivated to ask a GP to refer them for carrier testing does not necessarily or readily discuss this experience and their eventual test results with close family members. Non-disclosure of test results to relatives who are potential carriers of genetic conditions is, in fact, a striking feature of other personal accounts of people whose lives have been affected by genetic conditions. Approximately 18 per cent of people with a parent who has Huntington's disease, a late-onset dominantly inherited condition, actually seek predictive genetic testing, despite the earlier prediction that uptake of testing would be as high as 80%, and, once tested, may be reluctant to communicate test results to relatives because of the emotional and psychological burdens this carriers (Wright 1996: 7; Harper et al. 2000; Creighton et al. 2003). Those with favourable 'negative' results may feel guilty about being 'clear' when others are or may be carriers and so not communicate their results, or they may fear that knowledge of test results will prove divisive in the family, especially among relatives who remain at risk but are ambivalent about testing (Anon 1996; Madigan 1996). Thus, someone aware of familial risks may believe they have a sibling who is not interested in testing or is unconcerned about their risk, when in fact this sibling does worry and may seek testing, but does not talk about doing so with their parents or siblings.

Competitive fertility and stigma of compromised fertility

The issue of privacy with respect to genetic information also needs to be understood with reference to the fact that it affects and potentially stigmatises individuals and couples primarily in the context of marriage and childbearing. As the rapid uptake of techniques of assisted reproduction in both the developing and developed world indicates (Bharadwaj 2003; Inhorn 2006), children remain highly desired in many cultural contexts, including in Pakistan and South Asia where marriage is almost universal and the birth of children indicates the success of a marriage. People may thus be unwilling to accept that 'inherited factors' might compromise their child's marriage prospects or their own childbearing potential. During a discussion of carrier testing, Husnain told me that he did not agree with the idea of premarital genetic testing in relation to thalassaemia:

> You don't turn down a marriage for medical reasons, if you know you were carrying thalassaemia, if I knew I was a carrier, and the family knew, they

> would not want anyone else to know – they would not want it to get out. If my Mum was looking for a *rishta* for me, she is not going to tell them that I am a thalassaemia carrier. It will be the family's well-kept secret. If I had blood cancer, my parents would not tell anyone, because, if the other people where you are looking for a *rishta* know beforehand that you have a problem, they will say 'no' and bang, there goes the *rishta.*
> Would I tell them after the marriage? Well, my wife might understand, but the problem is that she might tell someone else and then it would get out and her relatives would start talking to my relatives and there would be a big split in the family and her relatives would stop talking to me. The other thing is that whatever the truth, they will blame the girl. They would never blame the son – they would blame the lady, even if the man had the problem ... Carrier testing could cause families to split. I go for the test, my Dad say's no, don't go, and I am not even married yet. I think it's worth telling them if there is a cure at the end of it: otherwise, why go for the test? Not even my Mum and Dad, no one understands what we went through with our daughter. In Pakistan they don't know. It would make them worried for nothing. In Pakistan, you have got black magic – they would say, *kālā jādū*, or something else like *nazar* (evil eye) or *jinn* (mischievous spirits). So it's best not to go into the arguments. The doctors in Pakistan, they say don't tell the ladies, the ladies don't need to know, the men make the decision. If we were in Pakistan, I would not tell her everything, I might tell my Dad, but not my Mum, and I would not tell my brothers ... A woman would not even tell her husband in Pakistan, in case he will remarry – she has to be careful because her husband might then taken another wife. Genetic? Well, if they say you have got this thing and we have to check your brother, I would not want to agree unless it is something they can cure. If I am going to die, what difference would it make? I would not even want her [indicating his wife] to know. I would not want her wailing and being upset.[2]

As this suggests, information about medical problems, as constituting a spoiled identity, may be withheld prior to a marriage as well as after it (Goffman 1990). This may be so even for married couples whose parents or other close kin such as siblings have played a part in arranging a marriage and have an interest in ensuring its success; the couple may also want to protect any close relatives who had been involved in arranging the marriage from feeling responsible and from being criticised by other kin, as well as to protect themselves from receiving unsolicited advice or criticism – which is usually directed at the woman. In Sofia's case, her mother-in-law had suggested that Sofia's visiting her brother at night had caused malicious spirits to harm the baby, resulting in miscarriage; Nadia had heard from a neighbour that it might be because she had slept curled up with a knife in her hand during an eclipse when pregnant that her daughter has limb defects; Basharat was told by her husband and her own parents that she had drunk too little water in pregnancy and this had reduced the amniotic fluid around her baby, causing her baby's kidney problem. Relatives are also likely to offer advice and suggestions about using such therapies as those prescribed by *hakīms* (practitioners of Unani medicine) and homoeopaths. Moreover, evidence of repeated, unsuccessful pregnancies may result in implicit and sometimes explicit criticism, usually of the woman, which, as in Sofia's case, may constitute ground for in-laws suggesting a new marriage. As a result, couples may try to conceal evidence of actual or potential reproductive failure even from close relatives living in the same household. A late stillbirth or newborn death cannot be hidden, but parents can withold details of the genetic cause and the circumstances of the death or of any other distressing features such as genital ambiguity, or other physical abnormalities, when reporting their loss within the family. Just as the desire for children can override fears of having another affected child, awareness of the social consequences of revealing knowledge of an inherited problem within the family can inhibit discussion of genetic risk with close relatives.

While conditions causing pregnancy loss or infant death compromise a couple's reproductive success, those marked by long-term medical or intellectual problems also spoil parents' hopes of having 'perfect' children – despite the belief that that the birth of such children is a blessing from God. Parents of children with relatively minor birth abnormalities may take pains to disguise the imperfection from enquiring neighbours and relatives. Certain problems, such as those involving genital ambiguity, are particularly stigmatising. Miriam did not tell her parents that the sex of her stillborn baby was unknown; the doctors told her that she could choose the reported sex, and so she told her parents and relatives in Pakistan that the baby was a boy. The condition in Najma's family includes, in females, a slightly enlarged clitoris which can be surgically corrected. For Najma's niece, this surgery was carried out, without any other family members knowing; a similar scenario seemed likely with the new affected baby girl. In this case, Najma told me:

> The condition was diagnosed right away, and the parents have consented to an operation on the clitoris, but my sister [the baby's mother] has not told anyone apart from us sisters and my niece. Perhaps if I was in the same situation I would do the same, but it is more of a shame factor – she is ashamed to tell anyone. The trouble is, we won't accept an imperfection. Our kids can be nothing less than perfect. It is so difficult to accept that they might not be.
>
> My niece is just absolutely gutted. It has got to the stage when she is having counselling. People are saying to her, 'There are worse conditions, and you only have to take tablets, it's not like you are handicapped.' But that is not the point. The biggest thing, the main problem, is that her Mum has never spoken to her about it. All these years, what has been bottled up inside her

is coming out. The counsellor asked her, 'Do you blame your Mum?' My niece told her, 'I don't blame her for the condition, but I do blame her for hiding it.' They have been having some huge rows about it. Her condition was diagnosed when she was four, and when she was six she had a small operation on her enlarged clitoris. No one said why; it was just done. All this has hit her now. What she knows now is only what she knows through her own research and she is strong and speaks out – she is a biology graduate – and she was always the best in our family for getting As.

My sister who has just had the affected baby is now behaving just like my other sister. She does not want anyone in the family to know about her child's condition. The other day she said, 'What if people find out about this condition? What if they notice something?' I told her, 'All you have to say is it's the condition our niece and nephew have. That's all you need to say, and as far as anyone else is concerned it's just a matter of taking a couple of tablets.' But she is afraid that people will notice that her baby is different. She wants her to have the operation so people don't stare, so that she can be as normal as possible. She won't take the baby to see our grandmother in Pakistan. She hasn't even told our Mum.

Her husband knows all about the condition; his brother is my niece's father, but he, too, is saying nothing. It makes my niece very angry. She says, 'It's OK to hide your own child, but you know about me. It is so hypocritical – to know that this is in the family, and then to hide your own child.' My sister, she isn't going to have any more children now. It has totally put her off. She had wanted to have four. My husband does not even know about the new baby's condition, and I find this very hard, because, when I am upset about it, I cannot talk to him, because I have promised my sister I won't.

Recently, my niece said to me, 'Now you understand why I suffered so much when you said you didn't get tested before you got pregnant … Waiting for your results was the longest time in my life … I was worrying that your daughter would have to go through what I had gone through.'

To an extent, the secrecy in this case reflects the particular nature of the condition. Genetic conditions involving genital ambiguity or genital reassignment surgery are particularly likely to lead to concealment and non-communication (Clarke et al. 2005). These issues are also linked to wider debate over the medical management of intersex conditions (see, for example, Fausto-Sterling 2000). More generally, secrecy in such cases reflects parents' concerns about the social impact of the condition, in the perceptions of others, and this is not restricted to conditions involving genital ambiguity. The secrecy highlights the shame generally felt by parents about any imperfection; as Najma put it, 'Our kids can be nothing less than perfect. It is so difficult to accept that they might not be.' This, too, is part of the reason why parents may withhold genetic risk information from other members of the family, at least where aspects of the condition can be hidden. Parents' reasons for not discussing genetic risk within the family are thus informed by a desire both to protect themselves and others from the stigma associated with a genetic problem.[3]

Even where many aspects of a condition involving long-term medical or learning problems cannot be concealed, parents may be reluctant to discuss the genetic implications for fear of compromising that child's and other children's marriage prospects. As Husnain said, 'If my Mum was looking for a *rishta* for me, she is not going to tell them that I am a thalassaemia carrier. It will be the family's well-kept secret.' Zahida, who had had a genetic prenatal test for the condition that affects her fourth child, had not discussed carrier testing with any of her relatives and did not know if her eldest daughter, now studying medicine, had sought a carrier test. She thought she might check her eldest son's carrier status, as he is approaching marriageable age, not because she is considering a *rishta* from within the family but because she will be looking outside it, since:

> there isn't a girl his age in the family, either here or in Pakistan ... Maybe he will marry an English girl – I mean, a Pakistani Muslim girl who knows English, brought up here and not from Pakistan – but it is difficult to find a girl here because most of them are not from Pindi side but are from Mirpur. We only have my husband's brothers and sisters here – the Mirpuris won't agree to give a girl to Pindi people.

As this suggests, the question of a person's carrier status may be more likely to emerge explicitly when people are considering introducing someone new to the family (see also Featherstone et al. 2006); in contrast, where *rishta*s are sought within the family, either in the U.K. or in Pakistan, it may be more likely that the issue is 'brushed under the carpet', as Hamid Ullah, who carries a balanced translocation, put it. Hamid married a first cousin from Pakistan and sought genetic testing for his children after their birth, while his university-educated younger brother, who also carries a balanced translocation, came with his U.K.-raised fiancée to seek genetic advice before their marriage.

Practical ethics: 'why worry them?'

The non-disclosure of genetic risk information is also a matter of making practical ethical decisions about whether or not it is appropriate to inform other family members about genetic risk, as has been shown for familial breast cancer and for some other genetic conditions (Richards 1996c; Hallowell 1999; Featherstone et al. 2006). For families in this study, similar processes were at work, against the backdrop of competitive fertility described above. After his son's sudden death, Khalida's husband went to the coroner's office to collect the death certificate, and his brother accompanied him. His brother therefore probably knew that the stated cause of death was cardiomyopathy, and also that genetic counselling was recommended for the parents, as this was written on the certificate. But, Khalida said,

> The rest of the family – they don't tend to think you're telling the truth anyway. We said bluntly that it is when the heart swells up and stops. And with our daughter, we said about the polycystic kidney that the kidneys did not develop. But I don't think they know that it is a genetic thing. I don't see any point in telling them.

Khalida's reasons for thinking there is no point in telling the rest of the family that her son's death had a genetic cause are worth discussing in some more detail, because they were echoed by many other couples in my study with children diagnosed with genetic disorders. When this couple were told that their son's sudden death had a genetic cause, the clinician had also explained that mutation analysis would allow their unaffected children to have carrier tests in the future: 'When they are older they may want to find out, especially if they marry a close relative. In ten years' time, it will be easier to do carrier screening. The chance goes down considerably if they marry outside the family. The chance would go up if they marry a close relative.' She also mentioned the implications for other relatives, since she knew from the family tree that had been drawn up in the clinic that one of Khalida's brothers is married to one of her husband's sisters:

> This also applies to any of your brothers and sisters who have married a close family member. It is difficult to appreciate, but other relatives are at risk if they marry close family members. A one in four is a significant risk, even though there is a three in four chance that the baby is OK, and here there are two conditions. It's not anything that you have done wrong, it is something that happens to all of us.

Four months later, I talked with Khalida about these implications for her siblings. Her initial response was to tell me that, apart from her husband's brother, no one in the family knows about 'the genetic thing', and that, anyway, she herself was not convinced that the cause was genetic and not simply attributable to 'bad luck': 'It is all theory – the theory is that we lost him because of genetics, and so we have a theoretical risk.' She then elaborated on her thinking about the implications for relatives, in the process revealing a slightly more complex family tree than the one drawn up in the clinic because she had not previously mentioned a divorced sister.

> My oldest brother has finished his family, all are healthy, so there's no point telling him. My oldest sister has healthy children, all girls, and she is widowed and not going to have any more children so there is no point telling her. My youngest brother is married out of the family so I don't

> think he needs to know. My middle brother is married to my husband's sister. So they do have the same risk as us, but they have two healthy children – so why worry them? I do have another sister, but she is disowned by the family because she divorced my husband's brother. She has healthy children from her first marriage and two children from her second marriage, but there is no point telling her, since her husband is not even Pakistani.

Before letting the topic drop, I pressed Khalida a little more on the implications for these relatives, because the fact that all her siblings have so far had healthy children does not rule out the possibility that they are carriers. She responded with a reflection on modern society that that echoes contemporary sociological discussion of risk and modernity:

> AS: Does it worry you that perhaps you know something that they need to know?
> K: No. I don't think they need to know. If they asked us, we would tell them. But I don't think they have to worry about something that doesn't happen.
> AS: You mean, that hasn't happened to them?
> K: Well yes, and probably won't happen. I don't see any point in telling them. It has got nothing to do with them anyway, unless they ask. The trouble is, once you have got into it – this high technology medicine – and into thinking about risk and the options, it is hard to get out of it. My husband says I should just put it out of my mind.

Khalida and her husband continued to attend their genetics appointments and consented to mutation research for the cardiomyopathy, hopeful that it might be useful diagnostically and therapeutically in the event of the birth of another affected child, for they would not consider terminating an affected pregnancy. They also consented to relatives being told of results should they ask. They therefore continued to be engaged with the clinicians and with clinical research, and to be hopeful of a useful result, while simultaneously retaining a degree of scepticism that the disorders are 'in the family', and considering it pointless to introduce the idea of genetic risk to relatives who don't already have affected children. Khalida's view was, 'If it happens, it happens; until then they don't need to know,' to which her husband added, 'They would not believe it anyway.'

Seeking carrier testing: 'Only if I have to'

Despite the view that siblings only need to know 'if it happens', brothers and sisters of people who have or whose children have genetic conditions do sometimes seek carrier testing on the basis of their family history, as we saw in Najma and

Nadeem's case and with Ikra's elder brother. Nonetheless, the proportion of people who seek carrier testing on the basis of a family history appears to be small in relation to the number of people diagnosed with genetic conditions. It may be that 'at-risk' individuals and couples have the information they need and have chosen not to come forward for carrier testing – at least until they feel they need to. Individuals who are aware of their risk of carrying a dominantly inherited genetic disorder such as Huntington's disease may live with this uncertainty for years, only seeking testing when reaching the age at which symptoms of this late-onset condition usually appear (Anon 1996). In relation to risk for recessive disorders, people may not feel they need to establish their carrier status until they 'need' to, and this need may not be felt until they marry, or are considering having children, or are pregnant, or have had a child and are planning another, or have had an affected child. It was a puzzle for the genetics clinic in Birmingham, England, why couples from extended Pakistani families with a family history of a recessive condition who have access to Urdu-speaking genetic counsellors often seek carrier testing only when they are already pregnant. This pattern of 'late referral' represents a failure from the perspective of genetic service provision, because clinicians would have liked to extend carrier testing to such couples in time for them to decide 'whether or not to start a family' (Canham et al. 2002). In my study, I observed directly only five genetics referrals that were for carrier testing in connection with a family history of a genetic condition (three concerning recessive conditions and two concerning chromosome anomalies, all five associated with long-term medical and learning problems). In two consultations, the sibling of an affected person was planning to marry (in one case, within, and in the other case, outside the family), while three referrals concerned already married couples who were either in the early stages of pregnancy or already had an unaffected baby. As we saw, Ikra's older brother sought a carrier test after he got married. Similarly, her younger brother sought carrier testing after his marriage. As Ikra told me:

> In fact, it was only when his wife got pregnant that he went to the doctors. He was quite worried, because he knew that I had thalassaemia and my brother was quite educated and wanted to know if he could be a carrier. They did the test on him, and found he was a carrier, and on his wife, and they were told they have a one in four risk. They were really worried with the first baby. Now they know their oldest child is a carrier, and the younger one is not, and they won't risk having any more children now.

What Ikra's brother and the other people in my study who sought carrier testing have in common is personal experience of the condition that is in their family, through their relationship with an affected sibling or other close relative such as a niece or nephew. While marriage, pregnancy and childbirth provide contexts for seeking a genetics referral, the experience of having an affected relative, in the context of their close relationships with them, provides the impetus for actually having the test. The test itself may in turn provide an opportunity for further discussion of the genetic aspects of the condition that may have gone unexplored when the condition was first diagnosed. It was not until her younger brother had a carrier test that Ikra herself fully appreciated the implications of her diagnosis for other relatives:

> What made him get the test is that he is very close to me. He has seen all that I have to go through. He could not take the thought that one of his children might have the same problems as me. All this happened about eight years ago, when I was fourteen. They gave my brother all this information, and he then explained it for everyone. After that my sister got tested, and her husband – though they don't have any children. It was only then that our parents understood. Up to then, I had gone for treatment without understanding that this was a genetic thing, with implications for other relatives.
>
> My father must have been told, years before, but he had not told my brother that he might be a carrier. My father must have known, but also he did not want to know. But my Mum did not know. My father did not say anything to her, and my Mum did not read anything, because she is illiterate.

Najma's sister and brother-in-law, as parents of two affected children, had not spoken about the genetic nature of their children's condition with their parents, now elderly first generation migrants, or with their siblings, even though all were married to first cousins. It was only on the insistence of her affected niece, by then a biology graduate, that Najma requested a risk assessment:

> Actually, when we married, I didn't really understand that the risk was quite high. I always knew that my niece and nephew took medication and had some condition, but as a child I never thought anything of it. It was just a way of life for us. No one said this is it, [names the condition], and this is how it happens, and this is the risk. But when I wanted a baby I spoke to my niece because I am close to her in age – there are only five years between us. She told me about the risk and she was quite insistent that we should get tested before we started planning for a baby. Yes, it was my niece, not her Mum, who talked about it. My sister has never spoken about it, never. But then I found I was already pregnant. Looking back, I can see that my niece was quite upset that we had not been tested first.
>
> Then I told the doctor about my niece and nephew, and that I might be at risk of having a similarly affected child. He said, 'You should think, if you go for carrier testing, what you would do if you were both carriers. Would you keep the baby?' We thought about it, and we thought either way we

> would keep the baby. 'So,' he said, 'in that case, wait till the baby is born before you get the carrier test.'
>
> Now I know that is not the only choice, because, if you test positive in pregnancy with this condition, you can do something for a girl – she would still need to take tablets, but the effect on the genitals is less. My niece was not thinking of termination when she told me to get the test. She always said, 'You can get treatment.' She wanted me to have children. She just said, 'Don't bury your head in the sand. It can happen. It will happen.' She was right ... Anyway, this meant that our daughter was about six months old when we were eventually both tested at the clinic. The results took about six months. Now I know my husband is a carrier but I am not. And now I know what the risks are, I would definitely not marry my daughter within the family – at least, I would prefer if she did not marry in the family. It is a possibility, of course, who knows? But, at least, she should have the carrier test when she is older. My husband says she should have the test and, if the test shows she is a carrier, then she should not be married in the family, or, if she is, then the boy should be tested. But that's down to my niece opening my eyes – she was the driving force behind me getting tested.

Najma's experience of carrier testing reflected her close personal relationship with her affected niece, rather than any open discussion between herself and her sisters about the risk of this particular condition in the family. I asked Najma whether there was anyone else in the immediate family for whom the diagnosis of this condition has implications:

> Two of my sisters are carriers because they have affected children. My other sister has not been tested. Her two kids are both fine – but it is possible that she is a carrier, and that her husband is too. She is married to a cousin. Her husband is my Mum's sister's daughter, and that sister could be a carrier like my Mum. But she is burying her head in the sand. She has two healthy kids, and she says she is not having any more, so there is no need to find out. Her kids could be carriers – but she does not want to think about this. So, actually, it is only me and my husband who have had carrier tests. The sisters with affected children have not had their unaffected children tested yet. But I think they will. Hasina, she will make sure of that, when the time comes for it to matter.
>
> I know that, if we went to our Mum and said, 'This has passed from generation to generation,' she would not believe it. She would say, 'It is because you don't pray enough.' At least we know now. And I know that it's not just a question of not marrying in the family, because if I am a carrier I could marry someone who is not a relative but still a carrier of it. English people are carriers too. I think more has to be told about this. But I only know what I know because of my niece.

Najma's neice is unusual in that her condition does not involve any learning problems, and she has been the driving force behind her sister's seeking a carrier test. Ikra, too, suffered no learning problems, and her own understanding of the genetics of her condition facilitated communication about risk in her family. For Hamid and his brother, the close personal experience of living with siblings with long-term learning problems, which they learnt early on were not associated with parental consanguinity, prompted them to seek carrier testing. Where a condition is less 'visible', as with experiences of pregnancy loss or infant death, there are fewer available routes through which communication about risk can occur, but, here again, close personal relationships and the indirect experience gained through them may be crucial to communication about genetic risk. After Shakeera's painful experience of neonatal death, her sister told me that she and her husband (Shakeera's husband's brother) intend to seek carrier testing when they have another child, because her knowledge of the depth of her sister's suffering, combined with her sister's explanation of the genetic risk, has made her realise the seriousness of the possibility that she is a carrier: 'Now that I know, I would want to avoid this if I possibly could.'

Conclusion: communication and assumptions about cultural difference

When a genetic diagnosis is made, it implicates those believed to share the same DNA (or 'blood'). In this way, developments in genomic medicine and research have the potential to reinforce or renew an understanding of kinship as being rooted in biology and specifically in shared DNA or blood. Kaja Finkler claims that the 'new' genetics is transforming kinship by prompting Americans with hereditary breast cancer to renew contacts with blood relatives, so as to communicate genetic risk information: kinship is being put to work in extending the network of diagnosable people and is thus, she argues, being medicalised or pathologised (Finkler 2001). The novelty of such processes may be questionable, however, in that people were interested in tracking those they understand to be biological kin long before the use of new molecular genetic techniques in the 1970s and they do so for many reasons besides medical ones – in the pursuit, for instance of concerns with identity and family history. Recent academic interest in the impact of the 'new' genetics on kinship tends to give disproportionate emphasis to 'the genetic' at the expense of conveying a sense of the wider context of family and kinship and the complexities of people's conceptualisations of the relationship between biology and culture (Freeman and Richards 2006).

Claims about the geneticisation of kinship are also challenged by empirical work demonstrating that a genetic diagnosis does not everywhere lead to the communication of genetic risk information among biological kin. Katie Featherstone and colleagues (2006) have recently demonstrated how problematic the concept of disclosure of genetic risk information to close biological kin can be. Definitions of family or close kinship are shaped by social and cultural processes. In these processes, ties of blood or DNA are only one of many ways in which people understand kinship to be constituted, and people's understandings of blood ties do not always follow models of genetic inheritance. In family understandings of illness causality and inheritance, a medical condition may not be understood within the family to have a genetic cause and, even where it is recognised as 'running in the family', the implications of it being genetic may not be understood in ways that match the medical model. A particular presentation in a family where a condition seems to run 'though men' or 'through women' can mean that inheritance and risk are understood in these terms. For instance, the fact that most breast cancer referrals are of cases where there is a maternal history of breast cancer is often associated with the belief that breast cancer is only transmitted in females. It is thus important to recognise the variety of understandings of inheritance that people from all ethnic or cultural backgrounds are likely to bring to a genetics consultation and to their negotiations of the implications of a genetic diagnosis. Indeed, everyday ideas about inheritance are also likely to be important in other areas of contemporary culture besides testing for medical conditions, for example in paternity testing, in forensic use and in the construction of genealogies (Freeman and Richards 2006).

For British Pakistani couples, accepting any serious illness in a child, including a genetic condition, can also be complicated by the parents' fear of being stigmatised (by clinicians or in the wider society) for being consanguineously married or (by relatives or neighbours) for their apparent reproductive failure. The difficulties of accepting a genetic diagnosis and discussing it within the family are for some couples compounded by the challenges of communicating technical information across language barriers, by their and their relatives' prior understandings of how the condition is inherited and by scepticism of the 'consanguinity thesis'. Parents of affected children may consider it 'not their business' to inform and therefore worry potential carriers about genetic risk, especially if these relatives do not have any affected children. Clinicians, too, may hesitate to discuss explicitly the implications for close biological kin, particularly if there is diagnostic uncertainty or if carrier tests are not available for the disorder in question, preferring instead to note these implications in a letter to the parents that may be copied to a GP and filed for future reference. In this study, those who sought carrier screening and testing because of a family history of a genetic condition (often many years after the initial diagnosis was made) were of reproductive age – considering marriage or having children or having more children. A main trigger for these referrals was their experience of the condition, gained from being brought up with, or having a close friendship with, an affected relative, rather than their theoretical or probabilistic knowledge of genetic risk.

In this discussion of people's understandings of and patterns of communicating within the family about genetic risk, I have identified themes shared by British

Pakistani and white Anglo-British users of UK genetic services. In so doing, I have challenged assumptions about how cultural difference may shape these experiences. While it may be useful for counsellors to be aware of the possible patrilineal bias in South Asian understandings of inheritance, this bias cannot be assumed, but is only one of a range of understandings that British Pakistani clients may bring to their genetics consultation. Equally, while it is important for clinicians to recognise the often complex patterns of consanguinity and affinity that characterise extended Pakistani families, close kinship in itself – even where extended family members live under one roof- offers no guarantee that genetic risk information will be easily shared; on the contrary, an individual or couple's privacy with respect to genetic disorders in their children may be carefully guarded, and indications of any possible reproductive problems may be kept secret from even parents and close siblings. In addition, relatives' understandings of inheritance and the causality of the condition, the nature of the condition and the potential stigma attached to it, as well as context and timing, are all likely to shape whether and how information about a genetic condition 'in the family' is communicated. Such issues are also likely to influence the success of more proactive approaches to genetic counselling, whereby a clinician identifies carriers from the family tree and seeks the proband's (or their parents') consent to contact these potential carriers so as to offer them genetic counselling and, if appropriate, carrier or prenatal testing.

Notes

1. These calculations refer to nuclear DNA, which is contained in the nucleus of every cell, packaged into twenty-three pairs of chromosomes, of which one single set is inherited from the mother and one from the father. Each cell also contains extra-nuclear mitochondrial DNA that is inherited from the mother only.
2. As noted, the term carrier is ambiguous. Here, it became clear to me that Husnain understood a carrier of thalassaemia to be someone who would certainly develop the condition. The distinction between being an unaffected carrier of a recessive disorder (having one copy of the mutation) and having the disorder (by being 'homozygous' or having two copies) is frequently lost. In the booklets about being a carrier of thalassaemia that have been translated into Urdu, the same phrase is used to refer to both being a carrier and being affected (thalassaemia *men mubtalā honā*) (Shaw and Ahmed 2004).
3. Among Hasidic Jews in Brooklyn, New York, the results of Tay–Sachs carrier tests are given to matchmakers, not to the individual or family, to avoid stigmatising anyone found to be a carrier (Wilkie 1994: 114).

CHAPTER 8
GENETIC RISK IN CONTEXT

Five years after her referral to clinical genetics, Zobeen's case remains in the category of unknown conditions, despite the clinician's hunch that her problems are chromosomal and repeating the chromosome test with a new, more sensitive technique. Zobeen's blood sample has now been sent to a U.K. research group investigating the genes that may be implicated in one of her problems, but the flurry of medical activity that surrounded Zobeen's first eighteen months has quietened and her parents' anxieties about the causes and management of her problems now largely belong to the past. The birth of three other unaffected children has also helped to put Zobeen's problems in perspective. As Husnain proudly told me, Zobeen now has two brothers and one sister, all perfectly healthy.

The experience of risk in relation to the diagnosis of a genetic condition occurs not within a social vacuum but within the wider political, historical, socio-economic and religious context of people's lives, shaped by and shaping experiences of kinship, marriage and childbearing. This study has focused mainly on the experiences of British Pakistani adults referred to clinical genetics in connection with a problem diagnosed in pregnancy, an infant or a child, against a background of evidence of higher rates of infant mortality and childhood morbidity among British Pakistanis and debate over the public health implications of the elevated risk of recessive disorders associated with parental consanguinity. I have been less concerned with what it means to live with genetic conditions (for which see, for example, Ablon 1984, 1988, 1999) than with exploring how the experience of a clinical genetics referral is influenced by the wider contemporary discourse of genetic risk associated with consanguineous marriage. I have also shown how the experience of genetic risk splinters off into risks for such problems as pregnancy loss or infant death; minor birth abnormalities; serious, life-shortening medical problems; and long-term major or minor problems that are medical, intellectual or both. While the risks for these problems are in many (but not all) cases genetic or probably genetic, they are not always associated with recessive inheritance and are not specific to British Pakistanis but instead confront couples of all ethnic backgrounds in the wider population.

My intention has been not to deny the reality of the elevated risk of recessive conditions associated with consanguineous marriage or to suggest the evidence be ignored, but, taking a lead from the work of Mary Douglas, to point to the social and cultural shaping of both the perception and the experience of this particular risk in contemporary Britain (Douglas and Wildavsky 1982; Douglas 1985, 1992). The medical management of pregnancy and childbirth represents one element of risk management as a central concern of late modern society; highlighting in public debate the genetic risks of consanguineous marriage, rather than, say, the risk of Down syndrome associated with late childbearing, also reflects the structural position of Britain's Pakistani population, whose social and cultural non-conformity has for some time been a source of political concern. The media focus on the biological risks of cousin marriage that accompanied a Member of Parliament's suggestion in 2006 that this 'risky lifestyle' be controlled through legislation drew from and fed into broader concerns about cultural difference, including concerns that arranged transnational marriages are coercive, entail cultural incompatibility and inhibit the integration of Muslims in Europe. Debates over these issues are not new but have reclaimed public attention following the terrorist attacks in the U.S.A. on 11 September 2001 and the London bombings of 7 July 2005. Yet, from the perspective not of dominant epidemiological or political discourses but of the British Pakistanis arranging or participating in transnational marriages involving kin, these marriages can be understood as involving a balance of a range of other types of risk, including the social and emotional risks, especially for daughters, of marrying outside the family. In these considerations, the idea of genetic risk, as risk rooted in cellular architecture, is a relative newcomer among the understandings of illness causality from which my research participants draw and it plays a variable role in their understandings of particular genetic conditions.

A historical perspective on cousin marriage in Europe further highlights the temporal and cultural specificity and the historical roots of contemporary concern over the genetic risks of cousin marriage. As Mary Douglas suggests, the idea of being at risk, not just for genetic problems but generally, represents not so much a new phenomenon but a modern expression of perennial concerns with dangers of all sorts. In the nineteenth century, the dangers for children (and adults) of inheritable problems were serious concerns for scholars and physicians and some physicians came quite close to modern understandings of risk in the realisation that cousin marriages were not inherently problematic but required case-by-case assessments of possible biological harm to offspring. At that time, cousin marriage, which had constituted a significant minority marriage pattern across a wide range of social strata in industrialising Europe, was still popular among the Victorian gentry. This may explain why a parliamentary group rejected a proposal to include a question on cousin marriages in the 1871 census, despite growing concern over its possible adverse biological effects: as we saw, one Member of Parliament commented that such a question would only stigmatise cousin couples. The contemporary debate combines these historically rooted concerns about medical risk with more recent concerns about cultural difference, augmenting what is now a majority perception of cousin marriages as both socially problematic and medically risky. This perception, as I have shown, is indeed stigmatising: it inhibits clinical communication where cousin couples hesitate to seek a genetics referral for fear of professional disapproval or where it is assumed that consanguineous marriage has 'caused' a child's problem when this is not the case.

While concern over the possible biological ill effects of cousin marriage in the light of understandings of Darwinian evolutionary theory undoubtedly contributed to the decline of cousin marriage from the late nineteenth century onwards within Europe and America, the wide-reaching social and demographic changes already set in motion by industrialisation probably played a more important role, by reducing family size and so decreasing the availability of cousins as marriage partners. It remains to be seen what the effects on Pakistani marriage practices of current concern over the genetic risks of consanguineous marriages will be, in relation to demographic and other forces of social change. Besides the evidence of genetic risk and attitudes to this evidence, it will also be important to consider the socio-economic, cultural and demographic significance of transnational kin connections as well as the opportunities and challenges offered by modern prenatal, genetic and medical technologies.

Some South Asian and Muslim groups in the U.K. have taken up the arguments about the genetic risks of consanguineous marriage, but locally there is a culture of scepticism about the 'consanguinity thesis'. Reflecting incomplete understandings of the genetic risks, some British Pakistanis now believe genetics is 'what happens when you marry cousins', while others strongly resist the idea that cousin marriage 'causes' birth defects, medical problems or learning difficulties, a resistance informed by the accurate lay observation that most Pakistanis marry cousins without having children with disabilities and English people do not marry cousins but may still have affected children. Scepticism over 'genetics' as a cause of birth abnormalities exists against a background of alternative explanations that recognise environmental and spiritual factors, and in which the probabilistic rather than certain nature of modern notions of epidemiological and reproductive risk can be difficult to accommodate. Indeed, in these understandings, the notion of risk itself becomes one of the hazards of life in the West. As Sohrab's grandfather put it, 'there is more risk here than in Pakistan'. Stories also abound about the seeming unreliability of genetic risk information, confirming the belief that what happens is ultimately 'up to God'.

These stories are not fabrications but draw on elements of experience. One genetics referral concerned Khurshid, whose blue eyes, light brown hair and skin colouring mean he is frequently mistaken by fellow Pakistanis as a *gora* (white, or Englishman) but are in fact the phenotypic characteristics of a mild form of recessive albinism. Khurshid and his parents had understood that by seeking a *rishta* for him from outside the family they would avoid risk of the condition in their grandchildren and so, drawing on family networks, found a bride from an unrelated family in Pakistan. However, the couple now have two children with a stronger form of their father's condition, indicating that it was insufficient simply to 'marry out' to avoid the condition. Khurshid's Pakistan born and raised wife, a college graduate, had been unaware of the genetic implications of her husband's condition and of the theoretical possibility that she might be a carrier until after a genetics referral for the children established her 'obligate carrier' status. It also emerged from her family history that she had a grandfather affected by a stronger form of the condition. In theory, then, this couple's risk could have been identified if a thorough family history had been taken in a prenatal genetics consultation, or if a premarital or prenatal carrier test for the condition had been offered to Khurshid's wife.

Transnational cousin marriage, gender and family care

Khurshid's story illustrates another important dimension of genetic risk as it affects British Pakistani families, namely the fact that this risk is experienced across a transnational arena marked by global structural and infrastructural inequality. Connections between people in Pakistan and Britain are largely constituted through the practical and emotional ties of kinship and facilitated by modern travel and communications technologies, yet these ties are rarely symmetrical or evenly constituted across this arena, as the experience of genetic risk and access to genetic services illustrates.

In this research, I have not traced directly the engagements of British Pakistanis with genetic services in Pakistan or explored in detail their communication with Pakistan-based kin about the nature and implications of a genetic diagnosis, but my observations and conversations on these topics indicate processes of communication and engagement that are frequently partial and pragmatic. One young U.K.-raised mother relocating to Pakistan, where her husband's family is based, requested copies of all the diagnostic information about her son's genetic condition to take to a Karachi hospital. Another mother, Riffat, requested extra copies of an Urdu booklet about Down syndrome to send to her in-laws in Pakistan. In other cases, however, detailed discussions of the medical and genetic aspects of a particular condition seem to remain U.K.-based. Nadia's husband sent photographs to his parents and brother in Pakistan that showed their daughter's limb abnormalities and later sent post-operation photographs showing how much more normal her limbs are now, but he did not name the condition or discuss its genetic aspects, feeling that such information would be meaningless to their relatives in Pakistan. Sofia felt it would be inappropriate to worry her mother in Mirpur with the name of the recessive kidney condition that had caused two infant deaths. Khalida described features of the two conditions from which she had lost three babies during her most recent visit to her mother-in-law in rural northern Punjab, but did not mention the genetic risk; as her husband later commented, 'They would not believe it anyway.' More generally, while there is evidence of some policy-level concern in Pakistan about the genetic risks of consanguineous marriage, my research participants tell me that this issues does not much feature within dominant public or media discourses there: hence Sohrab's grandfather's perception that 'there is more risk here [in the U.K.] than in Pakistan'.

This association of genetic risk with the U.K. context is in turn relevant to the continuing popularity of transnational cousin marriages. Such marriages are central to the maintenance of Pakistani transnational networks, linking individuals, households and kin beyond the household and providing a mechanism through which gender inequalities and patriarchal family relations are both reproduced and challenged. Informed and influenced by the dominant discourse of consanguinity and risk in Britain, young British Pakistani adults may, increasingly, regard their British-based cousins as 'too close' to marry. Katharine Charsley suggests that the prospect of a transnational cousin marriage reintroduces an acceptable distance that makes Pakistani cousins acceptable as spouses, and the issue of genetic risk does not generally seem to feature among any reservations that kin in Pakistan might have concerning *rishta*s involving cousins living overseas. Young British Pakistani adults may sometimes utilise the discourse of risk to justify rejecting Pakistani *rishta*s that they do not want for other reasons and some British-based parents may wish to avoid cousin marriages for their children because of general concerns about genetic risk or because of family history of a genetic condition. Yet, as this and other recent work has demonstrated, there remain strong socio-economic, cultural and emotional reasons for favouring transnational cousin marriages, and the demographic characteristics of *birādarī* networks in Pakistan and elsewhere in the Pakistani diaspora usually mean that there is more than one potential spouse to choose from (Charsley 2003; Shaw and Charsley 2006).

A further and sometimes important motivation for such marriages is that they can provide fallback options precisely because there are medical or social problems in the family. If a British-based arranged or 'love marriage' has failed, where public knowledge of a young man or woman's medical or intellectual problems makes marriage outside the family difficult to arrange, or if a married man is widowed, the parents or other close kin are likely to consider suitable kin in Pakistan as spouses. It is widely held that marriage is necessary for men and women, but especially for a man. Additionally, parents' concerns for the well-being of a child with particular disabilities may mean that kin are actively preferred over strangers as spouses. As Riaz, whose wife – a first cousin once removed – is deaf, as are three of his children, put it: 'If a deaf woman's in-laws are also her relatives, they will be patient and not shout at her if she does something wrong. If she is married outside, there is more chance that she will be harshly treated.' In Pakistan, part of the motivation for arranging marriages within the family is to provide support for people with special needs, understood broadly as an extension of the principle of family care. In Pakistan, this is particularly important in the absence of state provisions and where, for women especially, there are few alternative routes to a secure social status than by means of kinship and marriage. British Pakistanis continue to negotiate these needs for family-based care across the transnational arena. In this context, the additional attraction of a route to 'first-world' citizenship for a prospective spouse and their kin in Pakistan may mean that a *rishta* is accepted that might otherwise be considered unattractive (Shaw 2004; Harriss and Shaw 2006: 259–74).

Since the domestic burden of care, rather than the expectation of financial support, conventionally falls upon women, there is often an explicitly gendered dimension to family care. Saleem Ullah, whose eldest son has moderate learning difficulties and is of school leaving age, plans to arrange his son's marriage in the next few years, provided the boy has sufficient maturity to hold down a routine job 'such as in Tesco'. 'I will keep him with me; he will have this house,' Saleem Ullah told me, adding that he expects his daughter, whose learning difficulties are milder, to manage to live independently. He expects to find a wife for his son from within the family and considers his son's difficulties unrelated to consanguineous marriage. He received no conclusive genetic explanation for his son's problems from clinical genetics and still considers a childhood immunisation was the most likely cause. As he told me, learning problems can be related to environmental factors, such as a home or school that is not conducive to learning, and do not always run true in families: 'My brothers and sisters all married relatives and don't have children with learning disabilities … People with learning difficulties can give birth to people who become doctors. For example, in my own family, a man born here whose mother had a learning problem and father was not well educated went on to become a doctor.'

Zahida, whose sixteen-year-old son has a recessive metabolic condition, intellectual problems and very difficult behaviour, hopes to arrange his marriage to a girl from Pakistan. Zahida was confident that finding a girl would not be a problem. She understood that, to avoid risk of the condition occurring in any children, they should look outside the family, thus equating genetic risk with marrying in the family. However, she had clearly understood that this was a matter of risk, not of inevitability, and that the important thing would be to avoid marrying her son to a girl who is a carrier: 'He can marry a girl who is not a carrier and their children will not have the disease. This does not mean we won't marry in the family, but that we will do the test first: it is easy, all it involves is a blood test.' Her main worry was that although she and her husband would provide the couple with a house, her son's learning difficulties might mean he is denied a spousal visa:

> We will of course provide a home; there is not much mortgage on this house. He will get allowances and his wife will get allowances after marriage: income support, disability living allowance, mobility allowance and invalidity allowance for looking after him. If we can get such a girl, we will give him a house, but maybe there will be a problem with the visa.

The nature of the condition can thus affect the success of marriage plans. Akhtar's brothers have a rare recessive condition but no intellectual problems and

Akhtar successfully arranged for one of his brothers to marry a woman from Pakistan. In this instance, taking into account medical advice:

> We didn't look in the family because the doctors advised us not to. She is from a village where the women are not very educated. We told her he has problems. We explained to her and her family about the condition, and the role she would have. She would be like a nurse as well. We explained to her that your role is to help your husband, for example, you will have to give him a slight massage with olive oil, so that he will feel more nimble. And she accepted it, that role. But it turns out they were only interested in coming here. She is supposed to help, but she needs someone from outside the family like a doctor to advise her ... She was OK at first, but then people put ideas into her head that she should not be a nurse.

In the light of tensions that can arise with regard to expectations of care, Akhtar is now explicitly seeking nurses from Pakistan as wives for his other brothers and is prepared to look outside his ethnic group:

> We are looking for compatibility and for someone who will fulfil the role of nurse as well as the role of wife. The ones that are good nurses and good wives are from Peshawar but the problem is language: they speak Pashtu. We are going through family contacts and I asked my cousin in Pakistan – he knows Pathans from the Peshawar side. Some of their girls are very highly educated, with masters degrees. In that case, they may say they don't want this lifestyle. Two of them have said they don't mind. But we have to be certain that the *rishta* is compatible.

Occasionally, the gendered dimension of care is reversed when a man migrates to the U.K. for marriage to a kinswoman with a learning problem or physical disability of which, in some cases, the groom may not have been fully aware beforehand. This situation can augment the problems experienced by 'imported' husbands (Charsley 2003) but it does not inevitably result in the partial or complete breakdown of the marriage. The two husbands in such marriages in my study were also fathers of infants referred to clinical genetics, but remained committed to their marriages from a sense of family obligation, marital duty and emotional connection with their wives (who were cousins) and their in-laws (who were also their aunts and uncles), despite suggestions from friends and workmates that they should leave.

Using modern medical technology: religious morality, privacy and practical ethics

The modern identification of genetic risk does not mean that an adverse birth outcome is inevitable or that a couple should think they necessarily cannot have an unaffected child. Today, couples can be offered an estimate of the risk of genetic problems in their children, taking into account any parental consanguinity and history of genetic conditions in the family. These estimates are founded upon modern (post-1900) understandings of Mendelian genetics concerning how genes recombine in predictable ways in sexual reproduction. In addition, the recent and ongoing discoveries of the particular mutations associated with an increasing number of conditions means that couples with an established risk may also be offered prenatal genetic testing, the option of terminating a pregnancy and opportunities for carrier testing within the wider family (as well as, where appropriate, outside it) as ways of managing their risk. Such options were not available in the nineteenth century or in the first part of the twentieth century, even after the initial establishment of clinical genetics as a medical speciality. Today, a consanguineously married couple concerned about genetic risks to children, especially where there is a family history of consanguineous marriage or of a genetic condition would be best advised to ask their GP for a referral to clinical genetics.

Entering the system for managing reproductive risk entails further moral dilemmas. As Rayna Rapp (2000) has shown for women undergoing amniocentesis in America, so too I would argue that British Pakistani users of prenatal and genetic services are 'moral pioneers' traversing relatively uncharted moral territory. They navigate this territory by drawing on the resources of their family and their cultural and religious background; this profoundly shapes their engagement with and use of medical technologies. As we saw with Shakeera, whose first child's fatal problems were diagnosed in pregnancy and resulted in a traumatic childbirth and newborn death, young British Pakistani women may be terrified of having a, or another, child with major problems and may worry about the impact on their marriage, family life and prospects of returning to work, but equally may fear that it would be sinful according to Islam, besides inviting strong family and community disapproval, to take steps to end a pregnancy in these circumstances.

These dilemmas are experienced in relation to competing discourses of autonomy and control, changing expectations of work and marriage, especially for women, and competing Islamic discourses on the acceptability of contraception, prenatal diagnosis and termination of pregnancy. For some, the idea of managing risks in childbirth through prenatal genetic diagnosis, like the idea of controlling or planning pregnancy, represents a lack of faith in God and a fear of undertaking the tests God sets people in their lives. For others, contraceptive use, prenatal diagnosis and termination of pregnancy can be approached from an Islamic view that combines the idea of trust in God with recognition of human moral agency (*khilafah*). From this perspective, the exercise of *khilafah* entails taking responsibility for oneself and others by weighing up the harm and benefits of different courses of action in the light of particular circumstances and new biomedical knowledge. The exercise of *khilafah* is an important element in the scholarly and personal negotiation of *ijtihādī* issues – those on which the primary sources (the Qur'an and the Prophetic Traditions) are ambiguous. It allows, for instance, some negotiation with respect to termination of pregnancy and the moral status of the foetus, in that two Qur'anic verses and an authenticated Hadith recognise stages of foetal development and this provides a basis for the view that ensoulment occurs at 120 days. Locally, however, there is little explicit awareness of this discourse and thus little scope for negotiation, as Shakeera learnt by bitter experience. Shakeera had felt very isolated when confronting these issues in her first pregnancy. Literature in the local library – books such as *When Pregnancy Fails* (Borg and Lasker 1982) or *When a Baby Dies* (Kohner and Henley 1991) – had not helped her negotiate her dilemma, nor had they resonated with her experience as a Muslim. She is currently considering retraining as a paediatric nurse so that she can support other young mothers experiencing traumatic childbirth.

In practice, though, individuals and couples may or may not take Islamic teachings explicitly into account in their reproductive decisions. The issue of managing pregnancy and its outcomes involves such key concerns of people's lives – marriage and childbearing – that any departure from locally accepted norms and practices contains social and moral risks, even where it is rationalised and can be given Islamic justification. There is enormous social and moral pressure against taking steps to test a pregnancy, to end a pregnancy or to prevent another pregnancy, especially from older women who do not work outside the home and whose main roles revolve around family and marriage. Indeed, women who have taken such steps may be plagued by guilt even years later. Zahida now worries that the prenatal genetic test she had for the baby she was carrying when Mukhtar's recessive metabolic condition was diagnosed sixteen years ago might have harmed her fifth pregnancy because, although the genetic test result was negative, this child is currently not doing well at school. Although she considers Mukhtar's problems a 'blessing from God', she also worries that it was sinful to have had a sterilisation after her fifth child's birth and she fears the Judgement at which God will decide whether she will go to heaven or to hell. She would like to have another child and thinks it would be a good way of rebalancing her account with God to adopt an orphan from Pakistan.

In detailing some of the ways in which parents and prospective parents draw on the views of close relatives, religious experts and their understandings of Islam to negotiate the use of modern medical and genetic technology, my material illustrates the insight offered by recent feminist theory that autonomy is always relational, exercised in a social and moral context and the outcome not only of interactions with experts and professionals but of ongoing relationships that must be sustained with people such as close relatives (Mackenzie and Stoljar 2000). At the same time, the moral ambiguity associated with the use of modern medical and genetic technologies also means that the final decision that individuals and couples make may need to be kept private. The precise details of such a decision, the outcome of a problematic pregnancy or the genetic risks involved will not necessarily or easily be shared with other members of the family or community. The many cross-cutting ties of affinity and consanguinity that characterise a transnational Pakistani *birādarī* do not necessarily mean that risk information is communicated any more easily than within white Anglo-British families, either within a household or beyond it. On the contrary, there are some very strong cultural and emotional reasons why such information may remain a 'well kept secret', as Husnain put it.

These reasons concern marriage and childbearing, the competitive ethos surrounding fertility in marriage and the stigma of infertility and unsuccessful childbearing. For Pakistani Muslims, marriage generally marks the transition from child to adult (an unmarried woman or man may continue to be referred to as a girl or boy, even when they are in their thirties) and full adulthood is achieved with becoming a parent. A marriage is thus conventionally more secure once a child is born, while childlessness has negative implications for its stability and future. Infertility and unsuccessful childbearing, whether rooted in genetic or other problems, puts external pressures on the husband and wife. The man's parents are likely to blame their son's wife for the problems (as the consequence of her inappropriate action or behaviour when pregnant, for instance) and to suggest that their son takes another wife, polygamy being a conventional solution to infertility. Some couples in this situation have themselves considered separation and remarriage. Genetic explanations for a reproductive problem do not necessarily challenge these powerful cultural conventions. As we saw in Sofia's case, the fact that both parents must carry the mutation for a child to be affected by a recessive condition demonstrates that the condition is not the woman's fault, but is nonetheless compatible with the idea of taking another wife as a solution to the problems of childlessness and genetic risk.

Against such pressures, a medical or genetic consultation can offer couples opportunities for, or the hope of, an alternative solution to their problem. In pursuing this solution, couples may be particularly concerned to protect their marriage from potential interference by other family members. In other words, in this highly relational cultural context, a medical or genetic consultation may be significant for the privacy it offers a husband and wife as a couple, as separate from their in-laws, parents or siblings. Often, such couples may remain ambivalent about the use of prenatal diagnostic tests and about sharing genetic risk information within the wider family; individuals and couples engage in genetic diagnostic processes, including mutation research, most centrally because they want to solve their reproductive or health problem, rather than because they want to make use of genetic prenatal diagnostics or carrier testing. Ambivalence can mean that some couples 'drop out' of the system of genetic risk management, at least temporarily. Sofia and her husband eventually had a successful pregnancy, during which they did not contact the genetics clinic. When I heard from Sofia, she now felt that the genetic research was perhaps no longer necessary:

> Alison, there is something I must tell you. We have had a baby (*hamāre hān ek bachchā paidā huā*) and he is perfectly alright. So maybe we don't need to go ahead with the research. We were under the care of the obstetricians. I did not want to see the genetics department. But I did have a scan. I was thinking I would contact the genetics department but then he was born early. You shared my pain. I want you to come and see my baby.

Challenging geneticisation

Thus far, I have emphasised the relative novelty of modern understandings of genetic risk, particularly as these are experienced by British Pakistani patients against a strongly pro-natalist social and cultural background, in which Islamic values play an important role. In situating these experiences, I also want to make a point of more general relevance to arguments concerning the social effects of the use of the 'new' genetics. Increasingly, empirical evidence is challenging the view that an expanding genetics service and a widening repertoire of conditions whose genetic basis is known are necessarily or in any simple way resulting in a pervasive geneticisation, by which illness is seen as reducible to its underlying DNA (Lippman 1992; Nelkin and Lindee 1995), and that we are witnessing a corresponding medicalisation of kinship, by which the relatives of people with genetic conditions are seen as potentially affected (Finkler 2001). The processes involved both in the work of clinical geneticists and in how users of genetic services understand a genetic diagnosis seem to be much more complex than these theories allow.

Clinical geneticists are professionally committed to the pursuit of a genetic diagnosis, but differential diagnosis does not rule out other causes such as birth trauma, environmental agents or a complex aetiology involving genetic and non-genetic effects. In addition, the process of genetic diagnosis does not rest on the use of modern molecular technologies alone but draws on long-established skills of clinical observation and judgement (Shaw 2003b; Shaw et al. 2003). In their diagnostic work, clinical geneticists constantly shift between a perspective that focuses on the client as identifiable by one constituent part – the change or potential change in DNA sequence – and one that recognises their complexity as whole and unique persons (Latimer 2006).

There is growing evidence that patients attending genetics clinics accord varied and complex meanings to genetic information (see, for example, Rose and Novas

2004; Featherstone et al. 2006). For the participants in this study, a genetics referral was usually just one of many specialist routine NHS referrals (to paediatrics, orthopaedics, endocrinology, neurology, ophthalmology, obstetrics and so on) in connection with a problem with pregnancy or infant health. The 'genetic risk' aspects of the problem often seemed relatively unimportant in relation to parents' desires to secure a successful pregnancy or help their child. Doctors in genetics do offer some prognostic or therapeutic advice, make further referrals or suggest that clients consult patient support groups or other specialists, but they are mainly concerned with making an accurate diagnosis and assessment of recurrence risks and giving up-to-date information on reproductive options and risk management. Some patients also want to know their reproductive or carrier risks but most mainly desire a solution of their or their child's problem in the form of a treatment or cure. There can thus be a mismatch between clinicians' concerns with refining and managing genetic risk and patients' expectations of a genetics referral as a route to treatment or cure, even though this motivates client enrolment in endeavours to 'find the gene'.

Khalida and her husband wanted a large family. After having two healthy children, the next three pregnancies resulted in infant deaths. They then proceeded with another pregnancy, in the full understanding of their risk for two different recessive conditions. One condition is observable by prenatal ultrasound; the other is now detectable be a prenatal genetic test via amniocentesis or CVS, now that the causative mutation has been identified. Prenatal scans showed no signs of the first condition, and the parents chose not to risk a spontaneous abortion or otherwise harming the baby with a prenatal genetic test for the second condition, requesting instead a post-natal DNA test. If the test was positive, early knowledge of the genetic constitution would enable more accurate therapy and might reduce the risk of illness and sudden death. The post-natal test established that the baby has the genotype for this condition. He now receives a special diet and is taken regularly to London for specialist medical surveillance. Khalida acknowledges the impact of his presence on her other children and their family life, but remains clear that she would not have ended the pregnancy: 'English people will terminate if it's not convenient – I was born thirteen months after my brother and that was not convenient, but my mother would not have conceived of a termination.'

My informants often described their engagements with genetics with reference to Islamic ideals about the value of human life, and the pursuit of scientific knowledge for effecting treatments and cures, rather than for managing risk or 'convenience'. This desire for treatments or cures and the pursuit of various routes to this end are not unique to British Pakistani users of genetic services. They are also an increasingly prominent feature of the activities of some patient associations in America (Novas 2006). Through social events and newsletters, membership of such groups enables affected persons and their close kin and carers to share individual experiences and provides a mechanism for distributing up-to-date medical information including about the latest research (Rabinow 1992; Rapp et al. 2001). One patient association, founded by the parents of two children with a rare genetic disorder, engaged with biomedical research by fund-raising and coordinating research efforts, including through collecting blood samples from affected individuals, thus helping researchers find the gene associated with the condition (Novas 2006). This patient association is now collaborating with a biotechnology company to develop a prenatal genetic test, but also hopes that further research will illuminate the molecular pathways that lead to the condition and therefore assist the development of therapies to improve the health of affected persons. Thus, the hope for treatments and cures is 'not only an aspiration, but can also be thought of as having a political and economic materiality that seeks to bring to fruition the many future possibilities inherent in the science of the present' (Novas 2006).

As Novas and others recognise, however, there are marked structural inequalities in people's abilities to transform their desires for treatments and cures into strategies that may significantly shape medical research. Those who are most effective in engaging with research, by influencing what is investigated, how research is organised and how its benefits are distributed, particularly in an environment in which research efforts are driven mainly by commercial interests, are almost invariably white and middle-class; these are the people most likely to establish or participate in patient associations. For many participants in this study, participation in patients' associations was seriously constrained by factors that include: the rareness of many of the disorders; parents' or carers' inability to speak or read English fluently and a dearth of comprehensible translated materials; parents' or carers' fear that they or their child would feel 'out of place'; and hesitancy over using respite care. Nonetheless, some parents and carers expressed a desire to meet other parents caring for similarly affected children. Several families of older children with disabilities had benefited from contact with patient associations. Hamid Ullah had attended a U.K. meeting for people with his brother's chromosomal condition, at which he noticed that his brother was not as severely affected as some people are, and where he learnt about current research. Mukhtar's parents are now members of the U.K. branch of the a charity working to support those affected with metabolic conditions, and have twice attended their annual conferences – one of which was in Paris – doing so with financial assistance and encouragement from the society. They are now well informed about different forms of their son's condition and aware that some children are much more severely affected than their son. Akhtar's brothers, too, regularly receive and read newsletters from the society supporting people with their neurological condition and maintain an interest in the current research that they hope will eventually produce a cure. For most people, though, membership of such associations was only very indirectly a route towards engagement with medical research.

Nonetheless, hopes for treatments or cures remain high. Encouraged by the expectation that research would be under way in the U.S.A. into Bilaal's extremely rare disorder (for which no patients' association exists), Nighat and Nasir enlisted the help of a relative living in America to conduct an Internet search for a research group interested in finding the mutation causing Bilaal's possibly recessive condition, but this yielded no results. 'We were expecting to find a group in the U.S.A. doing something with this gene, but were surprised that there is none and the research that is happening is happening here in the U.K.,' Nasir said. His surprise reflects a local view of America as a possible source of cure because the now-adult children in another local Pakistani family are apparently receiving treatment from America for their problem, following the relatively recent discovery of a gene involved. Another local mother, whose child also has a – different – metabolic condition, remarked on this case that she thinks the affected children are taken to American for treatment; in fact, they receive medication via the local hospital. In another case, a father who has lost three infants to a very rare recessive condition travelled at his own expense to Japan to meet the researcher who first described the syndrome (and after whom the syndrome is named), and established Internet contact with other parents of similarly affected children from all around the world. But, for him, as for many other parents, the realities of therapy remain elusive, for there are considerable impediments to effective and sustained engagement with research into rare genetic disorders. Moreover, for many families, the demands of 'life as usual' – concerns about employment and housing, the demands of maintaining transnational lives, worries about the well-being, education and marriage of their affected and unaffected children and, for many, the births of further children – all tend to work against any sustained activity and engagement with medical research, despite the culture of hope and expectation that surrounds genetic research.

Alongside these concerns for treatments or cures, parents also have an often greater or more sustained concern (particularly given that effective cures have not been forthcoming) about their child's future, especially once their child has left the well-structured environment of the special school they are attending. Parents of younger children appeared to be generally quite satisfied with and grateful for current educational provisions for children with special needs, especially in contrast with the perceived lack of such facilities in Pakistan. Jobeen's five-year-old daughter has severe learning difficulties and some unusual physical features (but no genetic diagnosis). Jobeen said that, since her daughter has started attending a special school, she has began to move about, pulling herself up against the furniture, and now shows an interest in her environment that was absent before and might not have developed had she remained at home, without any specialist attention – such as a therapeutic pool, regular physiotherapy and consistent intellectual stimulation. Jobeen's husband disagreed with some other local parents' views that disabilities are more common in England than in Pakistan, by pointing out the infrastructural differences: 'You don't see disabled children in Pakistan, but this is not because they aren't there. A child like that would be kept at home, kept behind walls and not taken out to special schools, and so there they don't have all the opportunities they have here.'

Hamid Ullah's mother, who has cared for two boys with a chromosomal syndrome and severe learning difficulties, also commented on the facilities for children with disabilities in England: in Pakistan, she said, such children or adults would remain at home, cared for by their siblings or parents, or else would go out on the streets as beggars. (At this point in the conversation, her daughter-in-law added, seriously, that you see just as many people with disabilities in Pakistan as in England 'because families fight, people get into fights and cut off their arms and legs.') Riffat told me about one British Pakistani man who was so impressed with the provisions in the U.K. that he has since returned to Pakistan to establish a special school for children with disabilities in the town of Jhelum.

Yet, while parents are generally grateful for special educational provisions for school-age children in the U.K., they feel deep concerns as their children approach school leaving age about the options for day-to-day care for young adults with learning difficulties. In Pakistan, day-to-day care is conventionally provided by the family, and family care remains an ideal to which British Pakistanis often aspire, even though they also recognise that the reality of family care, both in Pakistan and the U.K., often falls short of the ideal, especially for people with special needs; as Hamid's wife put it, '*kahne men awr karne men faraq hai,*' meaning 'There's a difference between what people say and what they do.' In the U.K., extended family support is often very difficult to arrange or simply not available. The provisions for and expectations of day-to-day care are highly gendered: although there are many obstacles in these arrangements, parents may nonetheless plan a marriage to ensure that a son with disabilities has someone to care for him. Marriage is much less likely to be an option for daughters with serious medical problems or learning difficulties who are unable to look after themselves, let alone someone else. Parveen Akhtar, whose teenage daughter has learning difficulties of unknown origin and the intellectual ability of a much younger girl, reflected that, had the family been living in Pakistan, they might have felt able to rely on one of their sons and his wife to provide and care for their daughter, but in the U.K. this seems an unrealistic expectation because their sons are currently at university and no longer living at home. 'While we are alive, it is OK,' she said, 'but what will happen to her when I am dead?' Parveen's husband has recently become active in seeking to establish a Muslim care home for young adults with disabilities, with the support of doctors, lawyers and the local mosque, and considers this a key issue for the future. His concerns reflect an issue noted at national policy level: that there is evidence of cultural, linguistic and religious barriers to effective uptake by people of South Asian origins of community health and social services for adolescents and adults with learning difficulties, and to support for their carers (see, for example, Hatton et al. 1998; Croot 2005).

Cultural sensitivity and cultural competence: generic issues in delivering genetic services within culturally diverse populations

In this last section, I consider some implications of this extended case study for clinical genetics policy and practice in 'cross-cultural' contexts. How to provide 'culturally appropriate' or 'culturally sensitive' genetic services, or, as one volume puts it, 'genetic counselling across cultures' has been a matter of recent discussion in the U.K. (e.g. Clarke and Parsons 1997). These questions originate from the 1970s ideology of multiculturalism, which sought to recognise and respect the diversity of religious beliefs and cultural practices evident in Britain following the post-war New Commonwealth immigration. Multiculturalist approaches to cultural diversity have included interventions such as training in cultural difference for professionals in the fields of education and health; more recent initiatives promote cultural competence to enable health professionals to develop cross-cultural skills so as to become culturally sensitive practitioners (e.g. Papadopoulos 2006).

Defining cross-cultural skills or cultural sensitivity, however, is not straightforward. In what, exactly, should a health professional be skilled, or to what should he or she be sensitive? In an everyday sense, culture has an obvious meaning, its diversity evident all around us in the variation that exists in people's personal values, in the norms that govern marriage, kinship and family life, in how people think of themselves in relation to others, in the languages they speak and so on. This diversity is often sufficiently systematic to indicate not just individual but group characteristics, shared by kin and community, which can significantly influence interpersonal relationships. However, in attempts to capture 'culture' and incorporate it into policy and practice, 'culture' frequently becomes equated with 'difference' from the mainstream. The result is a tendency to stereotype particular ethnic groups or communities on the basis of a list of cultural characteristics and to downplay the socio-economic dimensions of structural inequality. Almost by definition, this view pays scant attention to the internal dynamics and disputes, cross-cutting allegiances and interests and processes of social and cultural change that characterise all communities, as Gerhard Baumann has demonstrated for multi-ethnic Southall (Britain's 'South Asian capital') in West London (Baumann 1996). It also conceals from view the transnational links that characterise many migrant populations, challenging the view that ethnic minority populations are bounded entities (Vertovec 2001). Conventional multiculturalism is, moreover, now ill-equipped to capture the sheer diversity present in contemporary Britain, with immigration including people from all over the world, not just South Asia and the Caribbean.

In reality, members of any so-called ethnic community do not all share the beliefs and values stereotypically associated with it within public discourse. A health professional therefore cannot assume in advance what any individual's values will be. As Aneez Esmail notes in his argument against the provision of faith-based health services for Muslims in the U.K., to provide 'special services for defined groups of people risks stigmatisation and stereotyping'; for example, to make the assumption that a woman with a Muslim name on a maternity ward 'will need to pray five times a day, have special dietary requirements and want to have her male child circumcised' does not allow 'for the fact that different Muslims conduct their lives in different ways' (Sheikh and Esmail 2007). As we have also seen, for a health professional to assume, for instance, that the idea of ending a pregnancy is unacceptable to a Muslim patient on religious grounds and so to withhold information about prenatal genetic testing represents not cultural sensitivity but a failure of clinical communication and an undermining of the principle of informed consent that governs prenatal and genetic service provision in the NHS (see also Modell et al. 2000). Attempts to 'culturally match' patients and practitioners, whereby, for instance, a Muslim patient is seen by a Muslim doctor, or a deaf patient is seen by a deaf doctor, are also, often, not just impractical but also exclusionary in their effects on both patients and professionals (see, for example, Middleton et al. 2007).

Nonetheless, a case can be made for fostering 'cultural sensitivity' among health professionals while seeking to avoid the pitfalls of a 'cultural compendium' approach emphasising boundaries and difference. What is needed is not a redefinition of culture so much as a critical appreciation of it as it applies to us all and a rethinking, in more general terms, of the issues that are important to effective service delivery within diverse populations. Health practitioners need to develop generic skills that will empower them to work with a diversity of patients. Such an approach would include factual information about the main dimensions of diversity with particular reference to health but should also empower professionals to respond to patients as individuals, to facilitate their access to services and to ensure effective communication. Part of this would include raising professionals' awareness of the socially and culturally shaped nature of their own values and practices, and of the potential for stereotyping or making ethnocentric judgements about patients whose values and practices differ (Kai 2003; Papadopoulos et al. 2004). Effective communication and access to services would include assessing patients' language needs, making technical medical information accessible and being aware of the need for adequate informed consent as well as of the potential relevance of patients' religious beliefs or ethical principles in the decisions they make about medical treatment.

These issues have a particular salience in clinical genetics because, as we have seen, a genetic diagnosis is unusual in several ways. It concerns information about the body that is located in cellular DNA (and, as such, is effectively immutable, except by gene therapy) and has implications both for an individual's reproductive future and for the health of their close relatives because biological kin share some of their DNA. Yet unfamiliarity with genetics and genetics services is widespread within mainstream American and British populations (Lewis et al. 2000; Wood-Robinson et al. 2000; Lanie et al. 2004) as well as within minority populations and across national boundaries. Understanding a genetic diagnosis and its implications can therefore be very challenging for patients regardless of their specific language needs or ethnic background. Moreover, people respond to genetic information not in a social and cultural vacuum but within the framework of their prior understandings of illness causality, relatedness and inheritance. These prior understandings may not match genetic theory but instead may invoke environmental or spiritual causes or entail other conceptualisations of blood ties between kin. White Anglo-British patients had 'well established beliefs and practices concerning the kindred and inheritance' (Featherstone et al. 2006: 141). The idea of blood being 'stronger' on the father's than the mother's side may be more common among people of South and East Asian backgrounds (Meiser et al. 2001).

Certain ideas about illness causality and risk may therefore be more likely to occur within some patient groups than others. Nonetheless, these ideas should be viewed not as fixed elements associated with any particular cultural background, but rather as numbering among many possible working hypotheses about how patients may understand genetics. In their consultations with individual patients, genetic doctors need to elicit, work with and, where appropriate and using due sensitivity, challenge these understandings where they differ from genetic theory in clinically significant ways (Davison 1996; Richards 1996b). It may rarely be sufficient simply to provide information in a single consultation, for patients may not fully appreciate the 'genetic' aspects of a diagnosis until well after a diagnosis has been made (Pembrey 1996: 77; Novas 2006: 293). It often takes considerable time for the genetic implications to sink in – for instance, in the somewhat counter-intuitive idea that both parents must be unaffected carriers of a mutation if their child has a recessive condition and that unaffected siblings of an affected child might be carriers too.

Within Western medicine, there is a fast-growing literature detailing the ethical issues that have emerged in clinical genetics practice, mostly concerning the dilemmas confronting genetics doctors and counsellors because of the particular nature of genetic information. For example, how much information about the implications of genetic test results should doctors provide for their patients' consent to be informed? Or, if a doctor needs access to a patient's relative's genetic test results to provide a patient with accurate risk information, but the relative does not want their test results disclosed, does the doctor have a right to override the relative's right to privacy or the need to obtain consent? While these types of clinical dilemmas relate to defining the boundaries of a clinician's responsibility, the dilemmas that confront patients more often concern the use of modern technologies for managing the often probabilistically calculated reproductive risks implied by a genetic diagnosis – the use, for instance of genetic carrier tests, or prenatal tests with the option of ending an affected pregnancy and, for some conditions, preimplantation genetic diagnosis. For all patients, use of these technologies raises practical ethical issues that patients may choose to navigate with reference to the views of relatives and friends, or by drawing on religious beliefs or ethical principles derived from religion.

As I have shown, for many British Pakistani men and women Islam is of central importance in providing the ethical bearings from which they navigate the novel moral territory of prenatal diagnosis, explore the permissibility of ending a pregnancy or withdrawing life support from an infant in special care, or worry about the management of childbirth where infant death is predicted. In local contexts, as this book has shown, there exist both diversity of opinion and a degree of uncertainty about 'what Islam says' on these issues; doctors thus need to appreciate that patients may need information on such topics as the acceptability of abortion in Islam. Significantly, given the generally Western bias in bioethics publications, a recent commentary in *Nature Genetics* discusses the Islamic ethical framework for genetic research and disease prevention and its relevance for genetic service delivery in the Muslim world and elsewhere (Al Aqeel 2007). It is also important for clinicians to be aware that some Muslims will make a decision on medical rather than religious grounds. Health professionals therefore need to be sensitive to the range of feelings and views surrounding the use of genetic and associated medical technologies, regardless of what may be seen to be the official religious discourse. A person's religious identity 'should not be taken as a proxy' for their attitudes (Ahmed et al. 2006b).

The familial nature of genetic information also raises generic questions about whether, how and when genetic information should be shared within the family. As we have seen, this can be a difficult issue to resolve; in contemporary clinical practice, the implications for relatives are sometimes simply noted in a letter to the family doctor. Within some families, after the initial flurry of activity associated with a diagnosis has quietened, the details of the inheritance of a condition may not be discussed again within the family, and family members may not appreciate the risks to other relatives until many years later, after the birth of further affected children (Featherstone et al. 2006: 93–94). For British Pakistani as for white Anglo-British families, clinical geneticists 'cannot assume that there will be "open" communication patterns among members of a kindred, any more than they can assume that what is transmitted between family members corresponds to the professionals' own intended meanings' (Featherstone et al. 2006: 147). Indeed, as I have documented in this book, there are good reasons why sharing information about genetic risk can at times be particularly difficult within some British Pakistani families, and the need for privacy over genetic information and its implications can be particularly acute. This is despite the dense, overlapping connections that characterise Pakistani kinship and the claim that these will facilitate cascade screening (Darr 1997). Communication about genetic information is context-dependent and contingent upon what kinship means in practice for the families concerned. Rather than assuming it will be either easy or difficult in any given case, clinicians need to discuss with their patients the most appropriate ways of supporting family communication and decision-making, including by offering opportunities for clinical follow-up at a later date. Such support is particularly important for consanguineous families in which a recessive condition has been diagnosed, because further marriages between people who may be carriers are likely to take place.

This brings me to another key issue that cuts across all aspects of patients' engagements with clinical genetics: that of language use and its impact on access to information and services. Genetic concepts are difficult to grasp for those untrained in genetics, as much for English patients during a genetics consultation conducted in English (the dominant language of clinical consultations in the U.K.) as it is for those who must access this information through interpreters. Appropriate language provision, ideally via trained interpreters who are familiar with genetics or bilingual genetics professionals, is essential to effective communication between doctors and patients. The act of translation presents considerable challenges because the interpreter needs to understand what the genetic concepts refer to if they are to explain them effectively (see, for example, Shaw and Ahmed 2004). One recent U.K. initiative is seeking to bring some consistency into the translation of genetic information into languages other than English and to make these resources freely available online (see http://www.gig.org.uk/). Given that it often takes time for a diagnosis to be reached, for a genetic test to become available and for the patients to assimilate the implications of a genetic diagnosis, language support should be viewed as a long-term need, extending beyond the moment of a clinical consultation.

Finally, I want to return to the 'foreshadowed problem' (Malinowski 1922: 9) of the elevated risk of genetic disorders that provided the initial impetus for this study. As I have shown, for consanguineous Pakistani Muslim couples in the U.K., the use of genetic services is itself overshadowed by a public discourse of genetic risk in cousin marriages. Professionals need to be sensitive to the tendency of some staff and some patients to prejudge a medical or genetic problem as 'caused by' cousin marriage, to misconstrue 'genetic' as 'what happens when you marry cousins' and to exaggerate the genetic risks of consanguineous marriages. Other misconceptions about cousin marriage need to be corrected: for example, that it is a specifically Muslim practice. As I have shown, although important in many Muslim communities, it is not restricted to them, nor is it required by Islam; on the contrary, the second Caliph is reported to have advised tribesmen whose children had become weak to stop marrying close relatives (see Chapter 1, also Al Aqeel 2007: 1294, note 6).

It would be doing a disservice to consanguineous couples to downplay the elevated risk for recessive conditions. Such a risk brings other costs such as the financial burden on health care systems of caring for people with serious genetic conditions and the social and psychological burdens on families and carers, usually women. For first cousins without a family history of consanguineous marriage, the risk (of about 4–6 per cent) is about twice the background risk of congenital or genetic problems in the children of non-consanguineous couples (2–3 per cent) and so is much less that the chance of having an unaffected child. However, this risk increases where marriages in previous generations are also consanguineous: thus, the Birmingham birth study found the risk of serious congenital or genetic problems in the children of British Pakistanis to be about 10 per cent (Bundey and Alam 1993). How should this risk be managed in the U.K.? Is it sufficient to provide risk information and allow reproductive choice, or should consanguineous marriages be actively discouraged?

As I have shown in this book, the singling out of consanguineous marriage for special public attention has reinforced a dominant public image of such marriages as emblematic of cultural difference. A community-education approach that focuses on the genetic risk seems likely to reinforce this dominant view and to alienate some potential users of genetic services. Moreover, to emphasise the genetic risks of cousin marriage may limit informed choice, by implying that the only way consanguineous couples can avoid the birth of affected children is by refraining from marrying or having children, thus diverting attention from the reproductive options currently available (Richards 1996b: 262; Shaw and Ahmed 2004). Just as the elevated risk of Down syndrome in babies born to women (of all ethnicities) over age thirty-five – which rises from about 1 per cent at age forty, to 2 per cent at age forty-three, and to 3 per cent at age forty-five (www.bbc.co.uk/health, accessed 6 December 2007) – is managed prenatally (via amniocentesis), so too the elevated risk for certain recessive conditions, either because they are associated with ethnicity (such as thalassaemia among South Asians) or because they are known to be 'in the family', can be managed through genetic carrier and prenatal tests. The number of conditions for which the mutations have been discovered is growing and medical technologies are, increasingly, enabling patients to make informed choices concerning the use of termination of pregnancy or preimplantation genetic diagnosis of embryos, particularly for serious or fatal conditions.

At this point, it may be instructive to step beyond the boundaries of the U.K. debate. Consanguineous marriages occur in about a fifth of the world's population, in parts of the Middle East, Africa and Asia (Bittles 2001). They are also important within ethnically diverse populations of North America, Western Europe and Australia, following significant recent migrations from countries where cousin marriage is practised (Port et al. 2005). Particular recessive conditions are known to be more common within certain consanguineous populations. In principle, a proportion of the elevated risk for recessive conditions can be managed by premarital or pre-conception carrier testing or else by, or in combination with, prenatal diagnosis and selective abortion. Carrier matching schemes in some orthodox Jewish and Muslim communities seek to reduce the birth of children with such conditions as Tay–Sachs disease, recessive forms of hearing loss and thalassaemia, without the use of prenatal diagnosis and selective abortion, by ensuring that only 'compatible' people marry (Ekstein and Katsenstein 2001; Raz and Atar 2004). In Palestine, obligatory premarital testing for beta thalassaemia has gradually reduced the number of carrier couples marrying and the number of affected children (Tarazi et al. 2007). In Saudi Arabia, mandatory premarital screening for thalassaemia and sickle-cell disease since 2004 has led to a decline in consanguineous marriage within the screening population (Alhamdan et al. 2007). In Iran, prenatal screening for thalassaemia is integrated with facilities enabling carrier couples to opt for early prenatal diagnosis (via CVS) and selective abortion, and this rather than the separation of carrier couples has led to a significant reduction in the births of babies with thalassaemia (Samavat and Modell 2004). Such approaches, working within the framework of culturally accepted forms of marriage, are generally considered more effective than 'preaching against consanguinity' (Raz and Atar 2004: 50) or declaring it a medical emergency.

In the U.K., risks for thalassaemia are now managed through routine prenatal carrier testing. Beyond this, there is currently little firm evidence that particular recessive conditions prevail among Pakistanis (or other minority groups) at frequencies to justify carrier testing on grounds of parental consanguinity or ethnicity without any relevant family history. Nonetheless, consanguineous couples may be particularly worried about the elevated risks associated with their consanguinity and may seek a genetics referral on these grounds alone. As for any other couple, the advice, screening and genetic tests that genetics professionals offer consanguineous couples should be based on a thorough family history and on their ethnicity (as carrier frequencies for particular disorders such as thalassaemia vary with ethnicity). Beyond this, however, no additional counselling or testing is recommended (Bennett et al. 2002): it is then for the individual, couple or family to weigh up the added recessive risks against the other considerations involved in marital and reproductive choices. Further, since the risks associated with parental consanguinity are mostly for a wide range of rare recessive conditions, rather than for a particular condition such as Tay–Sachs disease, a strategy such as carrier matching is unlikely to be appropriate, except perhaps on an individual or family basis where a particular condition has been diagnosed and the mutation associated with it has been identified. Even so, it is important to note that British Pakistani Muslims are a varied population in terms social characteristics and religious beliefs, including with respect to the acceptability of prenatal diagnosis and ending a pregnancy; a strategy effective among orthodox Ashkenazi Jews or the Bedouin Muslims of the Negev region of Israel, among whom marriages are arranged, will not therefore be appropriate in the U.K. Arranged consanguineous marriage is not the only form of marriage among British Pakistanis, the process of arranged marriage is itself changing and young adults are increasingly aware of the elevated genetic risks associated with consanguineous marriage. An individual and family-based approach to genetic risk management, as offered to all users of clinical genetic services, and one that is sensitive to cultural difference therefore seems most appropriate in the U.K. Because deaths from other causes are decreasing, genetic conditions are gaining significance within the overall spectrum of diseases, and as Western nations are increasingly ethnically diverse, parental consanguinity will continue to be a significant element within clinical genetics casework for the foreseeable future.

BIBLIOGRAPHY

Ablon, J. 1984. *Little People in America: the Social Dimensions of Dwarfism.* New York: Praeger Publications.

Ablon, J. 1988. *Living with Difference: Families with Dwarf Children.* New York: Praeger Publications.

Ablon, J. 1999. *Living with Genetic Disorder: the Impact of Neurofibromatosis 1.* Westport, Connecticut: Auburn House.

Abel, E.K. and C.H. Browner. 1998. Selective compliance with biomedical authority and the uses of experiential knowledge. In M. Lock and P. Kaufert (eds) *Pragmatic Women and Body Politics.* Cambridge: Cambridge University Press, pp. 310–26.

Abel Haleem, M.A.S. 1993. Medical ethics in Islam. In A. Grubb (ed.) *Choices and Decisions in Health Care.* Chichester, U.K.: John Wiley and Sons, pp. 1–20.

Abu-Lughod, L. 1986. *Veiled Sentiments: Honor and Poetry in a Bedouin Society.* Berkeley: University of California Press.

Abu-Lughod, L. 2002. The marriage of feminism and Islamism in Egypt: selective repudiation as a dynamic of postcolonial cultural politics. In J.X. Inda and R. Rosaldo (eds) *The Anthropology of Globalisation: a Reader.* Malden, MA: Blackwell, pp. 428–51.

Ahmad, I. (ed.). 1978. *Caste and Social Stratification among Muslims in India.* Delhi: Manohar.

Ahmad. W. 1993. Making black people sick: 'race', ideology and health research. In W.I.U. Ahmed (ed.) *'Race' and Health in Contemporary Britain.* Buckingham: Open University Press, pp. 1–33.

Ahmad, W. 1996. Consanguinity and related demons: science and racism in the debate on consanguinity and birth outcome. In C. Samson and N. South (eds) *The Social Construction of Social Policy: Methodologies, Racism, Citizenship and the Environment.* London: Macmillan, pp. 68–87.

Ahmed, S., M. Saleem, N. Sultana, Y. Raashid, A. Waqar, M. Anwar, B. Modell, K.A. Karamat and M. Petrou. 2000. Prenatal diagnosis of beta-thalassaemia in Pakistan: experience in a Muslim country. *Prenatal Diagnosis,* 20: 378–83.

Ahmed, S., J. Green and J. Hewison. 2005. Antenatal thalassaemia carrier testing: women's perceptions of 'information' and 'consent'. *Journal of Medical Screening,* 12 (2): 69–77.

Ahmed, S., K. Atkin, J. Hewison and J. Green. 2006a. The influence of faith and religion and the role of religious and community leaders in prenatal decisions for sickle cell disorders and thalassaemia major. *Prenatal Diagnosis,* 26, 801–9.

Ahmed, S., J.M. Green, J.M. and J. Hewison. 2006b. Attitudes towards prenatal diagnosis and termination of pregnancy for thalassaemia in pregnant Pakistani women in the North of England. *Prenatal Diagnosis*, 26: 248–57.

Al Aqeel, A.I. 2007. Islamic ethical framework for research into and prevention of genetic diseases. *Nature Genetics*, 39 (11): 1293–96.

Alhamdan, N.A., Y.Y. Almazrou, F.M. Alswaidi and A.J. Choudhry. 2007. *Genetic Medicine*, 9: 373–77.

Alkuraya, F.S. and R.A. Kilani. 2001. Attitudes of Saudi families affected with haemoglobinopathies towards prenatal screening and abortion and the influence of religious ruling (fatwa). *Prenatal Diagnosis*, 21, 448–51.

Anderson, N.F. 1986. Cousin marriage in Victorian England. *Journal of Family History*, 11 (3): 285–301.

Anon. 1996. Living with the threat of Huntington's disease. In T. Marteau and M. Richards (eds) *The Troubled Helix: Social and Psychological Implications of the New Human Genetics*. Cambridge: Cambridge University Press, pp. 23–26.

Armstrong, D. 1983. *Political Anatomy of the Body: Medical Knowledge in Britain in the Twentieth Century.* Cambridge: Cambridge University Press.

Aslam, N. 2004. *Maps for Lost Lovers*. London: Faber and Faber.

Atkinson, P. 1981. *The Clinical Experience: the Construction and Reconstruction of Medical Reality.* Farnborough: Gower.

Baily, J. 1993. Born in music: the Khalifa Muslim community in Britain. Paper read at the 32nd World Conference of the International Council for Traditional Music, Berlin, 16–22 June, cited in M. Böck and A.R. Rao (eds) *Culture, Creation and Procreation: Concepts of Kinship in South Asian Practice.* Oxford and New York: Berghahn Books.

Balarajan, R. and V. Soni Raleigh. 1992. A health profile of Britain's ethnic minorities. In A. Bittles and D.F. Roberts (eds) *Minority Populations: Genetics, Demography and Health. Proceedings of the Twenty-seventh Annual Symposium of the Galton Institute, London, 1990.* London: Macmillan, in association with the Galton Institute, pp. 119–42.

Balarajan, R., V. Soni Raleigh and B. Botting. 1989. Sudden infant death syndrome and postneonatal mortality in immigrants in England and Wales. *British Medical Journal*, 298: 716–20.

Ballard, R. 1987. The political economy of migration: Pakistan, Britain, and the Middle East. In J. Eades (ed.) *Migrants, Workers and the Social Order.* ASA Monographs, 26. London: Tavistock, pp. 17–41.

Ballard, R. 1990. Migration and kinship: the differential effect of marriage rules on the processes of Punjabi migration to Britain. In C. Clarke, C. Peach and S. Vertovec (eds) *South Asians Overseas: Migration and Ethnicity*. Cambridge: Cambridge University Press, pp. 219–49.

Banks, J.A. 1954. *Prosperity and Parenthood: a Study of Family Planning among the Victorian Middle Classes.* London: Routledge and Kegan Paul.

Barker, D.J.P. 1998. *Mothers, Babies and Health in Later Life.* Edinburgh: Churchill Livingstone.

Barth, F. 1954. Father's brother's daughter's marriage in Kurdistan. *South Western Journal of Anthropology,* 10: 164–71.

Baumann, G. 1996. *Contesting Culture: Discourses of Identity in Multi-ethnic London.* Cambridge: Cambridge University Press.

Beck, U. 1992. *Risk Society: Towards a New Modernity.* London: Sage Publications.

Bennett, R.L, A.G. Motuksly, A. Bittles, L. Hudgins, S. Uhrichs, D.L. Doyle, K. Silvey, C.R. Scott, E. Chang, B. McGillivray, R.D. Steiner and D. Olson. 2002. Genetic counselling and screening of consanguineous couples. *Journal of Genetic Counseling,* 11 (2): 97–119.

Berrington, A. 1994. Marriage and family formation among the white and ethnic minority populations in Britain. *Ethnic and Racial Studies,* 17: 517–46.

Berthoud, R. 2001. Teenage births to ethnic minority women. *Population Trends,* 104: 12–17.

Bharadwaj, A. 2003. Why adoption is not an option in India: the visibility of infertility, the secrecy of donor insemination. *Social Science and Medicine,* 56: 1867–80.

Bhopal, R., N. Unwin, M. White, J. Yallop, L. Walker, K.G.M.M. Alberti, J. Harland, S. Patel, N. Ahmad, C. Turner, B. Watson, D. Kaur, A. Kulkarni, M. Laker and A. Tavridou. 1999. Heterogeneity of coronary heart disease risk factors in Indian, Pakistani, Bangladeshi, and European origin populations: cross sectional study. *British Medical Journal,* 319: 215–20.

Bittles, A.H. 1990. *Consanguineous Marriage: Current Global Incidence and its Relevance to Demographic Research.* Research Report, No. 90–186. Ann Arbor: University of Michigan, Population Studies Center.

Bittles, A.H. 2001. Consanguinity and its relevance to clinical genetics. *Clinical Genetics,* 60: 89–98.

Bittles, A.H. and E. Makov. 1988. Inbreeding in human populations: an assessment of the costs. In C.G.N. Mascie-Taylor and A.J. Boyce (eds) *Human Mating Patterns.* Cambridge: Cambridge University Press.

Bittles, A.H., W.M. Mason, J. Greene and N.A. Rao. 1991. Reproductive behaviour and health in consanguineous marriages. *Science,* 252: 789–94.

Böck, M. and A. Rao. 2000. *Culture, Creation and Procreation: Concepts of Kinship in South Asian Practice.* Oxford and New York: Berghahn Books.

Bond, J., E. Roberts, G.H. Mochida, D.J. Hampshire, S. Scott, J.M. Askham, K. Springell, M. Mahadevan, Y.J. Crow, A.F. Markham, C.A. Walsh and C.G. Woods. 2002. ASPM is a major determinant of cerebral cortical size. *Nature Genetics,* 32 (2): 316–20.

Bond, J., S. Scott, D.J. Hampshire, K. Springell, P. Corry, M.J. Abramowicz, G.H. Mochida, R.C. Hennekam, E.R. Maher, J.P. Fryns, A. Alswaid, H. Jafri, Y. Rashid, A. Mubaidin, C.A. Walsh, E. Roberts and C.G. Woods. 2003.

Protein-truncating mutations in ASPM cause variable reduction in brain size. *American Journal of Human Genetics,* 73 (5): 1170–77.

Borg, S. and J. Lasker. 1982. *When Pregnancy Fails: Coping with Miscarriage, Stillbirth and Infant Death.* London: Routledge.

Bouquet, M. 1996. Family trees and their affinities: the visual impact of the genealogical diagram. *Journal of the Royal Anthropological Institute,* 2: 43–66.

Bourdieu, P. 1977. *Outline of a Theory of Practice,* trans. R. Nice. Cambridge: Cambridge University Press.

Bourdieu, P. 1990. *In Other Words. Essays towards a Reflexive Sociology.* London: Polity Press.

Bowler, I. 1993. 'They're not the same as us': midwives' stereotypes of South Asian descent maternity patients. *Sociology of Health and Illness,* 15 (2): 157–78.

Boyle, R.J., L. De Crespigny and J. Savulescu. 2003. An ethical approach to giving couples information about their fetus. *Human Reproduction,* 18 (11): 2253–56.

Bradby, H. 1996. Genetics and Racism. In T. Marteau and M. Richards (eds) *The Ttroubled Helix: Social and Psychological Implications of the New Human Genetics.* Cambridge: Cambridge University Press, pp. 295–316.

Brown, K.A., A.H. Janjua, G. Karbani, G. Parry, A. Noble, G. Crockford, D.T. Bishop, V.E. Newton, A.F. Markham and R.F. Mueller. 1996. Linkage studies of non-syndromal recessive deafness (NSRD) in a family originating from the Mirpur region of Pakistan maps DFNB1 centromeric to D13S175. *Human Molecular Genetics,* 5 (1): 169–73.

Bujra, J. 2000. *Risk and Trust: Unsafe Sex, Gender and Aids in Tanzania.* In P. Caplan (ed.) *Risk Revisited.* London: Pluto Press, 59–84.

Bundey, S. 1992. A prospective study on the health of Birmingham babies in different ethnic groups: interim findings. In A. Bittles and D.F. Roberts (eds) *Minority Populations: Genetics, Demography and Health. Proceedings of the Twenty-seventh Annual Symposium of the Galton Institute, London, 1990.* London: Macmillan, in association with the Galton Institute, pp. 143–55.

Bundey, S. and H. Alam. 1993. A five-year prospective study of the health of children in different ethnic groups, with particular reference to the effect of inbreeding. *European Journal of Human Genetics,* 1: 206–19.

Bundey, S., H. Alam, A. Kaur, S. Mir and R. Lancashire. 1991. Why do UK-born Pakistani babies have high perinatal and neonatal mortality rates? *Paediatric and Perinatal Epidemiology,* 5: 101–14.

Busfield, J. 2000. *Health and Health Care in Modern Britain.* Oxford: Oxford University Press.

Canham, N., A. Ahmad, A. Cooper and C.M. McKeown. 2002. More than just DNA analysis: carrier testing in a multiply consanguineous family. Spoken presentation, Clinical Genetics Society, Spring Conference.

Caplan, P. (ed.). 2000. *Risk Revisited.* London: Pluto Press.

Carsten, J. 2001. Substantivism, antisubstantivism and anti-antisubstantivism. In S. Franklin and S. McKinnon (eds) *Relative Values: Reconfiguring Kinship Studies.* Durham, NC: Duke University Press, pp. 29–53.

Cassidy, R. 2002. *The Sport of Kings: Kinship, Class and Thoroughbred Breeding in Newmarket*. Cambridge: Cambridge University Press.

Cecil, R. 1996a. Introduction: an insignificant event? Literary and anthropological perspectives on pregnancy loss. In R. Cecil (ed.) *The Anthropology of Pregnancy Loss: Comparative Studies in Miscarriage, Stillbirth and Neonatal Death*. Oxford: Berg, pp. 1–14.

Cecil, R. 1996b. Memories of pregnancy loss: recollections of elderly women in Northern Ireland. In R. Cecil (ed.) *The Anthropology of Pregnancy Loss: Comparative Studies in Miscarriage, Stillbirth and Neonatal Death*. Oxford: Berg, pp. 177–95.

Chandola, T. 2001. Ethnic and class differences in health in relation to British South Asians: using the new national statistics socio-economic classification. *Social Science and Medicine*, 52: 1285–96.

Chard, T. and M.P.M. Richards (eds). 1977. *Benefits and Hazards of the New Obstetrics*. London: Heinemann Medical Books.

Chard, T. and M.P.M. Richards (eds). 1990. *Obstetrics in the 1990s: Current Controversies*. Oxford: Blackwell Scientific.

Charsley, K. 2003. *Rishtas:* transnational Pakistani marriages. Unpublished PhD thesis, University of Edinburgh.

Charsley, K. 2005. Unhappy husbands: masculinity and migration in transnational Pakistani marriages. *Journal of the Royal Anthropological Institute*, 11 (1): 85–105.

Charlsey, K. 2006. Risk and ritual: the protection of British Pakistani women in transnational marriage. *Journal of Ethnic and Migration Studies*, 32 (7): 1169–87.

Child, G. 1862. On marriages of consanguinity. *The British and Foreign Medico-Chirurgical Review or Quarterly Journal of Medicine and Surgery*, Vol. XXIX, Jan–April. London: John Churchill.

Chitty, L.S. and R.M. Winter. 1989. Perinatal mortality in different ethnic groups. *Archives of Disease in Childhood*, 64, 1036–41.

Clarke, A. (ed.). 1994. *Genetic Counselling: Practice and Principles*. London: Routledge.

Clarke, A. and E. Parsons (eds). 1997. *Culture, Kinship and Genes: Towards Cross-cultural Genetics*. London: Macmillan.

Clarke, A., M. Richards, L. Kerzin-Storrar, J. Halliday, M.A. Young, S.A. Simpson, K. Featherstone, A. Lucassan, P.J. Morrison, O.W.J. Quarrel and H. Stewart. 2005. Genetic professionals' report of non-disclosure of genetic risk information families. *European Journal of Medical Genetics*, 13: 556–62.

Coleman, D.A. 1980. A note on the frequency of consanguineous marriages in Reading, England in 1972/1973. *Human Heredity*, 30: 278–85.

Connerton, P. 1989. *How Societies Remember*. Cambridge: Cambridge University Press.

Conrad, P. and J. Gabe (eds). 1999. *Sociological Perspectives on the New Genetics*. Oxford: Blackwell Publishers.

Cordle, C.J. and R.J. Prettyman. 1994. A two-year follow-up of women who have experienced early miscarriage. *Journal of Reproductive and Infant Psychology*, 12 (1): 37–44.

Cox, J.J., F. Reimann, A.K. Nicholas, G. Thornton, E. Roberts, K. Springell, G. Karbani, H. Jafri, J. Mannan, Y. Raashid, L. Al-Gazali, H. Hamamy, E.M. Valente, S. Gorman, R. Williams, D.P. McHale, J.N. Wood, F.M. Gribble and C.G. Woods. 2006. An SCN9A channelopathy causes congenital inability to experience pain, *Nature,* 444 (7121): 894–98.

Creighton, S., E.W. Almqvist, D. MacGregor, B. Fernandez, H. Hogg, J. Beis, J.P. Welch, C. Riddell, R. Lokkesmoe, M. Khalifa, J. MacKenzie, A. Sajoo, S. Farrell, F. Robert, A. Shugar, A. Summers, W. Meschino, D. Allingham-Hawkins, T. Chiu, A. Hunter, J. Allanson, H. Hare, J. Schween, L. Collins, S. Sanders, C. Greenberg, S. Cardwell, E. Lemire, P. MacLeod and M.R. Hayden. 2003. Predictive, pre-natal and diagnostic genetic testing for Huntington's disease: the experience in Canada from 1987 to 2000. *Clinical Genetics,* 63 (6): 462–75.

Cressey, G. 2006. *Diaspora Youth and Ancestral Homeland. British Pakistani/Kashmiri Youth Visiting kin in Pakistan and Kashmir.* Leiden: Brill.

Croot, L. 2005. Experiencing childhood disability: parenting children with high support needs in Pakistani families in Sheffield. Unpublished PhD thesis, University of Sheffield.

Cryer, A. 2005. First cousin marriages: a public health issue? *Bio News,* 337. http://www.bionews.org.uk/commentary.lasso?storyid=2843

Czeizel, A., L. Bodnar, G. Illei and A. Molnar. 1976. The occurrence of consanguineous marriages in Hungary. *Human Heredity,* 26, 110–12.

Dahya, B. 1972–73. Pakistanis in England. *New Community,* 2, (1): 25–33.

Dale, A., N. Shaheen, E. Fieldhouse and V. Kalra. 2002. Routes into education and employment for young Pakistani and Bangladeshi women in the UK. *Ethnic and Racial Studies,* 25 (6): 942–68.

Darr, A. 1997. Consanguineous marriage and genetics: a positive relationship. In A. Clarke and E. Parsons (eds) *Culture, Kinship and Genes: Towards Cross-cultural Genetics.* London: Macmillan, pp. 83–96.

Darr, A. 1999. The patient's perspective. In P. Rose and A. Lucassan (eds) *Practical Genetics for Primary Care,* Oxford: Oxford University Press, pp. 331–38.

Darr, A. and B. Modell. 1988. The frequency of consanguineous marriage among British Pakistanis. *Journal of Medical Genetics,* 25: 191–94.

Darwin, C. 1859. *On the Origin of Species by Means of Natural Selection, or the Preservation of Favoured Races in the Struggle for Life.* London: Murray.

Darwin, C. 1862. *On the Various Contrivances by which British and Foreign Orchids are Fertilised by Insects and on the Good Effects of Intercrossing.* London: Murray.

Darwin, C. 1877. *The Various Contrivances by which Orchids are Fertilised by Insects.* 2nd edition, revised. London: Murray.

Darwin, C. 1868. [2nd edition 1875]. *The Variation of Animals and Plants under Domestication,* 2 Volumes. London: Murray.

Darwin, C. 1871. *The Descent of Man, and Selection in Relation to Sex.* London: Murray.

Darwin, C. 1876. *The Effects of Cross and Self Fertilisation in the Vegetable Kingdom.* London: Murray.

Darwin, G.H. 1875. Marriage between first cousins in England and their effects. *Journal of the Statistical Society of London,* 38 (2): 153–82.

Davey-Smith, G. 2000. Learning to live with complexity: ethnicity, socioeconomic position, and health in Britain and the United States. *American Journal of Public Health,* 90 (11): 1694–98.

Davey-Smith, G., C. Hart, D. Blane and D. Hole. 1998. Adverse socio-economic conditions in childhood and cause specific adult mortality: prospective observational study. *British Medical Journal,* 316: 1631–35.

Davey-Smith, G., K. Charsley, H. Lambert, S. Paul, S. Fenton and W. Ahmad. 2000a. Ethnicity, health and the meaning of socio-economic position. In H. Graham (ed.) *Understanding Health Inequalities.* London: Open University Press, pp. 23–37.

Davey-Smith, G., N. Chaturvedi, S. Harding, J. Nazroo and R. Williams. 2000b. Ethnic inequalities in health: a review of UK epidemiological evidence. *Critical Public Health,* 10 (4): 375–408.

Davidoff, L. 2006. 'Close marriage' in the nineteenth and twentieth century middle strata. In F. Ebtehaj, B. Lindley and M. Richards (eds) *Kinship Matters.* Cambridge: Hart Publishers, pp. 19–45.

Davidoff, L. and C. Hall. 2002 [1987]. *Family Fortunes: Men and Women of the English Middle Class, 1780–1850.* Routledge: London and New York.

Davis-Floyd, R. 1992. *Birth as an American Rite of Passage.* Berkeley: University of California Press.

Davis, J. 1993. Reproductive technologies for prenatal diagnosis. *Fetal Diagnosis and Therapy,* 8 (suppl. 1): 28–38.

Davison, C. 1996. Predictive genetics: the cultural implications of supplying probable futures. In T. Marteau and M. Richards (eds) *The Troubled Helix: Social and Psychological Implications of the New Human Genetics.* Cambridge: Cambridge University Press, pp. 317–30.

Desmond, A. and J. Moore. 1991. *Darwin.* London: Penguin Books.

Devereux, G., L. Stellitano, C.M. Verity, A. Nicoll, R.G. Will and P. Rogers. 2004. Variations in neurodegenerative disease across the UK: findings from the national study of Progressive Intellectual and Neurological Deterioration (PIND). *Archives of Diseases in Childhood,* 89 (1): 8–12.

Donnan, H. 1985. The rules and rhetoric of marriage negotiations among the Dhund Abbasi of North East Pakistan. *Ethnology,* XXIV (3): 183–96.

Donnan, H. 1988. *Marriage among Muslims: Preference and Choice in Northern Pakistan.* Delhi: Hindustan Publishing Corporation.

Douglas, M. 1966. *Purity and Danger: an Analysis of Concepts of Pollution and Taboo.* London: Routledge.

Douglas, M. 1985. *Risk Acceptability According to the Social Sciences.* New York: Russell Sage Foundation.

Douglas, M. 1992. *Risk and Blame: Essays in Cultural Theory*. London and New York: Routledge.

Douglas, M. and A. Wildavsky. 1982. *Risk and Culture: an Essay on the Selection of Technical and Environmental Dangers*. Berkeley: University of California Press.

Doving, C.A. 2003. *Migration – Ritual Attrition?* Paper presented to the Pakistan Workshop, The Rook How, Lake District.

Dube, L. 1986. Seed and earth: the symbolism of biological reproduction and sexual relations of production. In L. Dube (ed.) *Visibility and Power: Essays on Women in Society and Development*. Oxford: Oxford University Press.

Duster, T. 2003 [1990]. *Backdoor to Eugenics*. New York: Routledge.

Eade, J. 1996. Nationalism, community and the Islamisation of space in London. In B. Metcalf (ed.) *Making Muslim Space in North America and Europe*. Berkeley, California. University of California Press, pp. 217–34.

Edwards J. 2000. *Born and Bred: Idioms of Kinship and New Reproductive Technologies in England.* Oxford: Oxford University Press.

Eglar, Z. 1960. *A Punjabi Village in Pakistan.* New York: Columbia University Press.

Ekstein, J. and H. Katzenstein. 2001. The Dor Yeshorin story: community-based carrier screening for Tay–Sachs disease. *Advances in Genetics,* 44: 297–310.

Farah, M. 1984. *Marriage and Sexuality in Islam: a Translation of Al-Ghazali's Book on the Etiquette of Marriage from the Ihya.* Salt Lake City: University of Utah Press.

Farrant, W. 1985. Who's for amniocentesis? The politics of prenatal testing. In H. Homans (ed.) *The Sexual Politics of Reproduction.* London: Gower, pp. 96–122.

Fausto-Sterling, A. 2000. *Sexing the Body: Gender Politics and the Construction of Sexuality.* New York: Basic Books.

Featherstone, K., P. Atkinson, A. Bharadwaj and A. Clarke. 2006. *Risky Relations: Family, Kinship and the New Genetics.* Oxford and New York: Berg.

Ferguson, N. 1998. *The House of Rothschild. Money's Prophets 1798–1848.* New York and London: Penguin Books.

Finkler, K. 2000. *Experiencing the New Genetics: Family and Kinship on the Medical Frontier.* Philadelphia: University of Pennsylvania Press.

Finkler, K. 2001. The kin in the gene: the medicalization of family and kinship in American society. *Current Anthropology,* 42: 235–63.

Firth, H.V. 1991. Severe limb abnormalities after chorionic villus sampling. *Lancet,* 337: 762–63.

Firth, H.V. and J.A. Hurst. 2005. *Oxford Desk Reference: Clinical Genetics.* Oxford: Oxford University Press.

Firth, R., J. Hubert and A. Forge. 1970. *Families and their Relatives: Kinship in a Middle-class Section of London.* London: Routledge and Kegan Paul.

Fischer, M. 1991. Marriage and power: tradition and transition in an urban Punjabi community. In H. Donnan and P. Werbner (eds) *Economy and Culture in Pakistan: Migrants and Cities in a Muslim Society.* Basingstoke: Macmillan, pp. 97–123.

Fischer, M. and W. Lyon. 2000. Marriage strategies in Lahore: projections of model marriage on social practice. In M. Böck and A. Rao (eds) *Culture, Creation and Procreation: Concepts of Kinship in South Asian Practice.* Oxford and New York: Berghahn Books, pp. 297–322.

Fleming, P.H. 1973. The politics of marriage among non-Catholic European royalty. *Current Anthropology,* 14 (3): 231–49.

Foucault, M. 1973. *The Birth of the Clinic.* London: Tavistock.

Foucault, M. 1979. *Discipline and Punish: the Birth of the Prison,* trans. A. Sheridan. New York: Vintage Books.

Fox, R. 1967. *Kinship and Marriage: an Anthropological Perspective.* London: Penguin Books.

Franklin, S. 1997. *Embodied Progress: a Cultural Account of Assisted Conception.* London: Routledge.

Franklin, S. 2001. Biologization revisited: kinship theory in the context of the new biologies. In S. Franklin and S. McKinnon (eds) *Relative Values: Reconfiguring Kinship Studies,* Durham, NC: Duke University Press, pp. 302–25.

Franklin, S. and S. McKinnon. 2001. Introduction. In S. Franklin and S. McKinnon (eds) *Relative Values: Reconfiguring Kinship Studies.* Durham, NC: Duke University Press, pp. 1–25.

Franklin, S. and C. Roberts. 2006. *Born and Made: an Ethnography of Preimplantation Genetic Diagnosis.* Princeton: Princeton University Press.

Freeman, T. and M. Richards. 2006. DNA testing and kinship: paternity, genealogy and the search for the 'truth' of our genetic origins. In F. Ebtehaj, B. Lindley and M. Richards (eds) *Kinship Matters.* Cambridge: Hart Publishers, pp. 67–95.

Gameltoft, T. 2001. Between 'science' and 'superstition': moral perceptions of induced abortion among young adults in Vietnam. *Culture, Medicine and Psychiatry,* 26: 313–38.

Gardner, K. 2002. *Age, Narrative and Migration.* Oxford: Berg.

Geertz, C. 1983. Common sense as a cultural system. In C. Geertz *Local Knowledge.* New York: Basic Books, pp. 73–93.

Giddens, A. 1991. *Modernity and Self-identity: Self and Society in the Late Modern Age.* Cambridge: Polity Press.

Glick Schiller, N., L. Basch and C. Szanton-Blanc. 1995. From immigrant to transmigrant: theorizisng transnational migration. *Anthropological Quarterly,* 68 (1): 48–63.

Goffman, E. 1990 [1963]. *Stigma: Notes on the Management of Spoiled Identity.* London: Penguin.

Goody, J. 1983. *The Development of the Family and Marriage in Europe.* Cambridge: Cambridge University Press.

Gould, S.J. 1980. Dr Down's Syndrome. In S. Gould *The Panda's Thumb: More Reflections in Natural History.* London: Penguin Books.

Gregory, M. 2006. Research with families with haemophilia. Cardiff/Cambridge Genetic Discussion Meeting. Centre for Family Research, University of Cambridge, 14 July.

Gunaratnam, Y. 2001. 'We mustn't judge people … but': staff dilemmas in dealing with racial harassment amongst hospice service users. *Sociology of Health and Illness*, 23 (1): 65–84.

Hallowell, N. 1999. Doing the right thing: genetic risk and responsibility. *Sociology of Health and Illness*, 21: 597–621.

Halpern, D. and J. Nazroo. 2000. The ethnic density effect: results from a national community survey of England and Wales. *International Journal of Psychiatry*, 46: 34–46.

Hamamy, H., L. Jamhawi, J. Al-Darawsheh and K.Ajlouni. 2005. Consanguineous marriages in Jordan: why is the rate changing with time? *Clinical Genetics*, 67: 511–16.

Harper, P.S., C. Lim and D. Craufurd, on behalf of the UK Huntington's Disease Prediction Consortium. 2000. Ten years of presymptomatic testing for Huntington's disease: the experience of the UK Huntington's Disease Prediction Consortium. *Journal of Medical Genetics*, 37: 567–71.

Harriss, K. 2004. Living with chronic illness: limiting ill-health, ethnicity and poverty. Paper presented to the Pakistan Workshop, The Rook How, Lake District.

Harriss, K. and A. Shaw. 2006. Family care and transnational kinship: British Pakistani experiences. In F. Ebtehaj, B. Lindley and M. Richards (eds) *Kinship Matters*. Cambridge: Hart Publishers, pp. 259–74.

Haslam, J. 2001. Harsh troth. *Guardian Society*, 14 March, 6–7.

Hatton, C., S. Azmi, A. Caine and E. Emerson. 1998. Informal carers of adolescents and adults with learning difficulties from the South Asian communities: family circumstances, service support and carer stress. *British Journal of Social Work*, 28, 821–37.

Hedgecoe, A. 1998. Geneticization, medicalisation and polemics. *Medicine, Healthcare and Philosophy* 1, 235–43.

Herbert, I. 2000. British Asians are warned over risks to children of inter-marriage. *Independent*, 5 May.

Hirsch, E. 1993. Negotiated limits: interviews in South-east England. In J. Edwards, S. Franklin, E. Hirsch, F. Price and M. Strathern (eds) *Technologies of Procreation: Kinship in the Age of Assisted Conception*. Manchester: Manchester University Press, pp. 67–95.

Holy, L. 1989. *Kinship, Honour and Solidarity: Cousin Marriage in the Middle East*. Manchester: Manchester University Press.

Home Office. 2001. *Control of Immigration: Statistics United Kingdom 2000*. London: Stationery Office.

Home Office. 2002. *Secure Borders, Safe Haven: Integration with Diversity in Modern Britain*. London: Stationery Office.

Hoodfar, E. and A.S. Teebi. 1996. Genetic referrals of Middle Eastern origin in a western city: inbreeding and disease profile. *Journal of Medical Genetics*, 33: 212–15.

Hosseini, K. 2003. *The Kite Runner.* London: Bloomsbury.

Howell, S. 2001. Self-conscious kinship: some contested values in Norwegian transnational adoption. In S. Franklin and S. McKinnon (eds) *Relative Values: Reconfiguring Kinship Studies*, Durham. NC: Duke University Press, pp. 203–23.

Hundt, G.L., J.M. Green, J. Sandall, S. Hirst, S. Ahmed and J. Hewison. 2006. Navigating the troubled waters of prenatal testing decisions. In A. Webster (ed.) *New Technologies in Health Care: Challenge, Change and Innovation.* New York: Palgrave Macmillan, pp. 25–39.

Huntington, R. and P. Metcalf. 1979. *Celebrations of Death: the Anthropology of Mortuary Ritual.* Cambridge: Cambridge University Press.

Hurst, J. 2005. Congenital abnormalities and genetic diseases among British Pakistanis from High Wycombe. Presentation to conference on Genetic Disorders and People from the Indian Subcontinent: Challenges for Clinical Services in the NHS, Wales Gene Park, Wales Milennium Centre, Cardiff, 23 November.

Hussain, R. 1999. Community perceptions of reasons for preference for consanguineous marriages in Pakistan. *Journal of Biosocial Science*, 31: 449–61.

Huth, A.H. 1887. *The Marriage of Near Kin Considered with Respect to the Laws of Nations, the Results of Experience and the Teachings of Biology.* London: Longmans, Green and Company. (First edition 1875, London: Churchill)

Illich, I. 1992. *In the Mirror of the Past: Lectures and Addresses 1978–1990.* New York: Marion Boyars.

Imaizumi, Y. 1987. Reasons for consanguineous marriages in Japan. *Journal of Biosocial Science*, 19: 97–106.

Imran, I. and T. Smith. 1997. *Home from Home: British Pakistanis in Mirpur.* Bradford: Bradford Heritage Recording Unit.

Ingstadt, B. and S. Reynolds-Whyte (eds). 1995. *Disability and Culture.* Berkeley: University of California Press.

Inhorn, M.C. 1994. *Quest for Conception: Gender, Infertility, and Egyptian Medical Traditions.* Philadelphia: University of Pennsylvania Press.

Inhorn, M.C. 2003. *Local Babies, Global Science: Gender, Religion and In-vitro Fertilisation in Egypt.* New York, London: Routledge.

Inhorn, M.C. 2004. Privacy, privatization, and the politics of patronage: ethnographic challenges to penetrating the secret world of Middle Eastern, hospital-based in vitro fertilization. *Social Science and Medicine*, 59, 2095–108.

Inhorn, M.C. 2006. Making Muslim babies: IVF and gamete donation in Sunni versus Shi'a Islam. *Culture, Medicine and Psychiatry*, 2006, 30: 423–35.

Iqbal, Z. 1997. *Khūn ke rishton ke mābīn shadī ke khatrāt* (Dangers of marriage between blood relatives). Daily Jang, London.

Irwin, A. and B. Wynne (eds). 1996. *Misunderstanding Science? The Public Reconstruction of Science and Technology*. Cambridge: Cambridge University Press.

Jaber, L., G.J. Halpern and M. Shohat. 1998. The impact of consanguinity worldwide. *Community Genetics*, 1: 12–17.

Jackman, C., H.M. McGee and M. Turner. 1991. The experience and impact of early miscarriage. *Irish Journal of Psychology*, 12: 108–20.

Jackson, A.P., D.P. McHale, D.A. Campbell, H. Jafri, Y. Rashid, J. Mannan, G. Karbani, P. Corry, M.I. Levene, R.F. Mueller, A.F. Markham, N.J. Lench and C.G. Woods. 1998. Primary autosomal recessive microcephaly (MCPH1) maps to chromosome 8p22–pter. *American Journal of Human Genetics*, 63: 541–46.

Jeffery, P. 1976. *Migrants and Refugees: Muslim and Christian Pakistani Families in Bristol*. Cambridge: Cambridge University Press.

Jeffery, P. 1979. *Frogs in a Well: Indian Women in Purdah*. London: Zed Press.

Jeffery, P. and R. Jeffery. 1996a. *Don't Marry Me to a Plowman!* Boulder: Westview.

Jeffery, P. and R. Jeffery. 1996b. Delayed periods and falling babies: the ethnophysiology and politics of pregnancy loss in rural North India. In R. Cecil (ed.) *The Anthropology of Pregnancy Loss: Comparative Studies in Miscarriage, Stillbirth and Neonatal Death*. Oxford: Berg, pp. 17–37.

Jenkins, R. (ed.). 1998. *Questions of Competence: Culture, Classification and Intellectual Disability*. Cambridge: Cambridge University Press.

Johnson, M. 1996. 'Something more than blood': Conflicting accounts of pregnancy loss in eighteenth-century England. In R. Cecil (ed.) *The Anthropology of Pregnancy Loss: Comparative Studies in Miscarriage, Stillbirth and Neonatal Death*. Oxford: Berg, pp. 197–214.

Jones, S. 1994. *The Language of the Genes*. London: Flamingo.

Kai, J. (ed.). 2003. *Ethnicity, Health and Primary Care*. Oxford: Oxford University Press.

Kalra, V. 2000. *From Textile Mills to Taxi Ranks: Experiences of Migration, Labour and Social Change*. Ashgate: Aldershot.

Kandela, P. 1994. Premarital examination in the Arab world. *Lancet*, 334: 1426.

Kay, L. 2000. *Who Wrote the Book of Life? A History of the Genetic Code*. Stanford, California: Stanford University Press.

Keller, E.F. 1992. Nature, nurture and the Human Genome Project. In D.J. Kevles and L. Hood (eds) *The Code of Codes: Scientific and Social Issues in the Human Genome Project*. Cambridge, MA: Harvard University Press, pp. 281–99.

Kelly, E. 1990. Transcontinental families – Gujarat and Lancashire: a comparative study of social policy. In C. Clarke, C. Peach and S. Vertovec (eds) *South Asians Overseas: Migration and Ethnicity*. Cambridge: Cambridge University Press, pp. 251–67.

Kessler, S. (ed.). 1979. *Genetic Counseling: Psychological Dimensions*. New York: Academic Press.

Kevles, D. 1985. *In the Name of Eugenics: Genetics and the Uses of Human Heredity*. Berkeley: University of California Press.

Kleinman, A. 1995. A critique of objectivity in international health. In A. Kleinman *Writing at the Margin: Discourse between Anthropology and Medicine.* Berkeley: University of California Press, pp. 68–92.

Knorr-Cetina, K. 1999. *Epistemic Cultures: How the Sciences Make Knowledge.* Cambridge: Harvard University Press.

Kohner, N. and A. Henley. 1991. *When a Baby Dies: the Experience of Late Miscarriage, Stillbirth and Neonatal Death.* London: Pandora Press.

Krimsley, S. and D. Golding (eds). 1992. *Social Theories of Risk.* Westport: Praeger.

Kuper, A. 2001. Fraternity and endogamy. The house of Rothschild. *Social Anthropology,* 9 (3): 273–87.

Kuper, A. 2002. Incest, cousin marriage, and the origin of the human sciences in nineteenth-century England. *Past and Present,* 174 (1): 158–83.

Lander, E.S. and D. Botstein. 1987. Homozygosity mapping: a way to map human recessive traits with the DNA of inbred children. *Science,* 236: 1567–70.

Lanie, A.D., T.E. Jayaratne, J.P. Sheldon, S.L. Kardia, E.S. Anderson, M. Feldbaum and E.M. Petty. 2004. Exploring the public understanding of basic genetic concepts. *Journal of Genetic Counseling,* 13 (4): 305–20.

Latimer, J. 2006. Appearance and essence, parts and wholes: gene medicine reaffirming the human. Paper presented to the European Association of Social Anthropologists, 19 September.

Latimer, J., K. Featherstone, A. Clarke, D.T. Pilz and A. Shaw. 2006. Rebirthing the clinic: the interaction of clinical judgment and genetic technology in the production of medical science. *Science, Technology and Human Values,* 31 (5) 599–630.

Latour, B. and S. Woolgar. 1979 [1987]. *Laboratory Life: the Social Construction of Scientific Facts.* Los Angeles: Sage.

Leach, E. 1967. Virgin birth, *Proceedings of the Royal Anthropological Institute,* pp. 39–49, reprinted in E. Leach, *The Structural Study of Myth.* London: Jonathan Cape, 1969.

Lee, C. 1997. *This Sceptred Isle.* London: Penguin.

Leung, W.C., E.C. Mariman, J.C. van der Wouden, H. van Amergongen and C. Weijer. 2000. Results of genetic testing: where confidentiality conflicts with a duty to warn relatives. *British Medical Journal,* 321 (7274): 1464–66.

Lévi-Strauss, C. 1969. *The Elementary Structures of Kinship,* trans, J.H. Belle and J.R. von-Sturmer, ed. R. Needham. Boston: Beacon. (Original French edition 1949)

Lewis, J., J. Leach and C. Wood-Robinson. 2000. All in the genes? – young people's understanding of the nature of genes. *Journal of Biological Education,* 34 (2): 74–79.

Lippman, A. 1992. Led (astray) by genetic maps: the cartography of the human genome and health care. *Social Science and Medicine,* 35 (12) 1469–76.

Lippman-Hand, A. and F.C. Fraser. 1979. Genetic counseling: parents' responses to uncertainty. In C.J. Epstein, C.J.R. Curry, S. Packman, S. Sherman and B.D. Hall (eds) *Risk, Communication and Decision Making in Genetic Counseling.* The National Foundation – March of Dimes. *Birth Defects: Original Articles Series,* XV (5C), pp. 325–39.

Lock, M. 1998. Perfecting society: reproductive technologies, genetic testing, and the planned family in Japan. In M. Lock and P. Kaufert (eds) *Pragmatic Women and Body Politics*. Cambridge: Cambridge University Press, pp. 206–39.

Lock, M. 2005. Eclipse of the gene and the return of divination. *Current Anthropology*, 46: S47–S70.

Lock, M. and P. Kaufert. 1998. Introduction. In M. Lock and P. Kaufert (eds) *Pragmatic Women and Body Politics*. Cambridge: Cambridge University Press, pp. 1–27.

Lubbock, J. 1870. *The Origin of Civilization and the Primitive Condition s of Man*. London: Longmans.

Mackenzie, C. and N. Stoljar (eds). 2000. *Relational Autonomy: Feminist Perspectives on Autonomy, Agency and the Social Self*. Oxford and New York: Oxford University Press.

MacPherson, A.G. 1968. An old highland parish register II, *Scottish Studies*, 12 (2): 81–111.

Madigan, J. 1996. Needing it like this. Huntington's disease. In T. Marteau and M. Richards (eds) *The Troubled Helix: Social and Psychological Implications of the New Human Genetics*. Cambridge: Cambridge University Press, pp. 7–22.

Mahler, S.J. and P. Pessar. 2001. Gendered geographies of power: analyzing gender across transnational spaces. *Identities: Global Studies in Culture and Power*, 7 (4): 441–59.

Maine, H. 1883. *Dissertations on Early Law and Custom*. London: J. Murray.

Malinowski, B. 1922. *Argonauts of the Western Pacific*. New York: E.P. Dutton.

Malinowski, 1929. *The Sexual Life of Savages*. London: Routledge.

Marmot, M.G., A.M. Aldstein and L. Bulusu. 1984. *Immigrant Mortality in England and Wales 1970–78. Causes of Death by Country of Birth*. London: Her Majesty's Stationery Office.

Marriott, M. and R. Inden. 1977. Towards an ethnosociology of South Asian caste systems. In K. David (ed.) *The New Wind: Changing Identities in South Asia*. The Hague: Mouton.

Marteau, T.M. 1991. Psychological aspects of prenatal testing for fetal abnormalities. *Irish Journal of Psychiatry*, 12: 121–32.

Marteau, T.M. and E. Anionwu. 1996. Evaluating carrier testing: objectives and outcomes. In T. Marteau and M. Richards (eds) *The Troubled Helix: Social and Psychological Implications of the New Human Genetics*. Cambridge: Cambridge University Press, pp. 123–39.

Marteau, T.M., M. Plenicar and J. Kidd. 1993. Obstetricians presenting amniocentesis to pregnant women: practice observed. *Journal of Reproductive and Infant Psychology*, (11): 3–10.

Maududi, M. 1974. *Birth Control*, trans K. Ahmad and M.I. Faruqi. Lahore: Islamic Publications.

McLennan, J.F. 1865 (1970 reprint). *Primitive Marriage*. Edinburgh: A.C. Black.

Meiser, B., M. Eisenbruch, K. Barlow-Stewart, K. Tucker, Z. Steel and D. Goldstein. 2001. Cultural aspects of cancer genetics: setting a research agenda. *Journal of Medical Genetics*, 38: 425–29.

Menski, W. 2002. Letter. *Anthropology Today*, 18 (3): 20.

Merzario, R. 1990. Land, kinship, and consanguineous marriage in Italy from the seventeenth to the nineteenth centuries. *Journal of Family History*, 15 (4): 529–46.

Middleton, A., F. Robson, L. Burnell and M. Ahmed. 2007. Providing a transcultural genetic counseling service in the UK. *Journal of Genetic Counseling*, 5: 567–82.

Miles, M. 1992. Concepts of mental retardation in Pakistan: towards cross-cultural and historical perspectives. *Disability, Handicap and Society*, 7: 235–55.

Miller, W.B. 1983. Chance, choice and the future of reproduction. *American Psychologist*, 38, 1198–205.

Modell, B. 1997. Kinship and medical genetics: a clinician's perspective. In A. Clarke and E. Parsons (eds) *Culture, Kinship and Genes*. London: Macmillan, pp. 27–39.

Modell B. and A. Darr. 2002a. Consanguineous marriage in the UK: proposal for a multidisciplinary national strategy. Conference paper presented at the Royal Society of Medicine, 4 February.

Modell B. and A. Darr. 2002b. Genetic counselling and customary consanguineous marriage. *Nature Reviews*, 3: 225–29.

Modell, B. and A.M. Kuliev. 1991. Social and genetic implications of customary consanguineous marriage among British Pakistanis. Paper presented to a meeting held at the Ciba Foundation on 15 January.

Modell, B. and M. Petrou. 1994 (first published 1989 by Wright, London). Thalassaemia screening: ethics and practice. In J.K. Cruikshank and D.G. Beevers (eds) *Ethnic Factors in Health and Disease*. Oxford: Butterworth-Heinemann, pp. 114–22.

Modell, B., R. Harris, B. Lane, M. Khan, M. Darlison, M. Petrou, J. Old, M. Layton and L. Varnavides. 2000. Informed choice in genetic screening for thalassaemia during pregnancy: audit from a national confidential enquiry. *British Medical Journal*, 320, 337–41.

Modood, T., R. Berthoud, J. Lakey, J. Nazroo, P. Smith, S. Virdee and S. Beishon. 1997. *Ethnic Minorities in Britain: Diversity and Disadvantage*. London: Policy Studies Institute.

Molloy, M. 1986. 'No inclination to mix with strangers': marriage patterns among Highland Scots migrants to Cape Breton and New Zealand, 1800–1916. *Journal of Family History*, 11 (3): 221–43.

Morgan, L.H. 1871. *Systems of Consanguinity and Affinity of the Human Family*. Washington: Smithsonian Institution.

Morgan, L.H. 1877. *Ancient Society: Researches in the Lines of Human Progress from Savagery through Barbarism to Civilization*. New York: Holt.

Mueller R.F. and D.T. Bishop. 1993. Autozygosity mapping, complex consanguinity, and autosomal recessive disorders. *Journal of Medical Genetics*, 30 (9): 798–99.

Murphy, R. and L. Kasdan. 1959. The structure of parallel cousin marriage. *American Anthropologist*, 58: 687–715.

Musallam, B. 1983. *Sex and Society in Islam*. Cambridge: Cambridge University Press.

Nazroo, J. 1997. *The Health of Britain's Ethnic Minorities: Findings from a National Survey*. London: Policy Studies Institute.

Nazroo, J. 1998. Genetic, cultural or socio-economic vulnerability? Explaining ethnic inequalities in health. *Sociology of Health and Illness,* 20 (5): 710–30.

Nelkin, D. and M.S. Lindee. 1995. *The DNA Mystique: the Gene as a Cultural Icon.* New York: Freeman.

Novas, C. 2006. The Political Economy of Hope: Patients' organisations, science and biovalue. *Biosocieties,* 1, 289–305.

Oakley, A. 1984. *The Captured Womb.* Oxford: Blackwell.

Office for National Statistics: www.statistics.gov.uk

Omran, A.R. 1992. *Family Planning in the Legacy of Islam.* London: Routledge.

O'Rahilly, S., S.S. Farooqi, G.S.H. Yeo and B.G. Challis. 2003. Minireview: human obesity – lessons from monogenic disorders. *Endocrinology,* 144 (9) 3757–64.

Ostor, A., L. Fruzetti and S. Barnett (eds). 1982. *Concepts of Person: Kinship, Caste and Marriage in India.* Cambridge, MA. Harvard University Press.

Ottenheimer, M. 1986. Complementarity and the structures of parallel-cousin marriage. *American Anthropologist,* 88: 934–39.

Ottenheimer, M. 1996. *Forbidden Relatives: the American Myth of Cousin Marriage.* Urbana and Chicago: University of Illinois Press.

Papadopoulos, I. 2006. *Transcultural Health and Social Care: the Development of Culturally Competent Practitioners.* Oxford: Elsevier.

Papadopoulos, I., M. Tilki and S. Lees. 2004. Promoting cultural competence in healthcare through a research-based intervention in the UK. *Diversity in Health and Social Care,* 2: 107–15.

Parker, M., R. Ashcroft, A.O.M. Wilkie and A. Kent. 2004. Ethical review of research into rare genetic disorders. *British Medical Journal,* 329: 288–89.

Parkin, R. 1997. *Kinship: an Introduction to Basic Concepts.* Oxford: Blackwell.

Parkin, R. and L. Stone (eds). 2004. *Kinship and Family: an Anthropological Reader.* Oxford: Blackwell Publishing.

Parsons, L., A. Macfarlane and J. Golding. 1993. Pregnancy, birth and maternity care. In W.I.U. Ahmed (ed.) *'Race' and Health in Contemporary Britain.* Buckingham: Open University Press, pp. 51–75.

Peach, C. 2005. Britain's Muslim population: An overview. In T. Abbas (ed.) *Muslim Britain: Communities under Pressure.* London: Zed Books, pp. 18–30.

Pearson, H. 2006. Genetics: what is a gene? *Nature,* 44 (7092): 399–401.

Pembrey, M. 1996. The new genetics: a user's guide. In T. Marteau and M. Richards (eds) *The Troubled Helix: Social and Psychological Implications of the New Human Genetics.* Cambridge: Cambridge University Press, pp. 63–81.

Pessar, P. and S.J. Mahler. 2003. Transnational migration: bringing gender in. *International Migration Review,* 37(3): 812–16.

Petrou, M., B. Modell, A. Darr, J. Old, E. Kin and D.J. Weatherall. 1990. Antenatal diagnosis: how to deliver a comprehensive service in the United Kingdom. *Annals of the New York Academy of Sciences,* 612: 251–63.

Pickering, A. (ed.). 1992. *Science as Practice and Culture.* Chicago: University of Chicago Press.

Port, K.E., H. Mountain, J. Nelson and A. Bittles. 2005. Changing profile of couples seeking genetic counseling for consanguinity in Australia. *American Journal of Medical Genetics*, 132 (2), 159–63.

Press, N. and C.H. Browner. 1997. Why women say yes to prenatal diagnosis. *Social Science and Medicine*, 45 (7): 979–89.

Press, N., C.H. Browner, D. Tran, C. Morton and B.L. Master. 1998. Provisional normalcy and 'Perfect Babies': pregnant women's attitudes towards disability in the context of prenatal testing. In S. Franklin and H. Ragoné (eds) *Reproducing Reproduction: Kinship, Power and Technological Innovation*. Philadelphia: University of Pennsylvania Press, pp. 46–65.

Price, F. 1996. Now you see it, now you don't: mediating science and managing uncertainty in reproductive medicine. In A. Irwin and B. Wynne (eds) *Misunderstanding Science? The Public Reconstruction of Science and Technology*. Cambridge: Cambridge University Press, pp. 84–106.

Pryce, H. 1993. *Native Law and the Church in Medieval Wales*. Oxford: Clarendon Press.

Rabinow, P. 1992. Artificiality and enlightenment: from sociobiology to biosociality. In J. Crary and S. Kwinter (eds) *Incorporations*. New York: Zone Books, pp. 234–52.

Rahman, F. 1980. *Major Themes of the Quran*. Minneapolis: Bibliotheca Islamica.

Rahman, F. 1982. The status of women in Islam: a modernist interpretation. In H. Papanek and G. Minault (eds) *Separate Worlds: Studies of Purdah in South Asia*. Delhi: South Asia Books, pp. 285–310.

Rao, P.S.S. and S.G. Imbaraj. 1979. Inbreeding effects on fertility and sterility in southern India. *Journal of Medical Genetics*, 16: 24–31.

Rapp, R. 2000. *Testing Women, Testing the Fetus: the Social Impact of Amniocentesis in America*. New York: Routledge.

Rapp, R., D. Heath and K.S. Taussig. 2001. Genealogical dis-ease: where hereditary abnormality, biomedical explanation, and family responsibility meet. In S. Franklin and S. McKinnon (eds) *Relative Values: Reconfiguring Kinship Studies*. Durham, NC: Duke University Press, pp. 384–409.

Ratcliff, K.S. 1989. Health technologies for women: whose health? Whose technology? In K.S. Ratcliff, M.M. Ferree, G.O. Mellow, B.D. Wright, G.D. Price, K. Yanoshik and M.S. Freston *Healing Technologies: Feminist Perspectives*. Ann Arbor: University of Michigan Press, pp. 173–220.

Raz, A.E. and M. Atar. 2004. Cousin marriage and premarital carrier matching in a Bedouin community in Israel: attitudes, service development and educational intervention. *Journal of Family Planning and Reproductive Health Care*, 30 (1), 49–51.

Reid, R.M. 1988. Church membership, consanguineous marriage, and migration in a Scotch-Irish frontier population. *Journal of Family History*, 12 (4): 397–414.

Resnick, D.B. 2003. Genetic testing and primary care: a new ethic for a new setting. *New Genetics and Society*, 22 (3): 245–56.

Richards, M.P.M. 1975. Innovation in medical practice: obstetricians and the induction of labour in Britain. *Social Science and Medicine*, 9 (11/12): 592–652.

Richards, M.P.M. 1993. The new genetics: some issues for social scientists. *Sociology of Health and Illness,* 15: 567–87.

Richards, M. 1996a. Sickle cell disease: a father's view. An interview with Alexander Mottoh. In T. Marteau and M. Richards (eds) *The Troubled Helix: Social and Psychological Implications of the New Human Genetics.* Cambridge: Cambridge University Press, pp. 51–59.

Richards, M. 1996b. Families, kinship and genetics. In T. Marteau and M. Richards (eds) *The Troubled Helix: Social and Psychological Implications of the New Human Genetics.* Cambridge: Cambridge University Press, pp. 249–73.

Richards, M. 1996c. Daily life and the new genetics: some personal stories. In T. Marteau and M. Richards (eds) *The Troubled Helix: Social and Psychological Implications of the New Human Genetics.* Cambridge: Cambridge University Press, pp. 3–59.

Richards, M.P.M. and J. Green. 1993. Attitudes towards prenatal screening for fetal abnormality and detection of carriers of genetic disease: a discussion paper. *Journal of Reproductive and Infant Psychology,* 11: 49–56.

Richards, M.P.M. and M. Ponder. 1996. Lay understanding of genetics: a test of an hypothesis. *Journal of Medical Genetics,* 33: 1032–36.

Roberts, A., R. Cullen and S. Bundey. 1996. The representation of ethnic minorities at genetics clinics in Birmingham. *Journal of Medical Genetics,* 33: 56–58.

Robinson, G.E., R. Stirtzinger, D.E. Steward and E. Ralevski. 1994. Psychological reactions in women followed for one year after miscarriage. *Journal of Reproductive and Infant Psychology,* 12 (1): 31–36.

Rose, N. and C. Novas. 2005. Biological citizenship. In A. Ong and S.J. Collier (eds) *Global Assemblages.* Oxford: Blackwell, pp. 439–63.

Rose, S., R.C. Lewontin and L.J. Kamin. 1984. *Not in Our Genes: Biology, Ideology and Human Nature.* Penguin: Harmondsworth.

Rothman, B.K. 1986. *The Tentative Pregnancy: Prenatal Diagnosis and the Future of Motherhood.* New York: Viking.

Rozario, S. and S. Gilliat-Ray. 2007. Working Paper 93: Genetics, religion and identity: a study of Bangladeshi Muslims in Britain. Cardiff University, School of Social Sciences. http://www.cardiff.ac.uk/socsi/resources/wrkgpaper-93.pdf

Rudan, I., D. Rudan, H. Campbell, A. Carothers, A. Wright, N. Smolej-Narancic, B. Janicijevic, L. Jin, R. Chakraborty, R. Deka and P. Rudan. 2003. Inbreeding and risk of late onset complex disorders. *Journal of Medical Genetics,* 40: 925–32.

Rudan, I., H. Campbell, A.D. Carothers, N.D. Hastie and A.F. Wright. 2006. Contribution of consanguinity to polygenic and multifactorial disease. *Nature Genetics,* 38: 1224–25.

Sacks, K. 1979. *Sisters and Wives.* Westport, CO: Greenwood.

Sagan, S.D. 1993. *The Limits of Safety: Organizations, Accidents and Nuclear Weapons.* Princeton: Princeton University Press.

Samad, Y. and J. Eade. 2002. *Community Perceptions of Forced Marriage.* London: Community Liaison Unit, Foreign and Commonwealth Office.

Samavat, A. and B. Modell. 2004. Iranian national screening programme. *British Medical Journal,* 329: 1134–37.

Scherper-Hughes, N. 1991. Social indifference to child death. *Lancet,* 337: 1144–47.

Scherper-Hughes, N. 1992. *Death without Weeping: the Violence of Everyday Life in Brazil.* Berkeley: University of California Press.

Schneider, D. 1968 (1980 reprint). *American Kinship: A Cultural Account.* Chicago: University of Chicago Press (Reprinted by Prentice-Hall, Englewood Cliffs, NJ).

Shafik, V. 2001. Prostitute for a good reason: stars and morality in Egypt. *Women's Studies International Forum,* 24: 711–25.

Shaikh, S. 2003. Family planning, contraception, and abortion in Islam: undertaking *khilafah.* In D.C. Maguire (ed.) *Sacred Rights: the Case for Contraception and Abortion in World Religions.* Oxford: Oxford University Press, pp. 102–28.

Shaw, A. 2000a. *Kinship and Continuity: Pakistani Families in Britain.* London and Amsterdam: Routledge and Harwood.

Shaw, A. 2000b. Conflicting models of risk: clinical genetics and British Pakistanis. In P. Caplan (ed.) *Risk Revisited.* London: Pluto Press, pp. 85–107.

Shaw, A. 2001. Kinship, cultural preference and immigration: consanguineous marriage among British Pakistanis. *Journal of the Royal Anthropological Institute,* 7 (2): 315–34.

Shaw, A. 2003a. The impact of genetic risk on U.K. Pakistani families. http://www.wellcome.ac.uk/en/genome/geneticsandsociety/hg14f005.html

Shaw, A. 2003b. Interpreting images: diagnostic skill in the genetics clinic. *Journal of the Royal Anthropological Institute,* 9: 39–55.

Shaw, A. 2004. British Pakistani elderly without children: an invisible minority. In P. Kreager and E. Shroeder-Butterfill (eds) *Ageing Without Children: European and Asian Perspectives on Elderly Access to Support Networks.* Oxford and New York: Berghahn Books, pp. 198–222.

Shaw, A. 2006. The contingency of the 'genetic link' in constructions of kinship and inheritance: an anthropological perspective. In J. Spencer and A. Pedain (eds) *Freedom and Responsibility in Reproductive Choice.* Cambridge: Hart Publishers, pp. 73–90.

Shaw, A. n.d. *Maqool Javab Den: Letters to the Problem Page of an Urdu Weekly.* Unpublished manuscript.

Shaw, A. and M. Ahmed. 2004. Translating genetics leaflets into languages other than English: lessons from an assessment of Urdu materials. *Journal of Genetic Counseling,* 13 (4): 321–42.

Shaw, A. and K. Charsley. 2006. Rishtas: adding emotion to strategy in understanding British Pakistani transnational marriages. *Global Networks: a Journal of Transnational Affairs,* 6, (4): 405–21.

Shaw, A., J. Latimer, P. Atkinson and K. Featherstone. 2003. Surveying 'slides': clinical perception and clinical judgment in the construction of a genetic diagnosis. *New Genetics and Society*, 22 (1): 3–19.

Sheikh, A. and A. Esmail. 2007. Should Muslims have faith based health services? *British Medical Journal*, 334: 74–75.

Sherridan, E. 2005. Familial cancer among South Asians. Conference presentation. Genetic Disorders and People from the Indian Subcontinent: Challenges for Clinical Services in the NHS, Cardiff, Wales Millennium Centre, 23 November.

Shihol, S. 1996. Decision-making in the context of genetic risk. In T. Marteau and M. Richards (eds) *The Troubled Helix: Social and Psychological Implications of the New Human Genetics*. Cambridge: Cambridge University Press, pp. 82–103.

Simmons, D. and M.J. Powell. 1993. Metabolic and clinical characteristics of South Asians and Europeans in Coventry. *Diabetic Medicine*, 10: 751–58.

Simpson, R. 2004. Acting ethically, responding culturally: framing the new reproductive and genetic technologies in Sri Lanka. *The Asia Pacific Journal of Anthropology*, 5 (3): 227–43.

Simpson, R. 2006. Scrambling parenthood: English kinship and the prohibited degrees of affinity. *Anthropology Today*, 22 (3): 3–6.

Slade, P. 1994. Predictions of the psychological impact of miscarriage. *Journal of Reproductive and Infant Psychology*, 12: 5–16.

Smaje, C. 1996. The ethnic patterning of health: new directions for theory and research. *Sociology of Health and Illness*, 18: 139–71.

Snowdon, C. and J. Green. 1994. *New Reproductive Technologies: Attitudes and Experiences of Carriers of Recessive Disorders*. Cambridge: Centre for Family Research.

Sobo, E.J. 1995. *Choosing Unsafe Sex: Aids Risk Denial among Disadvantaged Women*. Philadelphia: University of Pennsylvania Press.

Spiro, M. 1968. Virgin birth, parthenogenesis and physiological paternity: an essay in cultural interpretation. *Man*, 3: 242–62.

Statham, H. and J.M. Green. 1994. The effects of miscarriage and other 'unsuccessful' pregnancies on feelings early in a subsequent pregnancy. *Journal of Reproductive and Infant Psychology*, 12 (1): 45–54.

Stoltenberg, C. 1998. *Birth Defects, Stillbirth and Infant Death: Epidemiological Studies of the Effects of Consanguinity and Parental Education on Births in Norway 1967–1995*. Oslo: Statens institutt for folkehelse.

Stoltenberg C., P. Magnus, R.T. Lie, A.K. Daltveit and L.M. Irgens. 1997. Birth defects and parental consanguinity in Norway. *American Journal of Epidemiology*, 145 (5): 439–48.

Strathern, M. (ed.). 1987. *Dealing with Inequality: Analysing Gender Relations in Melanesia and Beyond*. Cambridge: Cambridge University Press.

Strathern, M. 1992. *After Nature: English Kinship in the Late Twentieth Century*. Cambridge: Cambridge University Press.

Strathern, M. 1997. The work of culture: an anthropological perspective. In A. Clarke and E. Parsons (eds) *Culture, Kinship and Genes: Towards a Cross-Cultural Genetics,* London: Macmillan Press, pp. 40–53.

Svendsen, M.N. 2006. The social life of genetic knowledge: a case-study of choice and dilemmas in cancer genetic counselling in Denmark. *Medical Anthropology,* 25: 139–79.

Tapper, N. 1981. Direct exchange and brideprice: alternative forms in a complex marriage system. *Man,* 16: 387–407.

Tarazi, I., E. Al Najjar, N. Lulu and M. Sirdar. 2007. Obligatory premarital tests for beta-thalassaemia in the Gaza Strip: evaluation and recommendations, *International Journal of Laboratory Hematology,* 29 (2): 111–18.

Taylor, J.S. 1998. Image of contradiction: obstetrical ultrasound in American culture. In S. Franklin and H. Ragoné (eds) *Reproducing Reproduction: Kinship, Power and Technological Innovation.* Philadelphia: University of Pennsylvania Press, pp. 15–45.

Teebi, A.S. and H.I. El-Shanti. 2006. Consanguinity: implications for practice, research, and policy. *Lancet*: 370: 970–71.

Teebi, A.S. and T.I. Farangi (eds). 1997. *Genetic Disorders among Arab Populations.* New York: Oxford University Press.

Thompson, C. 2001. Strategic naturalizing: kinship in an infertility clinic. In S. Franklin and S. McKinnon (eds) *Relative Values.* Durham, NC: Duke University Press, pp. 175–202.

Tillion, G. 1983 [1966]. *The Republic of Cousins: Women's Oppression in Mediterranean Society,* trans. Q. Hoare. London: Al Saqi Books, distributed by Zed Press (First published as *Les harem et les cousins* by Éditions de Seuil, Paris).

Tomalin, C. 1997. *Jane Austen: a Life.* London: Viking.

Tylor, E.B. 1889. On a Method of investigating the development of institutions; applied to laws of marriage and descent. *Journal of the Anthropological Institute,* 18: 245–72.

Vertovec, S. 2001. Transnational challenges to the 'new' multiculturalism, Paper presented to the ASA conference held at the University of Sussex, 30 March-2 April 2001. Transnational Communities Programme Working Paper Series, WPTC-01–06.

Weatherall, D.J. 1985. *The New Genetics and Clinical Practice,* 2nd ed. Oxford: Oxford University Press.

Wedgwood, J.C. 1909. *A History of the Wedgwood Family.* London: St Catherine Press.

Weiner, A. 1976. *Women of Value, Men of Renown: New Perspectives in Trobriand Exchange.* Austin: University of Texas Press.

Wembah-Rashid, J.A.R. 1996. Explaining pregnancy loss in matrilineal Southeast Tanzania. In R. Cecil (ed.) *The Anthropology of Pregnancy Loss: Comparative Studies in Miscarriage, Stillbirth and Neonatal Death.* Oxford: Berg, pp. 75–93.

Werbner, P. 1990. *The Migration Process: Capital, Gifts and Offerings among British Pakistanis.* Oxford: Berg.

Werbner, P. 2002. Reproducing the multicultural nation. *Anthropology Today*, 18 (2): 3–4.

Wertz, D.C. and J.C. Fletcher. 1989. Ethical decision making in medical genetics: women as patients and practitioners in eighteen nations. In K.S. Ratcliff, M.M. Ferree, G.O. Mellow, B.D. Wright, G.D. Price, K. Yanoshik and M.S. Freston *Healing Technologies: Feminist Perspectives.* Ann Arbor: University of Michigan Press, pp. 221–41.

Wertz, D.C., S.R. Janes, J.M. Rosenfield and R.W. Erbe. 1992. Attitudes toward the prenatal diagnosis of cystic fibrosis: factors in decision making among affected families. *American Journal of Human Genetics*, 50: 1077–85.

Westermarck, E. 1891. *The History of Human Marriage.* London: Macmillan.

Wexler, N. 1979. Genetic 'Russian roulette': the experience of being 'at risk' for Huntington's disease. In Kessler, S. (ed.). *Genetic Counseling: Psychological Dimensions.* New York: Academic Press, pp. 199–220.

Wilkie. T. 1994. *Perilous Knowledge: the Human Genome Project and its Implications.* London: Faber and Faber.

Wolfram, S. 1987. *In-laws and Outlaws: Kinship and Marriage in England.* London: Croom Helm.

Woods C.G., S. Stricker, P. Seemann, R. Stern, J. Cox, E. Sherridan, E. Roberts, K. Springell, S. Scott, G. Karbani, S.M. Sharif, C. Toomes, J. Bond, D. Kumar, L. Al-Gazali and S. Mundlos. 2006. Mutations in WNT7A cause a range of limb malformations, including Fuhrmann syndrome and Al-Awadi/Raas-Rothschild/Schinzel phocomelia syndrome. *American Journal of Human Genetics,* 79 (2): 402–8.

Wood-Robinson, C., J. Lewis and J. Leach. 2000. Young people's understanding of the nature of genetic information in the cells of an organism. *Journal of Biological Education,* 35: 29–36.

Wright, S. 1996. It's a yo-yo- type of existence. Huntington's disease. In T. Marteau and M. Richards (eds) *The Troubled Helix: Social and Psychological Implications of the New Human Genetics.* Cambridge: Cambridge University Press, pp. 5–7.

Yoong, S.Y., R. Feltbower, N. Spencer and P.A. McKinney. 2005. Families affected by deafness: hospital services uptake in a multiethnic population. *Archives of Diseases in Childhood,* 90: 454–59.

Young, I.D. and M. Clarke. 1987. Lethal malformations and peri-natal mortality: a 10 year review with comparison of ethnic differences. *British Medical Journal,* 295: 89–91.

Zlotogora, J., H. Habiballa, A. Odatalla and S. Bargas. 2002. Changing family structure in modernizing society: a study of marriage patterns in a single Muslim village in Israel. *American Journal of Human Biology,* 14: 680–82.

INDEX